POSITIVELY beautiful

Published by Bay Books
61–69 Anzac Parade,
Kensington, NSW 2033.

National Library of Australia card number and ISBN: 1 86256 294 6

The Publisher wishes to thank the following for assistance during the production of this book: Bill Auton, Hamilton Laboratories Pty Ltd.

Photograph credits — Cover photo: Photo Library

Designed by Deb Johnston
Typeset by Savage Type Pty Ltd, Brisbane
Printed in Singapore by Toppan Printing Co.

BBC88

POSITIVELY beautiful

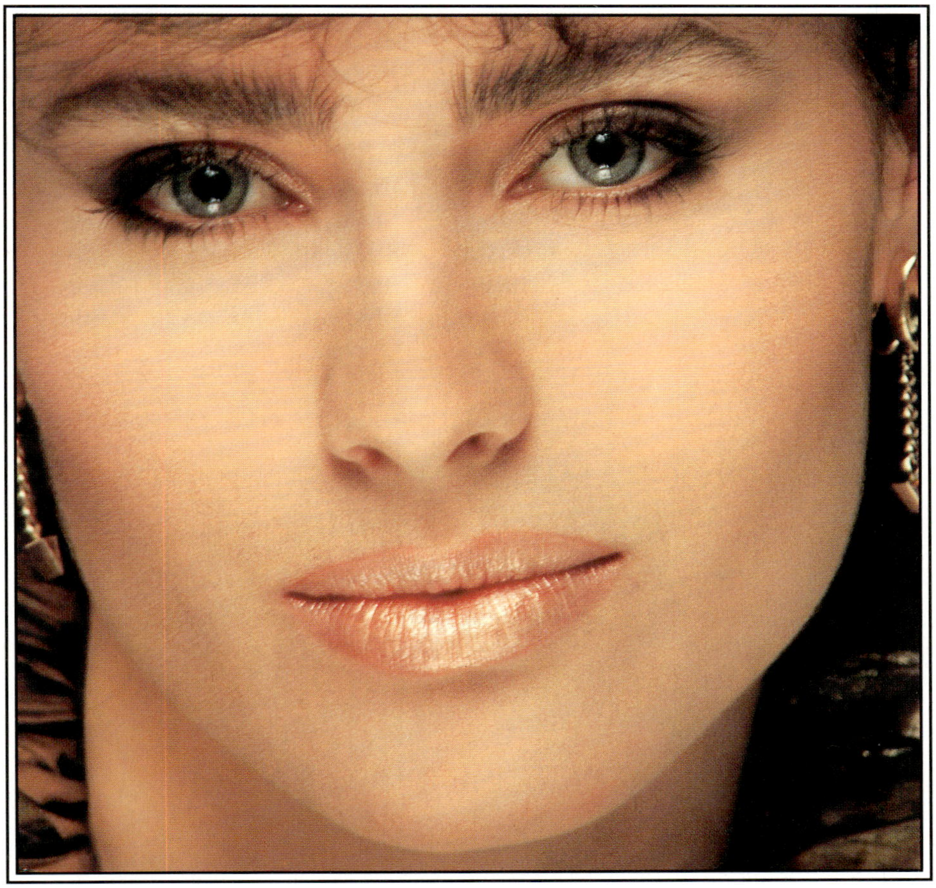

BAY BOOKS
Sydney and London

CONTENTS

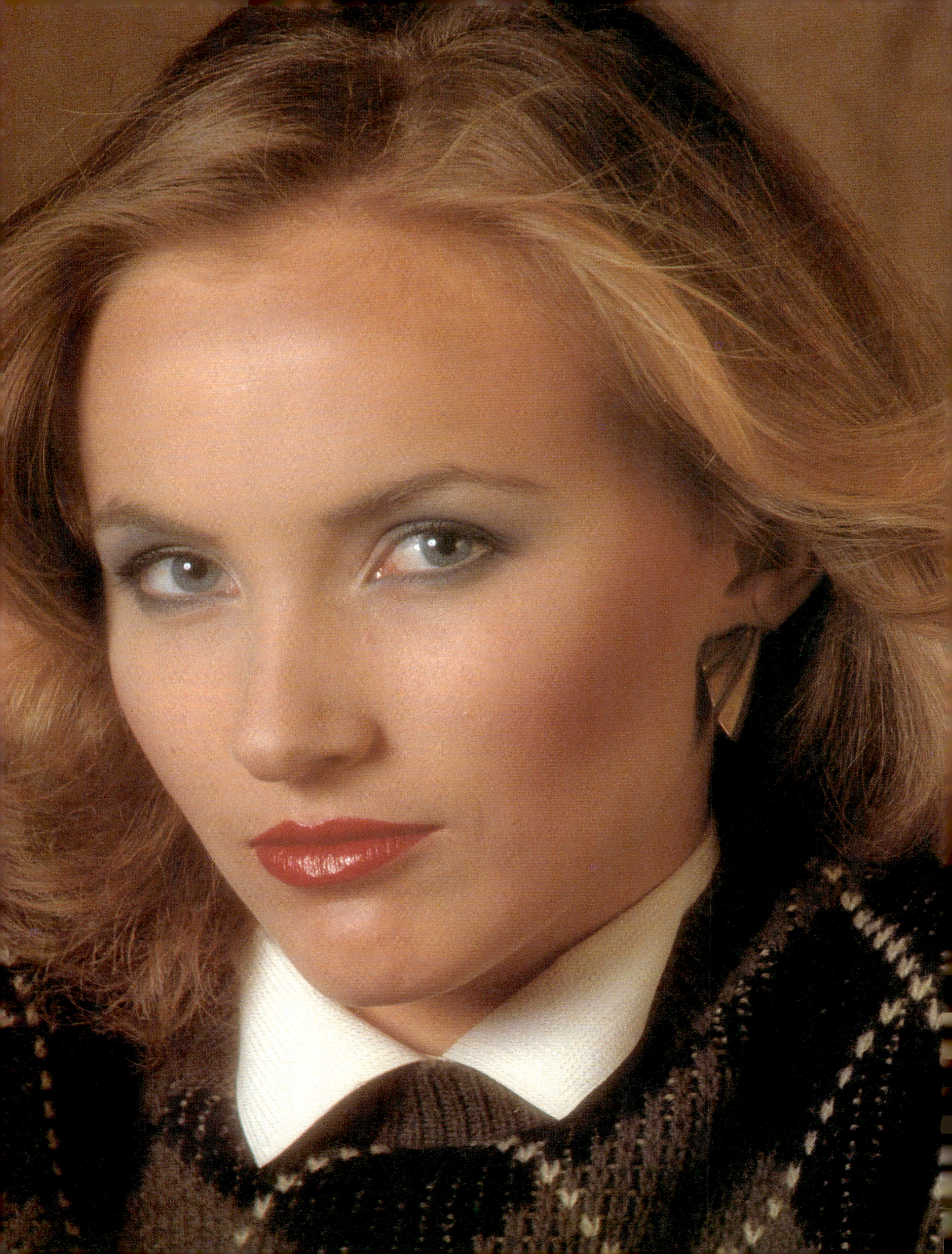

INTRODUCTION

Lissom bodies and lovely faces confront us every time we open a magazine, turn on the television or stare at an advertising billboard, but it's a cheering fact to learn that even these professional beauties have to work hard at their appearance to maintain their money-spinning good looks.

The blessed few who are born with natural beauty or a perfect body can, maybe, afford to rest on their laurels a year or two longer than the rest of us, but it's an unassailable fact that lasting health and good looks are inextricably linked and require a lifetime's dedication.

There's hardly a soul who hasn't registered shock and misery at the unexpected sight of themselves in a store's changing room mirrors, or shed bitter tears when trying on last summer's bikini for the first time in months.

Our physical appearance is often the barometer of our emotions and weight gain is frequently indicative of comfort eating to soothe a deeper malaise. Accordingly, when we take positive steps to address the problem with a healthy diet and an exercise regime which dissipates stress and anxiety as well as toning up our body, our battered spirits soar.

Weariness and lethargy are supplanted by a new vivacity, and self-esteem grows with the weight loss and regained bloom. All at once we feel happy, invigorated and in control of our lives again, so there is no doubting the old adage 'a healthy mind means a healthy body'.

Alas, the euphoria is often short lived; once our weight and fitness targets are reached, we slip back into our old bad habits and gradually regain all those lost kilos. The binge-then-starve syndrome is the scourge of our society and the obstacle that prevents many of us from maintaining a standard weight.

What we should be doing is adhering to a lifelong discipline of

Following a lifelong discipline of good eating and exercise is the key to beautiful, healthy looks.

Remember, even those born with natural beauty have to work hard at maintaining their appearances.

healthy eating and exercise and the first section of this book aims to guide you in precisely that direction. The very word 'discipline' tends to leave a nasty taste in the mouth but there is no reason why it should. As we point out in later chapters on nutrition and weight control, the diet you adopt to lose weight should merely be a slimmed-down version of your normal, healthy everyday eating habits.

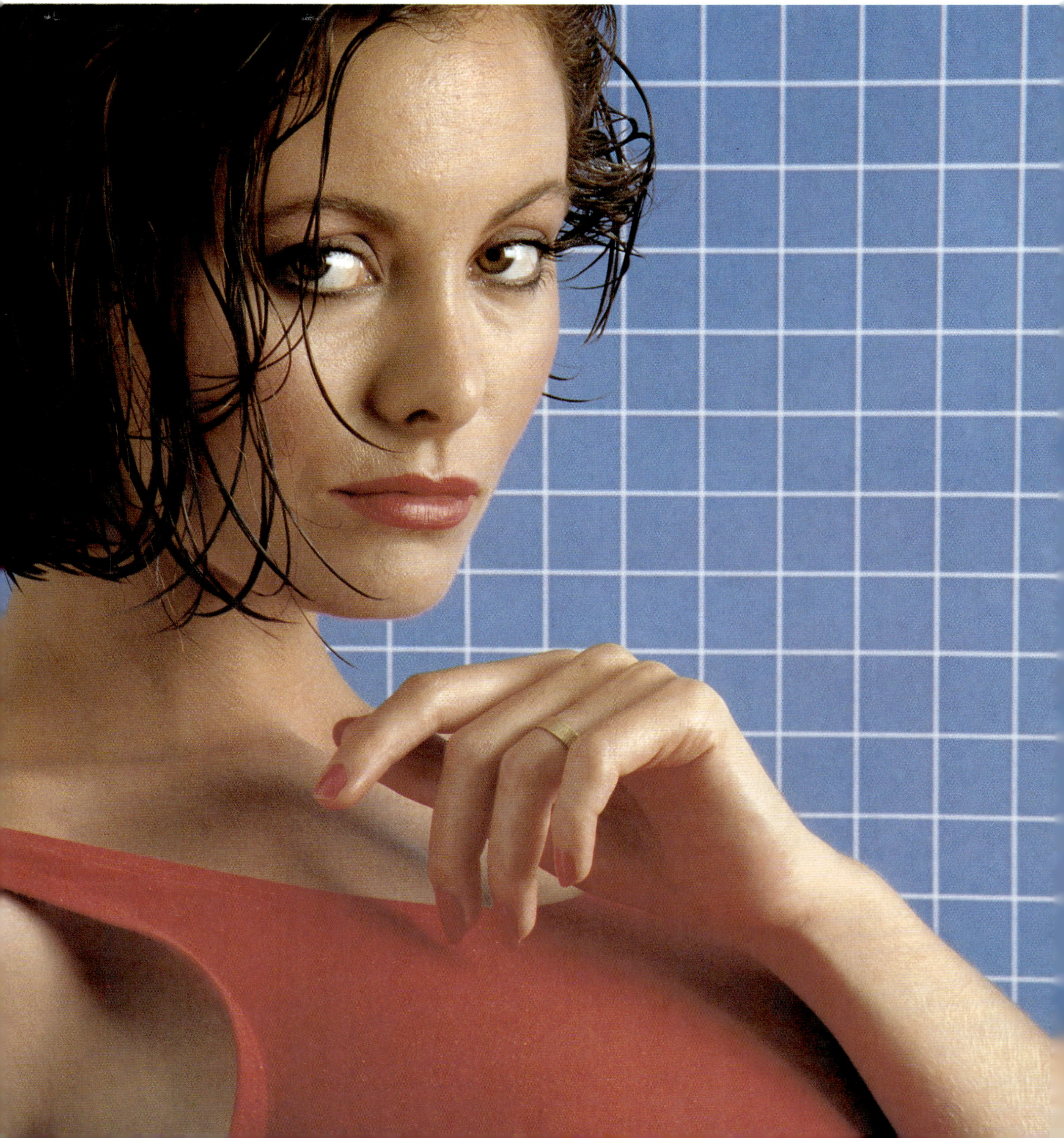

THE HEALTHY BODY

This comprehensive guide towards health and beauty should become a handbook you can use for life. Read it for all the information you will ever need on health and fitness and use it as a source of inspiration when you need to revamp your image. Styles and fashions may change, but our basic guides to shape, colour and care should remain worthwhile for years to come.

The first chapter outlines the healthy eating plan and an exercise program which is fun to follow! The diets in this section involve the use of wholesome, nutritious and bulky foods that satisfy both the appetite and the taste-buds. An added bonus is the fact that adherence to this diet achieves what many of us suppose to be impossible — it eventually turns us off sweet, stodgy and artificially titivated foods by re-educating our palate.

The benefits of launching into a regular exercise regime cannot be overstressed — apart from the improvements to breathing, circulation and in our energy levels, no one should overlook the potential for sheer fun. Many organised activities are extremely sociable, with limitless opportunities for meeting new people and even some of the more solitary pursuits, like jogging or swimming, can become companionable if you frequent the same routes or pools on a regular basis.

In the second section of the book, we have taken a detailed look at top-to-toe care, highlighting the common problems and showing how best to deal with them. Today's woman looks less to the naturopath and more to the laboratory for a solution. While products with a homeopathic or herbal element found favour a decade ago, today's consumer seems more adventurous, with a sophisticated interest in scientifically prepared products — hence the vast range of 'Ph balanced' shampoos, 'clinically formulated' skin creams and the like.

There are times in our lives when we must review the way we look, live and eat. Pregnancy is one key period; during this span our minds and bodies are subjected to the most enormous and demanding changes which are not always easy to accommodate. The third section of our book looks at the subject of pregnancy. We aim to help you anticipate the hurdles you are likely to face, bring you towards a closer understanding of your condition and encourage you to make the most of your great expectations. There are useful tips on diet, make-up, hair care, body care and exercises to help get you back in shape.

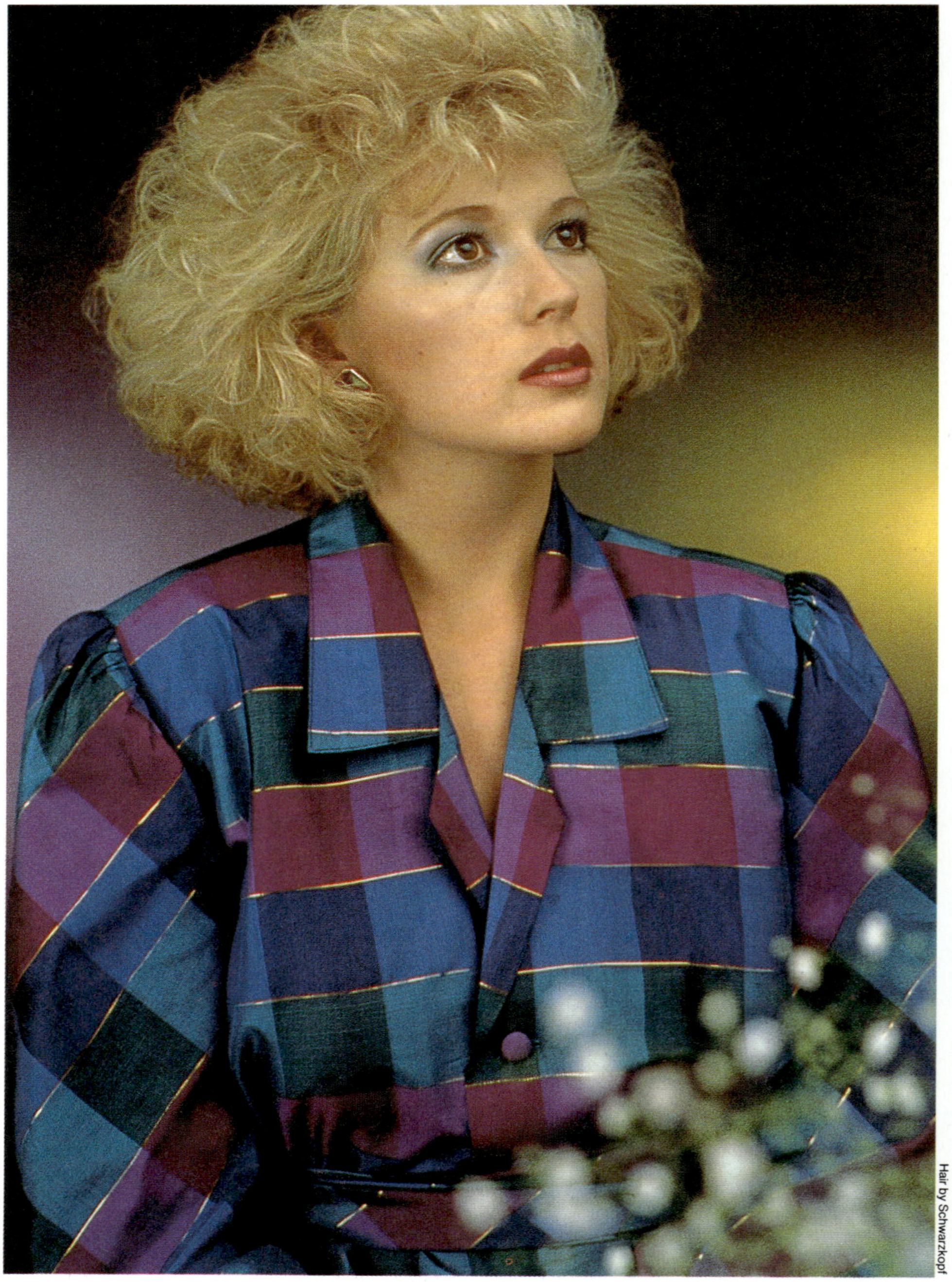

A top-to-toe health and beauty regimen should be followed by women through all stages of their lives.

the eye of the beholder

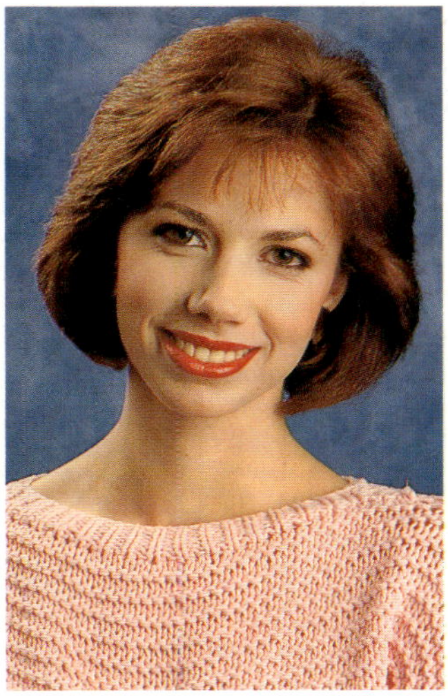

Accepting yourself as you are is half the battle won; you will make the most of what you have and won't try to set unrealistic goals.

An important factor in coming to grips with our health, weight and fitness is learning to accept ourselves for what we are, and not being blinkered by a pointless determination to aim for a shape or build far different from the one nature has given us.

Accepting yourself as you are is half the battle of gaining confidence and making the most of what you have.

We have, thankfully, moved away from the idealised 'Twiggy' shape of the 'sixties, but there is an unhealthy obsession with thinness that must, in part, be responsible for the binge-and-starve pattern that characterises our eating habits.

Unfortunately this attitude is enforced by the media with its devotion to glamour photographs of impossibly slim girls and a regular helping of gimmicky weight-loss routines. The anxiety engendered by this preoccupation is underwritten by the increase in diet-associated conditions like anorexia nervosa and bulimia among young women.

There is absolutely no virtue in embarking on an exercise regime that makes impossible demands on you, while struggling to stick to a near-starvation food allowance. Everyone lives for the moment when they can abandon *that* kind of punishment.

We cannot warn emphatically enough against all those gimmicky weight-loss schemes which exhort you to invest in costly meal replacements, or eat just fruit or, alternatively, a high-protein, low-carbohydrate diet.

Hopefully our chapter covering weight control should guide you to recognise your shape and build without setting impossible targets.

Of course, diet is only half the story in our quest for health and fitness. Regular exercise is a vital ingredient but again, it's a question of quality and quantity. As we very thoroughly explain in our chapter on exercise, no purpose is served by engaging in vigorous sport on an occasional basis — it is far kinder to subject the body to gentler activities in a regular pattern.

Stress and anxiety are great destabilisers and stand in the way of our health and general peace of mind, which is why we have considered it so important to deal with the art of rest and relaxation. The effects of stress will make their mark on our face and body perhaps more than anything else, and learning to cope with it is a skill more and more of us need to acquire.

All aspects of achieving health and beauty from the inside are covered in the first section of the book and there is no doubt that a healthy diet, regular exercise programme and the ability to control our anxieties give us firm foundations for looking good. However, care from within is just not enough to counter the effects of our modern environment. Harsh weather conditions, air pollution, stress, exhaustion and overwork all take their toll on our physical appearance.

In response, there is now an astonishing range of cosmetics, creams, treatments and professional care available with the alleged cure-all ability to deal with skin, hair, eye, dental and nail problems. The $64 000 question is — do any of them truly work?

Most of us are now aware of the need to take proper care of our skin from a very early age; confusion arises with the conflicting advice on the best cleansing, toning and moisturising routine. Should we avoid soap and water?

Will the alcohol in a toner give us broken veins or result eventually in open pores? Is an expensive moisturiser necessarily the best? There is also much anxiety about skin conditions, the effects of sunbathing and the ageing process. The chapter with our simple, no-frills guide to sensible skin care should answer all your questions.

While diet and exercise do a lot for our health and general shape, many areas of our body need special attention which cannot be achieved from within — for instance, action to deal with unsightly veins, hard skin, fungal infections caused by sweatiness, and spots or wrinkles caused by over-exposure to the elements. Our chapter on the body provides a battle plan for all the extremities and also deals very thoroughly with the issue of unwanted hair. It is often considered a taboo subject, so we all have unanswered questions on the topic of whether waxing is a better solution than plucking and in what context we might consider bleaching or electrolysis.

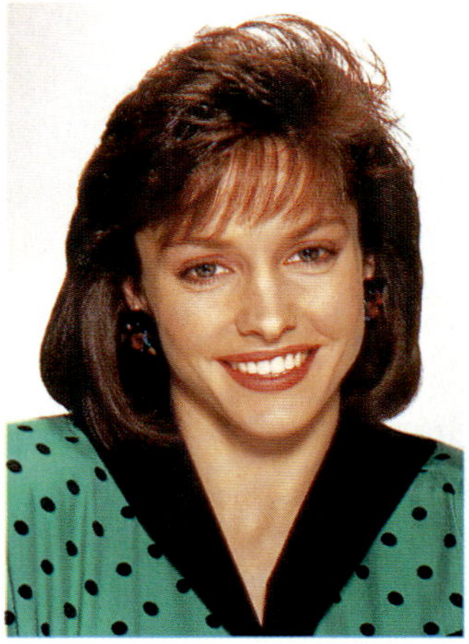

Having a healthy diet, following a good exercise program and mastering stress are the fundamentals for looking good.

Teeth are an increasingly important area, since modern dental care means there is really no need for us to lose them and face up to the prospect of wearing dentures. Accordingly, we have detailed the range of health-orientated treatments which should help keep your teeth and gums in tip-top condition, as well as the techniques which can dramatically improve the cosmetic appearance of your mouth.

As the face is so much the focal point of our appearance, we have devoted an entire chapter to highlighting and dealing with the dilemmas associated with our key features, and to creating a variety of 'looks' catering for every woman and every type of occasion.

The conflicts of current fashion and your opinion of what best suits you can make the business of choosing a 'look' rather overwhelming. Our step-by-step guide should give you the confidence to keep up with and adapt trends to fall in with your own style.

Advancing maturity also presents occasions when we should stand back and take a cool look at our shape, hair and general style. As we grow older, our metabolism tends to slow down and there's a risk that we might gradually start putting on weight, so we may need to adjust our food intake. Similarly, our activity level may well also drop, compounding the problem. The solution is to review any weight gain and physical shape on a regular basis. In our chapter on ageing, we have tackled the problems of advancing years, including the topics of hair and skin care together with different make-up styles. It is generally true to say that the eyeshadows and lipstick tones that flattered you as a teenager are unlikely to do so in your fifties. There's nothing more likely to date your looks as an old-fashioned style, so we have aimed to guide you towards make-up routines that, while geared to make the most of an older face, still make use of modern colours and techniques.

Nothing changes a woman's everyday appearance as dramatically as a new hair style. Whether it's long or short, curly or straight, dry or greasy, hair styling continues to perplex us. Now the trend is to wash our locks daily, a whole new range of problems has appeared: For instance, the question of what to do with dry hair accompanied by an oily scalp, the risks of over-treating hair and whether or not to use conditioner every time you wash your hair. Whatever the problem, this chapter should enable you to come up with a solution and help you choose from a variety of hairstyles and treatments that may suit you.

With proper skin care the rewards are great; a healthy, glowing complexion free of blemishes. It's worth investigating the range of skin care products available, and finding one that suits your skin.

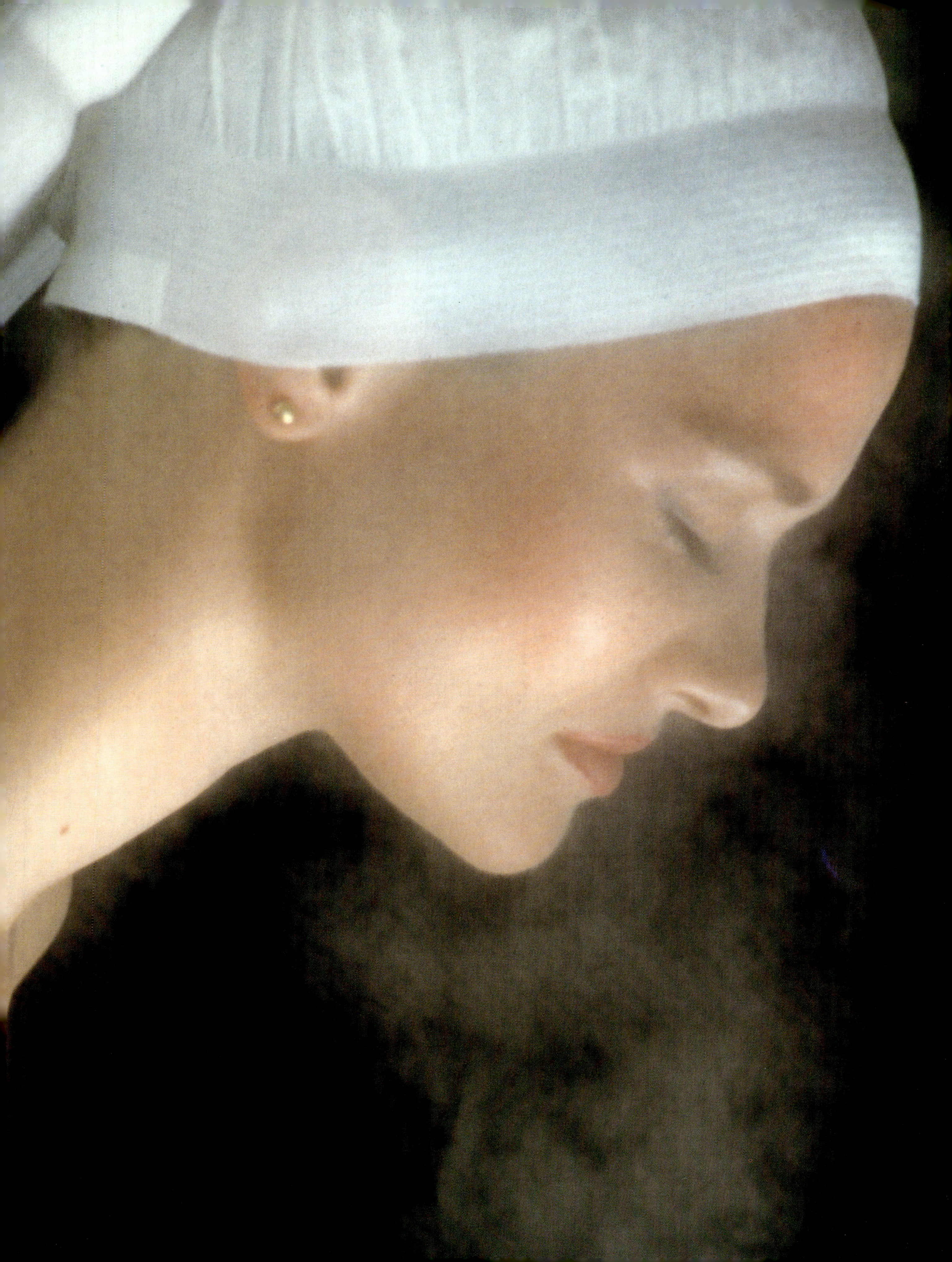

a taste of life

We are what we eat, so we are told. The right kind of diet is essential for health, beauty and a slim figure, as well as playing an important role in preventing disease and contributing to a longer life expectancy.

Times have changed and so has our attitude to food. Even nutritionists and teachers are having to rethink their guidelines. So what's good and not so good about our diet in the 1980s and are you up to date on the newest nutritional recommendations?

EATING FOR HEALTH

First step towards a better eating regime is to understand the different foods and how they fulfil our dietary needs. For a healthy diet, choose the right amount of foods from the basic food groups and drink plenty of water.

Food guide for good health

FOOD GROUP	NUTRIENT	SERVES
Bread and cereal group Bread, ready-to-eat and cooked cereal, rice, macaroni and spaghetti	Carbohydrates	4 servings each day; select wholegrain products for preference
Vegetables and fruit group Dark green, yellow vegetable or fruit (e.g. leafy greens, broccoli, carrots, pumpkin, apricots, rockmelon, mangoes) Citrus, tropical or berry fruits, or tomatoes Any other vegetables or fruits	Vitamins and minerals	1 serving each day 1 serving each day 2 servings each day
Meat and meat alternatives group Beaf, veal, lamb, pork, poultry, eggs, fish, dried peas and beans, lentils, nuts, or peanut butter	Protein	1 serving each day
Milk and milk products group Fluid, evaporated or powdered full-cream milk, yoghurt or cheeses	Protein	Each day — 300 mL for adults; 600 mL for children and expectant and nursing mothers 1 cup (250 mL) full-cream milk = ¼ cup powdered milk or ½ cup evaporated milk or 1 cup yoghurt or 3 cm cube cheese (30 g)
Fats and oils group Butter or table margarine Cream can be occasionally substituted	Fat	1 tablespoon each day 2 tablespoons cream = 1 tablespoon margarine
Extra servings of the food groups depend on your size, activity and age		

Source: *Dietary Guidelines for Australians*, Australian Government Publishing Service, Canberra, 1982.

A taste of life is a taste for healthy eating.

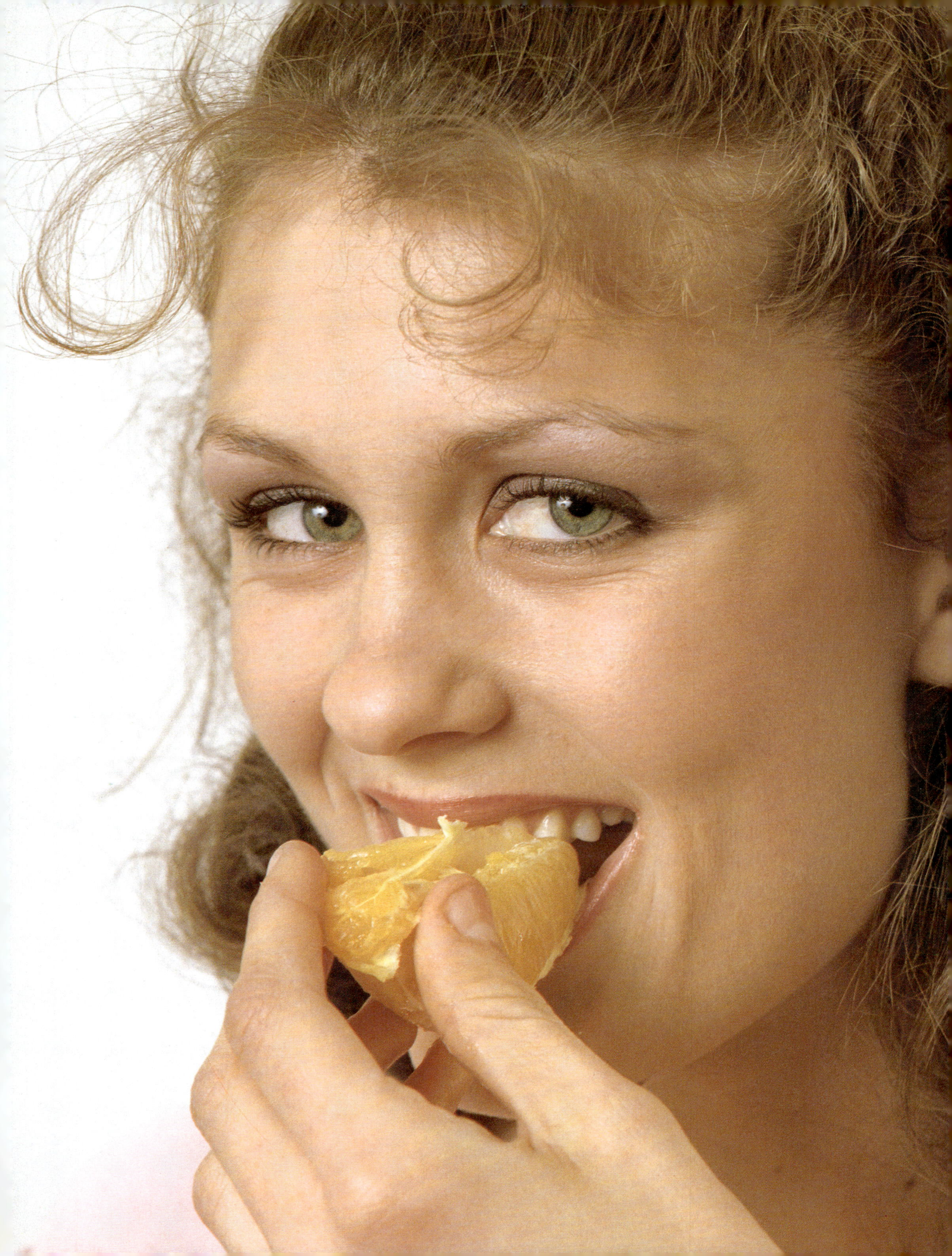

Fats and oils

Alas, over-indulgence is the national problem here — who can resist buttery breakfast muffins, sizzling chips from the lunchtime takeaway or the fast fry-up for supper? For good health we should restrict ourselves to just one tablespoon of butter, margarine or the equivalent each day. Most of us, unfortunately, are used to eating that much or more in the course of just one meal!

The problem with fats and oils is that they push up your cholesterol level (increasing the risk of heart disease, circulatory problems and strokes) and almost all are high in kilojoules, which encourage weight gain. While we can benefit from some of the ingredients in fats and oils — they provide energy and are a source of vitamin A — the message is that we should use all of them sparingly.

Breads and cereals

Gone are the days when every fashionable diet warned us off such carbohydrate-rich foods. Australian health guidelines now advise us to take four servings from this group *each day* and bread and cereals are thankfully losing their undeserved reputation as stodge sources.

The high dietary fibre content of these products (particularly the wholemeal varieties) is a great boon as it provides vital roughage which aids digestion and reduces the risk of dietary disease. So long as we steer clear of sugary bread or those with rich fillings and buttered or richly sauced rice or pasta dishes, they are also lower in kilojoules, gram for gram, than fatty meats and cheeses. Due to the high bulk of breads and cereal, research has shown that it fills us up faster than many other foods, so we eat less — a handy tip for dieters!

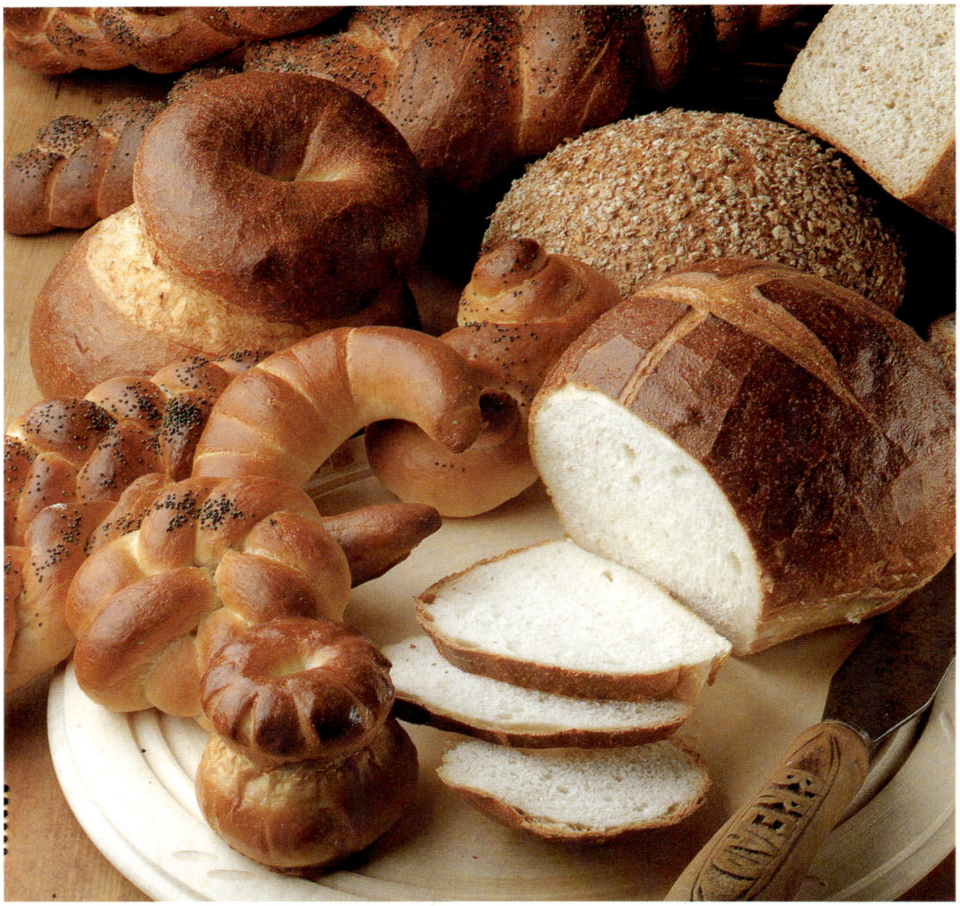

Breads and cereals group.

Vegetables and fruit

Apart from being an unbeatable source of minerals and vitamins, fruit and vegetables are also valuable providers of dietary fibre and energy, while pleasingly low in kilojoules. Official advice is that we should have four fruit and vegetable portions per day, but to vary our selection to ensure the widest range of nutrients.

Colour can be the clue here — for instance, we should aim for one serving that is either dark green, yellow or orange, such as leafy greens, broccoli, carrots, pumpkin, rockmelon, apricots and mangoes for vitamin A, while we can obtain vitamin C from one serving from the citrus fruit group, tropical or berry fruits or tomato. The other two portions are just a matter of choice.

Vegetables and fruit group.

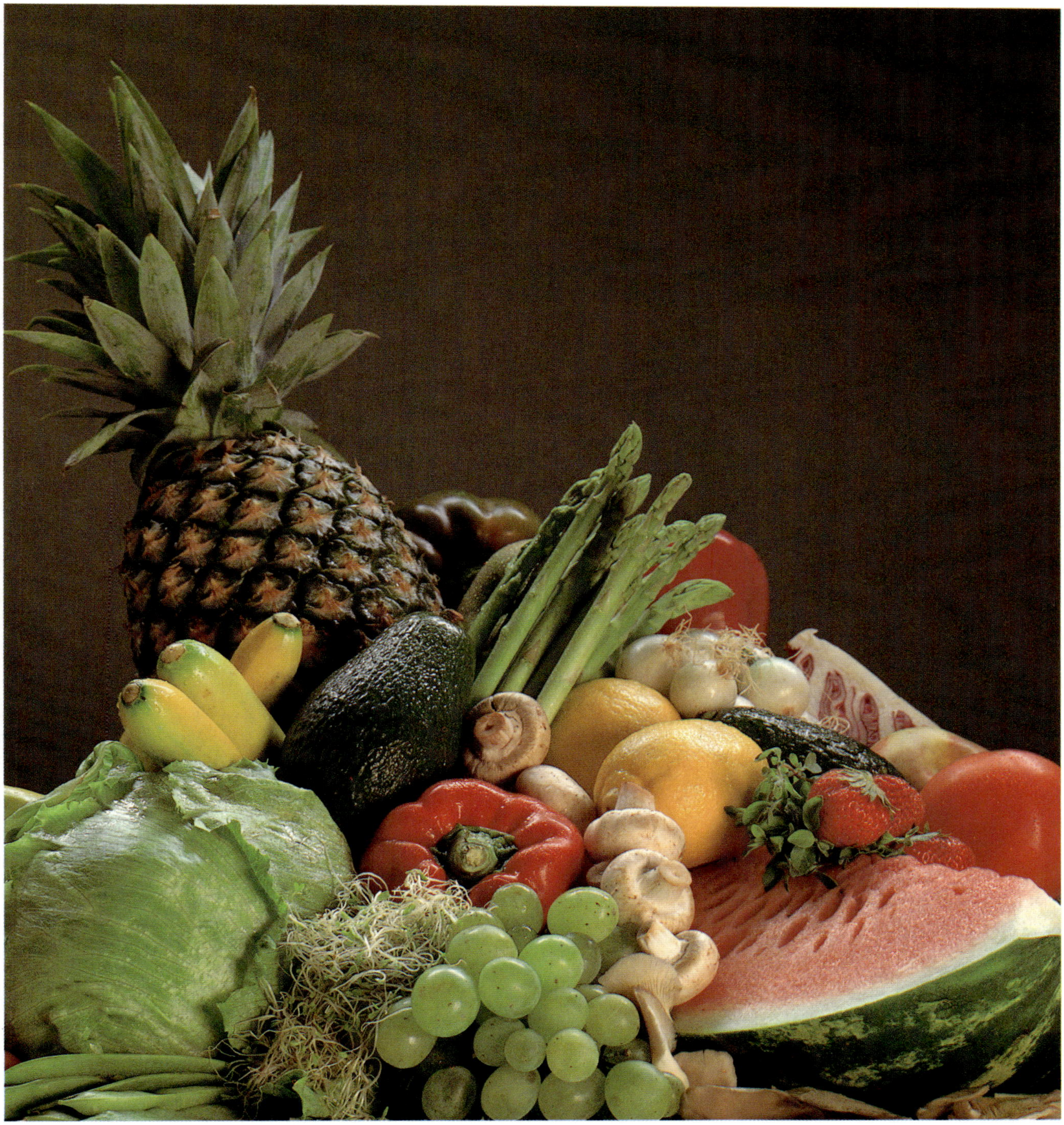

Meat and meat alternatives group

The official line now is we only need *one* serving per day of food in this category — a far cry from the traditional three-square-meals-a-day approach which encouraged meat, fish or eggs at every sitting. While the proteins and other nutrients they provide are vital for good health, ability to fight disease and energy, the disadvantages are that they are often fairly high in fat and therefore push up our cholesterol level (putting us at risk of heart disease) and boosting our kilojoule count, encouraging weight gain. Vegetable proteins are a good alternative as they generally don't have the fat and kilojoules that tend to come with meat, but it's important to pick the right balance to ensure a good spread of nutrients; the proteins of beans and wheat are complementary, making baked beans on toast a healthy combination.

Milk and milk products

While nutritionists now advise us to limit our intake of the fattier milk products like cream and full-cream milk, as well as richer cheeses, all foods in this category are an invaluable source of calcium, necessary for development of strong bones.

This is especially important for infants, children and thus indirectly nursing mothers and pregnant women. Milk products are also rich in proteins and vitamins necessary to promote our healing processes.

Meat and meat alternatives group.

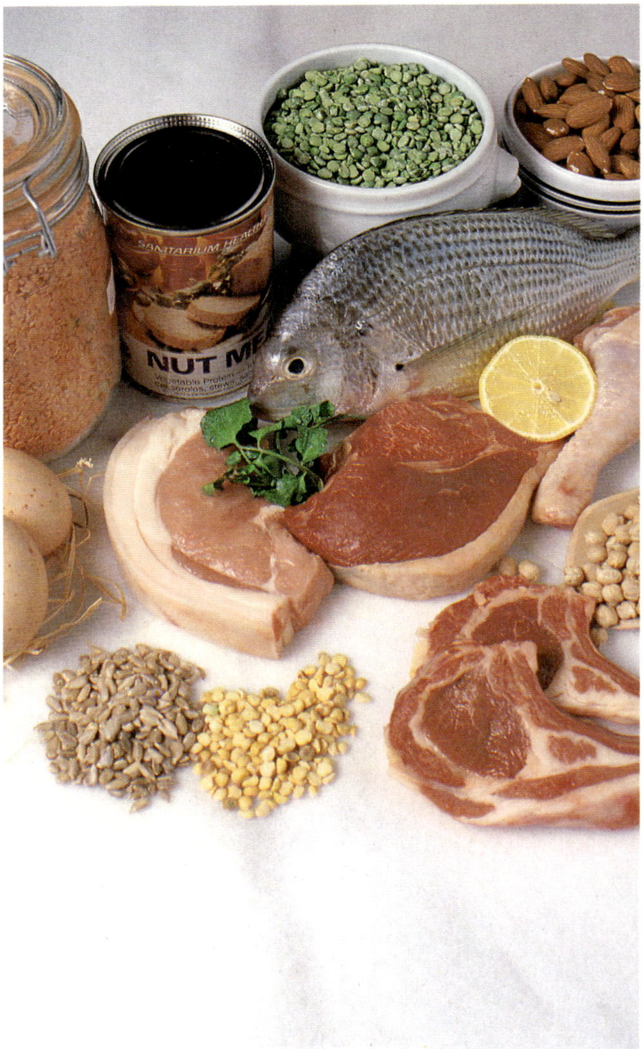

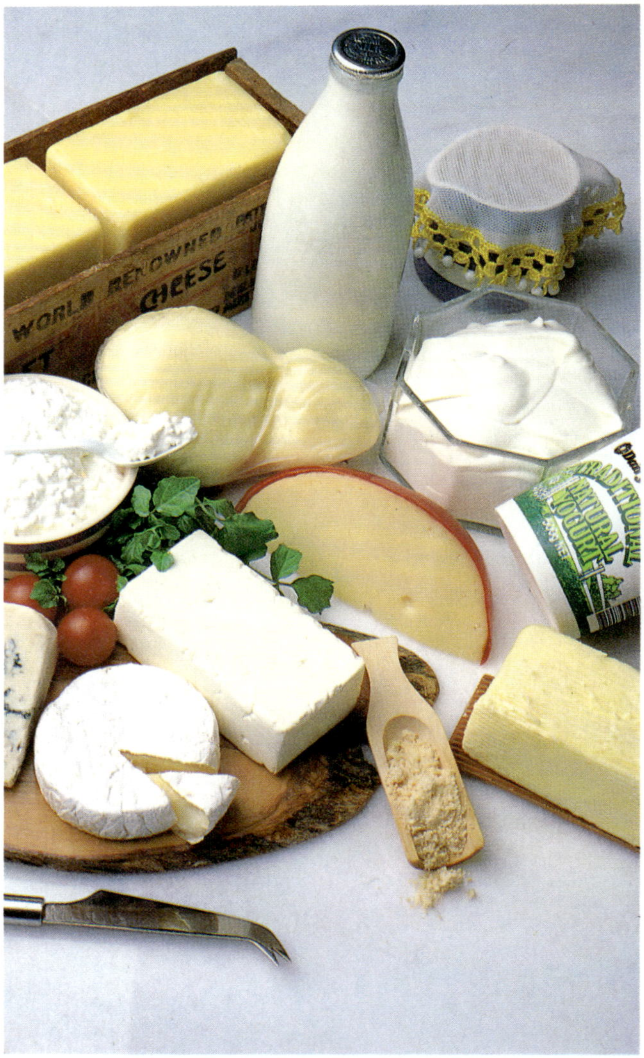

CUT DOWN ON SUGAR

Pure, white and deadly is the famous description of refined sugar, placed firmly on the list of dietary undesirables, and this is one area where times haven't changed! This sweet carbohydrate has long been thought unnecessary for a healthy diet and, because it is high in kilojoules without having any other nutrient benefits, it needs to be restricted on any slimming plan.

In the last hundred years, the amount of carbohydrate in our diet has gone down, but the amount of sugar has gone up, detrimental both to our figures and our teeth.

Doctors are advising us to halve our intake, restricting sugar in the form of confectionery, soft drinks and snacks as much as possible.

Sugar stimulates the body to lay down fat, say some experts. A diet high in sugar is directly associated with adult-onset diabetes, and although the exact role of sugar in contributing to coronary heart disease is not clear, obesity and diabetes are associated with heart disease and sugar may have an additional effect.

The more sugar you eat, the more dental problems you are likely to incur. The bacteria in plaque (a substance which forms on teeth quite soon after brushing and which gradually thickens into a sticky layer containing millions of bacteria) changes sugar into acid which dissolves and eventually makes holes in the outer enamel layer of the teeth.

After about one to two hours, the saliva in the mouth is able to neutralise the acid. But the more frequently sugar is eaten, the more often the teeth come under attack. So keep any sweet treats to mealtimes and try not to consume sugary snacks throughout the day.

Sugar is hidden in everything from baked beans, sauces and soups to cereals, crispbreads and even baby rusks. Sweets are the biggest offenders. A chocolate bar is more than 50 per cent sugar, some pickles and chutneys are 30 per cent, tomato sauce has 22 per cent sugar, ice-cream about 20 per cent and even a cola drink contains 10 per cent.

Read labels As contents are in descending order, if sugar is listed near the beginning, there is a lot in the food. Look out for sugar-free muesli, canned fruit in natural juice and low-kilojoule diet drinks.

Stop adding sugar If you cannot do without some sweetening in tea, coffee, fruit or cereal, try artificial sweeteners.

Cut down Try reducing your intake of sweets, chocolates, cakes, biscuits, puddings and sweet drinks. Use fruit for desserts — cubes or balls of melon mixed with strawberries, raspberries or other soft fruit, for example, or sliced bananas tossed in lemon juice with black or green grapes. Do not peel apples, pears or grapes because the skin is a valuable source of fibre.

Energy boosters We sometimes crave an ice-cream, cake or biscuit when we are feeling low and need a quick energy boost. But for every sugar 'high', there's a corresponding 'low' when the blood sugar levels return to normal. For a slow, steady and healthier increase in energy, nutritionists advocate complex carbohydrates such as bread, pasta and beans. And new research has shown, surprisingly, that some carbohydrates can raise blood sugar levels faster than a chocolate bar, and that an apple or orange has the same effect on blood sugar as an ice-cream!

According to American tests, ranking foods *in order* according to their effect on blood glucose levels, it would seem to be wiser to reach for a carrot than a toffee! The foods absorbed most quickly into the bloodstream were: parsnips, carrots, honey, cornflakes, white rice, wholewheat bread, instant potatoes, white bread, a candy bar, brown rice, raisins, bananas, sugar, apples, ice-cream, yoghurt, tomato soup, pasta, baked beans, chickpeas, lentils and peanuts.

Milk and milk products group.

A *sweet tooth* is another way of saying you have a sugar craving, which has been many a dieter's downfall. Like any other habit, it can be hard to break. One way is to give yourself a sugar holiday: give up *all* sugar, and anything sweet for a week, and try to experience the real taste of food. Then keep to natural fruit and fruit juice for adding a touch of sweetness.

The healthy diet pyramid

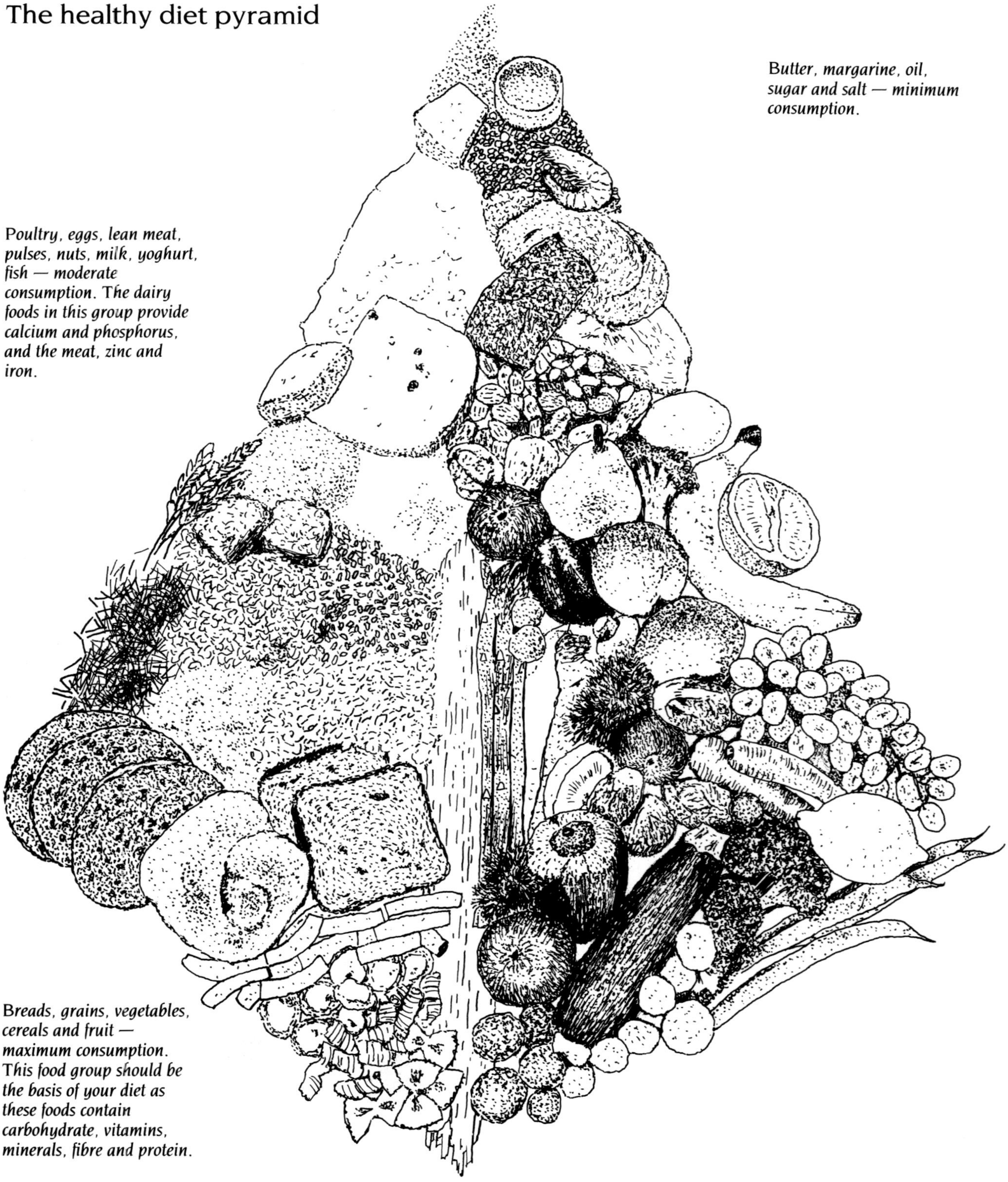

Butter, margarine, oil, sugar and salt — minimum consumption.

Poultry, eggs, lean meat, pulses, nuts, milk, yoghurt, fish — moderate consumption. The dairy foods in this group provide calcium and phosphorus, and the meat, zinc and iron.

Breads, grains, vegetables, cereals and fruit — maximum consumption. This food group should be the basis of your diet as these foods contain carbohydrate, vitamins, minerals, fibre and protein.

Reprinted with the permission of the Australian Nutrition Foundation Inc.

TAKE LESS SALT

The evidence is growing that too much salt can be a health risk because of its link with high blood pressure — and we eat about 20 times more salt than we need.

A high intake of salt can give rise to hypertension in some people (particularly if there is a family history of it) and it has been estimated that as many as one-third of the population could be affected.

High blood pressure develops over a number of years without noticeable symptoms. It is accepted as one of the major health risks (along with excess weight, smoking and lack of exercise) leading to a higher incidence of strokes and heart disease. In fact, the World Health Organization recommends that people should try to have their blood pressure checked regularly from childhood onwards. More than half of those found to have high blood pressure were unaware that they had a problem — and thus did not take steps to control it.

Too much salt in childhood might well lead to high blood pressure in later life, it is feared, so it is not a good idea to add salt to baby foods. A bland diet is probably better so children don't get a taste for salty foods.

Salt is more of a risk to women with a family history of hypertension, but also to women who are overweight or have passed the menopause, when the protective effects against heart disease of the hormone oestrogen have ended.

As salt is contained in so many packaged and instant foods, it is often impossible to know just how much salt you are eating. Labelling the sodium content would be useful. In the meantime, try to banish salt from the table and use less when preparing food.

Cut down on salty foods such as bacon, salted peanuts, cheese, cooked ox tongue, ham, luncheon meat, chopped pork, salami and sausages. Other foods with a very high salt content are: cereals, smoked cod, smoked salmon, shellfish, instant potato, olives in brine, pickles, tomato sauce, stock

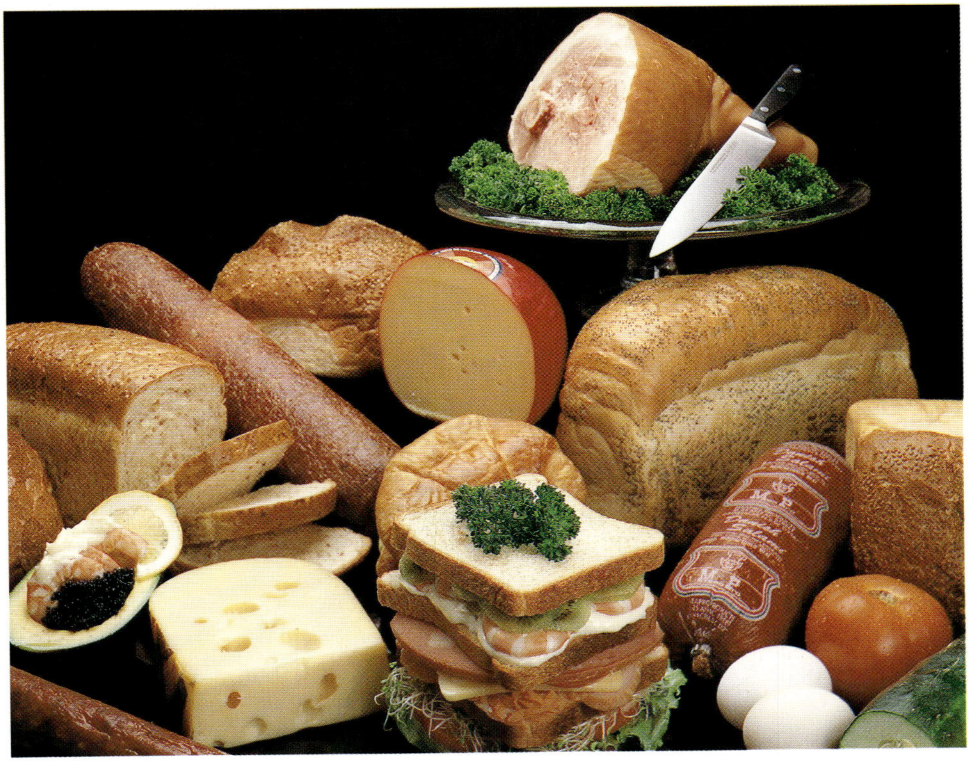

They may look yummy to eat but all these foods are high in salt. Too much salt leads to high blood pressure, hypertension and coronary diseases.

cubes and baking powder. Even custard powder, self-raising flour and bread contain salt, and it can be found in everything from beefburgers to butter; water biscuits and spaghetti. A reasonable helping of some breakfast cereals provides about a quarter of your daily needs.

Look at labels because, although the law does not insist on salt being listed, you can sometimes tell there is a salt content if it contains the following: baking powder, baking soda, sodium bicarbonate or bicarbonate of soda, brine, monosodium glutamate, sodium benzoate, sodium sulphite, sodium hydroxide, sodium cyclamate or sodium alginate.

One thing that may help protect against salt-induced hypertension is to increase the intake of potassium. Found in many fresh foods such as citrus fruits, watercress, all green leafy vegetables, potatoes, bananas, and even asparagus, potassium counteracts the effects of sodium.

EAT MORE FIBRE

Dietary fibre is the indigestible part of fruit, vegetables and cereals — a residue of plant cell walls that gets passed straight through the body. Doctors believe we should eat more fibre-containing foods to help prevent bowel disease, constipation and possibly heart disease, gall bladder disease, varicose veins, piles and obesity.

Fibre adds bulk to your meals and acts as a bulking agent during digestion, helping to prevent constipation, but leaving behind very few kilojoules. Because fibre is only partly digested, most of it passes through the intestines unchanged, where it absorbs water, increases the bulk of the undigested food and helps the muscles of the colon to work efficiently.

There's fibre and fibre. Bran is one form of lignin, which is effective in relieving constipation. Another — the gums and mucilages found in peas, beans and lentils — helps to control blood sugar. This is important both to diabetics and slimmers because it gives a feeling of fullness, which is useful if you are overweight. The pectins are natural gelling agents found in fruits and are said to be helpful in reducing cholesterol in the bloodstream.

Too much added bran can be harmful because you risk reducing mineral absorption (zinc, iron and calcium) into the body, because bran as well as being high in fibre, is also a source of phytate, a substance known to prevent some minerals from being absorbed. One to two tablespoons of bran have been shown to reduce calcium absorption. This is worrying for older people, since not only are they more likely to get constipation, but also osteoporosis, a bone disease found in the elderly, especially women after the menopause, which can be caused or aggravated by calcium deficiency.

So the healthiest way to increase fibre in your diet is to eat more wholefoods such as fruit and fresh vegetables, wholegrain cereals and pulses. Such a diet is much more healthy than a more typical western diet rich in fat, milk foods, sweet cakes, biscuits and refined foods and low in fibre. Simply adding a sprinkling of bran may add a little fibre, but it will not alter the unhealthy balance.

Bread and potatoes were wrongly classified as 'baddies' for years because of the popularity of low-carbohydrate diets, which are now considered the worst way to slim! Bread is an important source of fibre in our diet and all types contain useful amounts, although wholemeal bread provides more than three times the amount of fibre that white does.

Potatoes, besides being extremely important as a source of vitamin C, also contribute three to four per cent of our protein, and provide a useful amount of fibre, especially if you eat the skins.

Good sources of fibre to include in your diet: raspberries, baked beans,

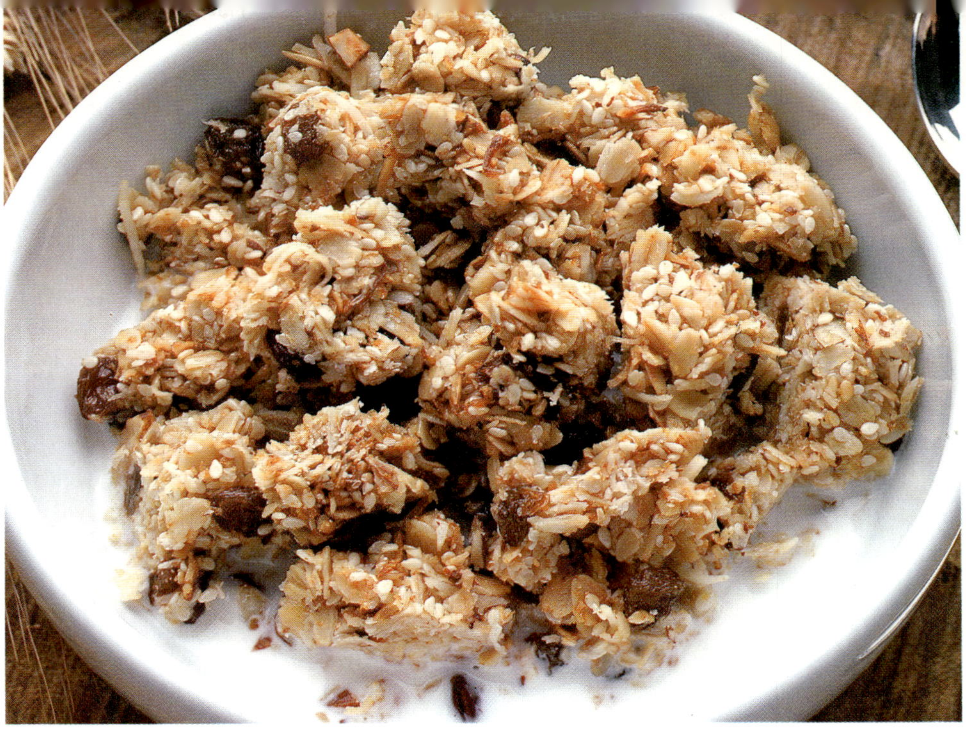

Fibre food is health food and it's good for you. However, as in most instances, too much of a good thing can reduce its benefits.

dried figs, wholewheat breakfast cereals or bran-based breakfast cereals, blackberries, stewed apricots, prunes, haricot and kidney beans, sweetcorn, spinach, nuts, pulses, wholewheat pasta, brown rice.

Wind warning! A sudden large increase in fibre can lead to flatulence, so increase the amount of fibre in your diet little by little over a period of time.

WHAT YOU SHOULD EAT

If you want to keep yourself and your family healthy and increase the fibre in your diet, what does it actually mean in terms of quantities and shopping?

Well, the 30 grams of fibre you should aim to eat in a day could come from a portion of wholewheat breakfast cereal, four small portions of leafy vegetables, one portion of peas, one medium potato and two or three slices of wholemeal bread.

Breakfasts

Instead of a cooked breakfast, introduce a variety of fibre-rich bran-based or wholewheat breakfast cereals. You could try making up your own muesli, or add dried apricots, raisins or sultanas to any mixture of cereals — you don't have to stick to just one type in your dish. Have a piece of fruit or fresh juice.

Lunch boxes

Packed lunches to take to work or school don't have to be boring and they can be ideal for slimmers because you control the kilojoules — you eat only what you take.

Always make sandwiches with wholemeal bread — not brown — and a scraping of low-fat spread (or polyunsaturated margarine).

The sandwich fillings depend on whether or not you are dieting. For instance, sardines and tomato, cottage cheese and cucumber, prawn and salad, egg and cress with a low-kilojoule dressing, are all about 1050 kilojoules a sandwich or less. Date and nut with low-fat cheese is about 1260 kilojoules. Peanut butter with prawns or chicken or raisins are also around 1260 kilojoules. Eat a piece of fresh fruit, too.

For a change, fill a small plastic container with salad and a low-kilojoule dressing. Take fresh fruit and a sugar-free fruit juice or low-fat drink.

For nibbling, take carrot, cucumber or strips of green capsicum.

Avoid pies or anything with pastry, chips, chocolate, biscuits and a lot of hard cheese (high in fat and kilojoules).

Evening meals

Enjoy wholewheat pasta dishes; try recipes using spinach, a good source of fibre. Its legendary iron content is rather a myth. Iron from meat is a better source, and more easily absorbed by the body if taken at the same time as vitamin C, from vegetables or fruit juice perhaps.

Use a baked jacket potato as the base for a meal, adding different ingredients, such as chicken and sweetcorn, pilchard and salad, scrambled egg and tomato. If you want to have salad, be a bit more imaginative about the ingredients.

For instance, the odd lettuce leaf or two, with cucumber, watercress and a shallot, won't give you much fibre. Try instead salads made with shredded white cabbage, carrot, chopped celery, Chinese cabbage leaves, mushrooms, chopped green capsicum, cauliflower sprigs, grated parsnips, diced turnip, beetroot, apple, cooked peas, new potatoes, sweetcorn, runner beans (cooked) or canned red kidney beans. Add shredded chicken or turkey, tuna or prawns, cottage cheese or ham. Use low-kilojoule salad dressings or make your own using tomato juice, low-fat natural yoghurt, and mustard, herbs, herb vinegars and lemon juice.

For desserts, mix up your own varieties of fruity yoghurts with low-fat natural yoghurt, artificial sweetener and fresh fruit such as raspberries, blackcurrants, a chopped apple, or raisins. Baked apples make good low-kilojoule, high-fibre puddings. Serve with cinnamon, dried apricots, dates, raisins or nuts, and honey. Stewed fruit is also a good choice.

Snacks

Baked beans are high in fibre (although they also contain quite a bit of sugar), so they are useful for quick cooking, served with wholemeal toast, mashed potato, a little grated cheese, mushrooms and eggs. Crispbreads containing a good percentage of bran are worth considering for a light meal, too.

Weekend and holiday eating

Eating together with your family or friends, the last thing you want to do is eat something different, or have the bother of making two kinds of meals. So if you work during the week and you are trying to lose weight, it could be better to be stricter on weekdays, and save more of your kilojoules to 'spend' at the weekend.

Start collecting recipes for low-fat sauces, soups and salad dressings. Since baked potatoes (or boiled), wholewheat pasta and brown rice are nutritious sources of healthy fibre, these can be made into family-filling dishes with lower fat sauces. Choose less fatty cuts of meat and cut off all visible fat.

If the family insist on chips, make bigger chips (less fat content) and cook them in polyunsaturated maize or sunflower oil at a very high temperature, drain, then blot on kitchen paper. Never cook with animal lard — it is a saturated fat. Don't keep a chip-pan of oil. Any oil which is continually reheated can become changed in composition, not for the better.

Always have plenty of fruit and vegetables available and buy wholemeal bread rather than white or brown.

On holiday, slimming and healthy eating can be difficult if you are at a motel. But if you are self-catering, you can shop for just what you want.

But a few weeks out of your year don't really matter, if you go back to a healthy, nutritious way of eating once you get back home.

weighing it up

YOUR SHAPE

The way you look has a lot to do with your ancestors, your nutrition and your environment. Our genetic inheritance is far from simple, but like still produces like, and if you come from a long line of small, fairly tubby people, you are probably not going to resemble a tall, slender model. Nutrition also affects your average height. Environment, the third factor, is particularly important in your early years: children brought up in love and security will

Living in a happy, loving and secure environment does affect the way we look.

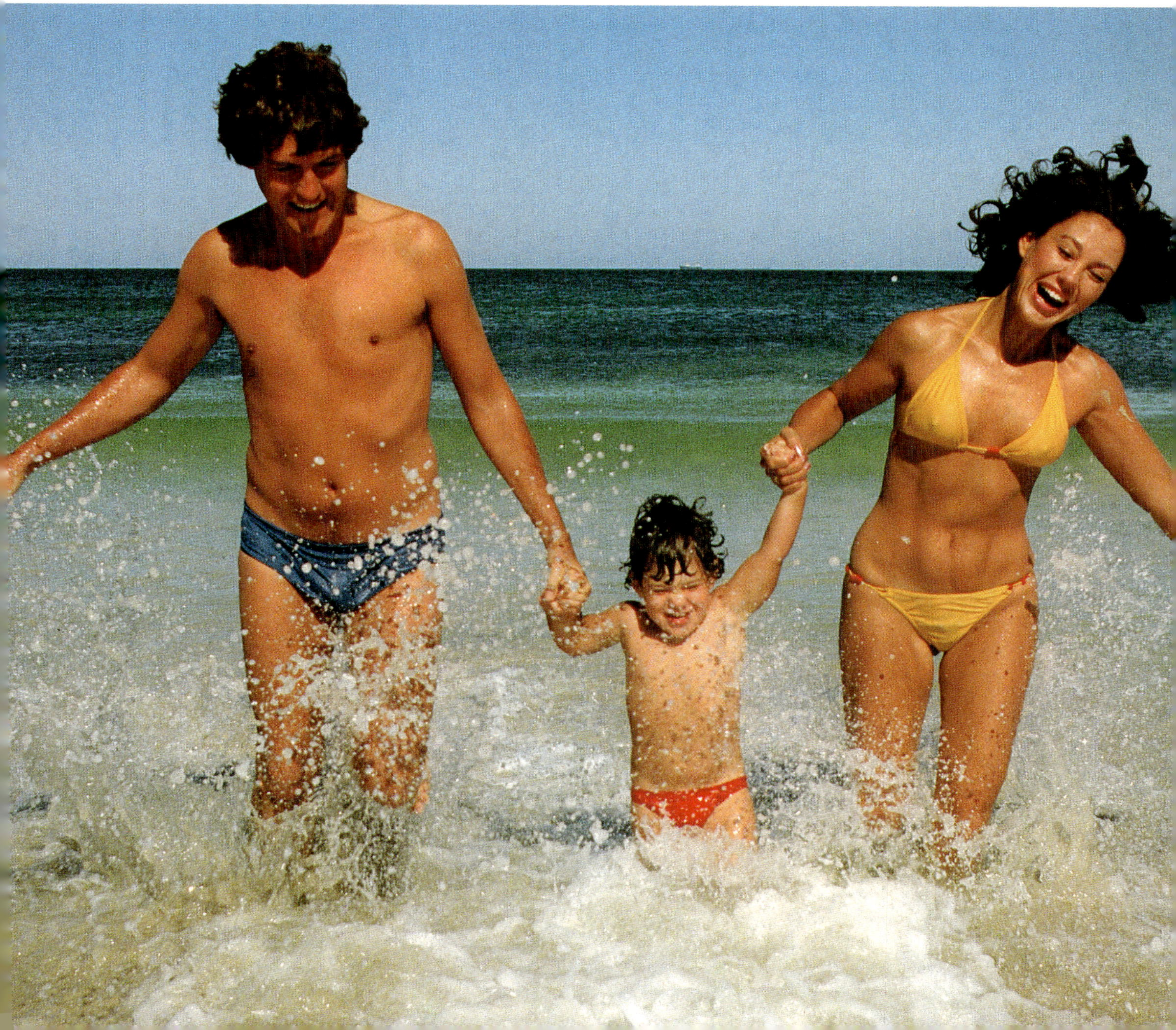

grow more than those on a similar diet but with fewer emotional advantages.

Body types fall into three basic categories.

The endomorph has a rounded shape (including the head), a heavy build and a lot of fat. Even if not obese, the endomorph will always be softly rounded, and is supposed to be easy-going and relaxed.

The ectomorph is sharp and thin, with spindly legs and arms, narrow shoulders and hips, not much muscle or fat. Ectomorphs are said to be sensitive and tense.

The mesomorph is more athletic, with a lot of bone and muscle but not much fat. This type has a large head, broad shoulders and relatively narrow hips, and tends to be aggressive and competitive.

Most of us, of course, are a combination of the three types, with a slant towards one particular shape. Your body type stays with you all your life, and although you can change the amount of fat under your skin and your general all-over plumpness or leanness, you will never alter your basic shape. A well-balanced diet combined with exercise can, however, improve your muscle-tone and make the very best of what nature has given you.

YOUR WEIGHT

It's easy to fool yourself into thinking you are not overweight. 'Heavy bones' 'nicely covered', 'generous proportions' are all phrases that we use to disguise the fact of our fatness. But in order to lose weight and, having lost it, maintain your ideal level, you must learn to assess yourself honestly. So how can you tell whether you're deceiving yourself?

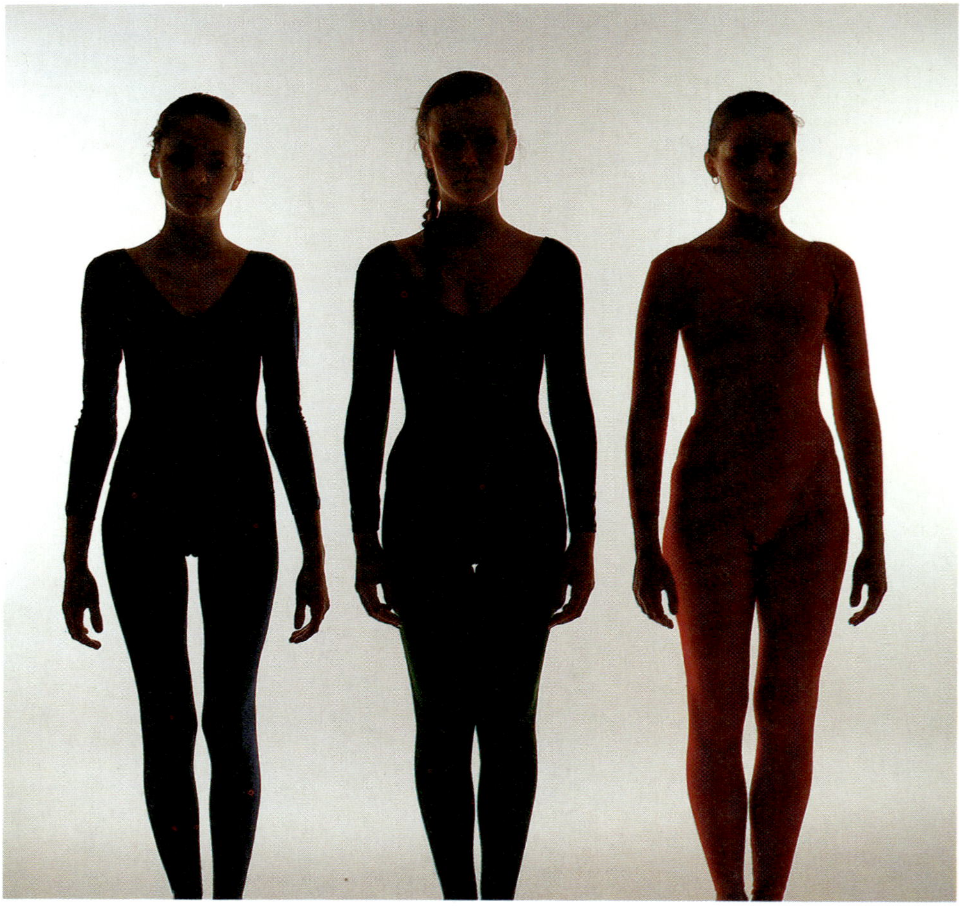

Weidenfeld & Nicolson Ltd

Left to right, an ectomorph, a mesomorph and an endomorph. Most people are a combination of the three body types.

Look at yourself

Stand naked in front of a full-length mirror and look at yourself from the front, back and sides. Take the shades from your eyes and face the truth of the situation. Does your flesh wobble and seem dimpled? Can you see the bulges? Are your thighs very thick? Does your stomach stick out?

Try the pinch test

Although this is most accurate when done by doctors or slimming experts using skinfold calipers, it's still a good indication of excess weight, and easy to do. Pinch a fold of skin at the back of your upper arm (halfway between your elbow and shoulder), 2.5 centimetres above your waist (in the front), and on the side of your leg where the hip meets the thigh. If the thickness of the pinched skin in any of these places is more than 2.5 centimetres, you are overweight. Bear in mind that the average healthy woman has 22 per cent body weight as fat; the average woman has more like 32 per cent body fat. If you can pinch the 2.5 centimetres then roughly 18 kilograms of your body weight is fat. That doesn't mean that you have to lose all of it, because the subcutaneous fat under your skin is what pads out your body and gives you womanly curves. But it does mean you have some weight to lose.

Weigh yourself regularly

Weight tables are a good but not infallible guide. The target table here is based on several expert sources and is more realistic than many of the tables produced by insurance companies, which usually seem to give very generous weight allowances. Try to weigh yourself about once a week at the same time of day, and preferably without clothes. Make sure your scales are standing on a smooth, flat surface — carpets can make weighing machines inaccurate and cause fluctuations.

This table is a general guide. Determine your type of frame by measuring your wrist. If it is 140 mm or less, you have a small frame; 140–160 mm, a medium frame; more than 160 mm, a large frame. The weights given are without clothes, and height should be measured without shoes.

Be realistic

Have you ever taken a smaller size in clothes? How do you look in a swimsuit? Could you wear a bikini? Have any of your clothes become too tight for you? Remember that when you can't do up the zip of your jeans one day, it does not necessarily mean that your trousers have shrunk.

What is your ideal weight?

WOMEN				MEN			
Height	**Small Frame**	**Medium Frame**	**Large Frame**	**Height**	**Small Frame**	**Medium Frame**	**Large Frame**
cm	kg	kg	kg	cm	kg	kg	kg
143	42–44	44–49	47–54	155	51–54	54–59	57–64
145	43–46	45–50	48–55	158	52–56	55–60	59–65
148	44–48	46–51	49–57	160	53–57	56–62	60–67
150	45–49	47–53	51–58	163	55–58	58–63	61–69
153	46–50	49–54	52–59	165	56–60	59–65	63–71
155	48–51	50–55	53–61	168	58–62	61–67	64–73
158	49–53	51–57	55–63	170	60–64	63–69	67–75
160	50–54	53–59	57–64	173	62–66	64–71	68–77
163	52–56	54–61	59–66	175	64–68	66–73	70–79
165	54–58	56–63	60–68	178	65–70	68–75	72–81
168	55–59	58–65	62–70	180	67–72	70–77	74–84
170	57–61	60–67	64–72	183	69–74	72–79	76–86
173	59–63	62–69	66–74	185	71–76	74–82	78–88
175	61–65	63–70	68–76	188	73–78	76–84	81–90
178	63–67	65–72	69–79	190	74–79	78–86	83–93

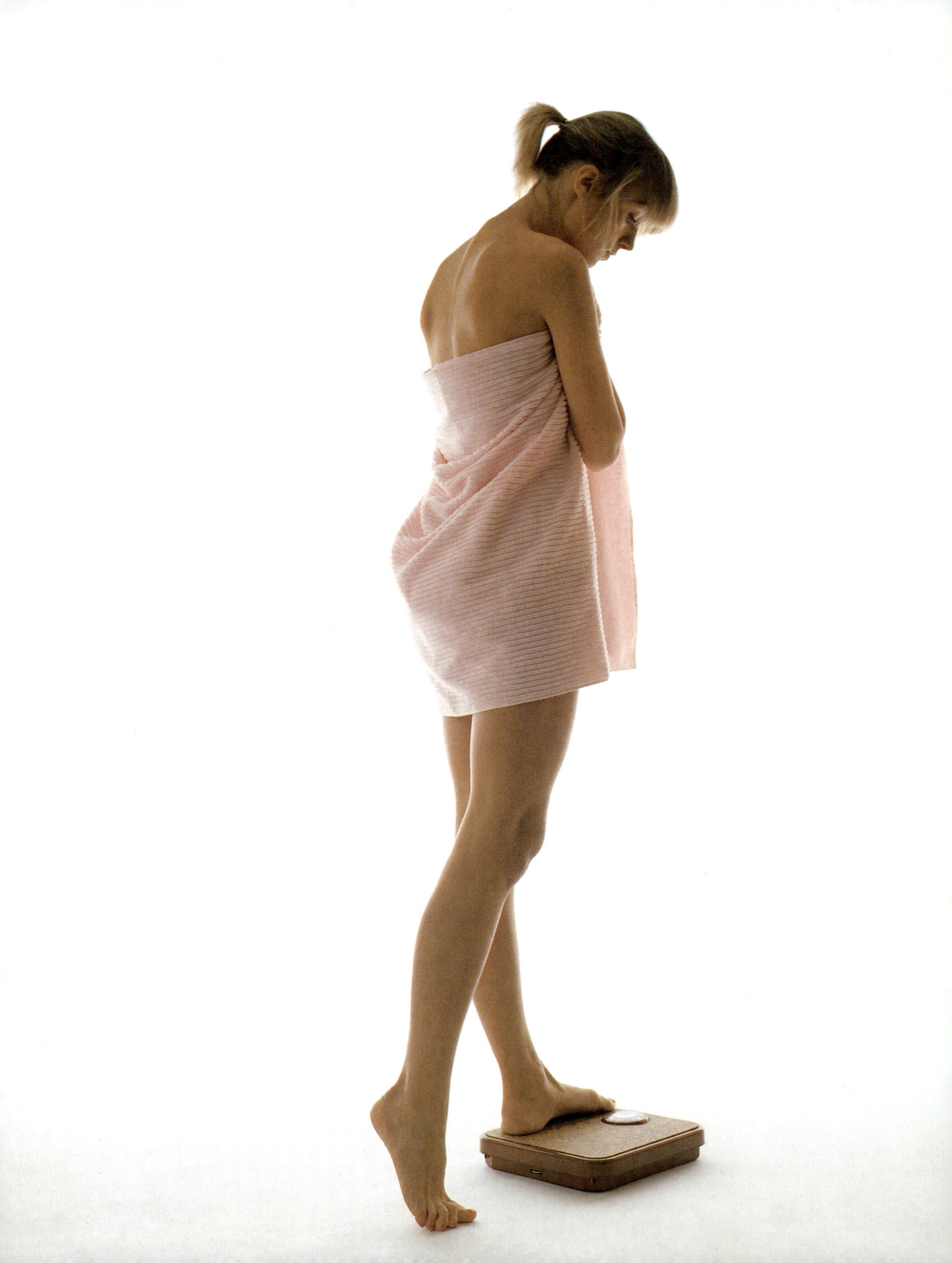

FAT TIMES OF YOUR LIFE

Being overweight seems to run in families, probably because everyone is eating the same kind of diet and, genetically, they are not good 'burners' of energy. Today, you won't find the chubbiest baby winning the Beautiful Baby competition because doctors know that it is wrong to encourage fatness in children. An overweight baby often becomes an obese adult; and the first 12 months are crucial.

Babies Bottle-fed babies may run a greater risk of becoming too fat than breastfed babies, because the mother may measure out food inaccurately and add cereals too early.

Children Although overeating, combined with less utilisation of energy, leads to fatness, fat children do not necessarily overeat. Often they simply use less energy than slimmer children because their movements are slower and they are less active. Fat children are not as popular at school as thinner, more athletic children; they are usually not good at games and feel embarrassed stripping down to sports clothes: all reasons to encourage a sensible eating pattern.

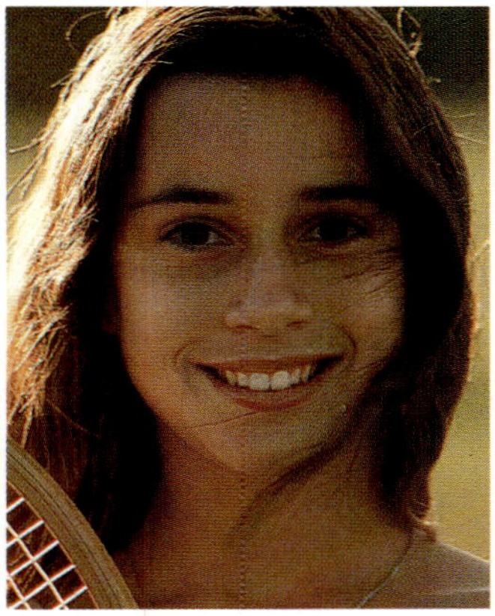

Teenage girls experience a lot of body changes. A sensible eating and exercise programme will help them during this difficult time.

Teenagers Hormonal changes at adolescence mean that girls put on fat and change shape in a pattern which isn't pleasing to them. Being teased is wounding, emotionally. But childhood fatness can also leave scars physically, when stretched skin leaves stretch marks even when the fatness has gone. It's an unwise mother who says 'Eat up and ignore it — it's only puppy fat'. A relaxed but sensible attitude towards family eating can help to win the battle of the bulges before it gets out of control.

Marriage Cooking for a husband, having a settled life, trying to produce interesting meals, giving dinner parties, shopping, more time to nibble . . . all these can lead to putting on weight. For some women, alas, going to the altar satisfies an ambition, and standards drop afterwards because they've lost their incentive to food discipline.

Motherhood A mother of young children seems to be surrounded by food all day long. Eating up left-overs is very tempting, and the opportunities to nibble are endless.

Getting older Generally, the older we become, the less active we are, and older people need fewer kilojoules from food. You should make a positive effort to get more exercise or, if that's not possible, reduce the amount you eat.

There are also factors other than age which can affect your weight at certain times.

The pill The hormones in birth control pills could encourage the body to retain more liquid and to lay down more stores of fat. Discuss any tendency to put on weight with your doctor, who may prescribe a different kind of pill.

Your state of mind The reason for a sudden spurt of weight may be a psychological one. You might find that when you feel more relaxed you increase your appetite. Or you could be the kind of person who overeats when depressed, as compensation; if being overweight depresses you, you could find yourself caught in a vicious circle that's hard to break.

Some women find that being in love takes away their appetite. They have other things in mind than food! An unhappy love affair, however, may lead to self-indulgence.

Weigh yourself regularly, without any clothes on. Keeping the scales on a bare floor rather than a carpet or rug helps to ensure accuracy of measurement.

Giving up smoking The oral satisfaction of a cigarette could be hard to give up and as smoking can dull your appetite, you may well find you have a healthier appetite when you quit. But do *not* be put off and certainly do not use any weight gain as an excuse to carry on smoking. Lots of people give up and don't put on weight. If you need something in your mouth chew one of the slimmers' chewing gums, without sugar, or eat a carrot.

WHY YOU SHOULD SLIM

Doctors consider you to be obese if you are more than 15 per cent heavier than your ideal weight for your height and build. Obesity affects about one in five people; many more are simply a little overweight. Most people go on diets purely for cosmetic reasons: they want to look better, feel more attractive, be able to wear the latest fashions. There are, however, very strong medical reasons for taking off that excess weight.

☐ The more overweight you are, the higher your chances of getting high blood pressure, diabetes, gallstones, bronchitis, arthritis, varicose veins, and heart attacks. Very obese people may also have a high level of cholesterol in the bloodstream, which may be closely linked with heart disease.

☐ Fat people are more prone to accidents. They find it difficult to move quickly or easily.

☐ Life insurance companies regularly load the policies of fat people because statistics show that anyone who is 20 per cent more than ideal weight has a greater chance of dying earlier than a person of the same age but normal weight.

☐ Surgeons will find it more difficult to operate on you if you are obese.

☐ Your bones and joints will take greater strain when you are very obese, which leads to other problems.

☐ Psychologically, being overweight leads to feelings of inadequacy and depression; it can ruin your love-life, destroy self-confidence and self-esteem. The image of the fat, jolly, easy-going person is not necessarily true. It could be a front, put up in self-defence.

☐ Fatness stops you being fit. You cannot exercise easily, will find it difficult to run. The fatter you are, the more difficult it is to move, which means your heart does not get the chance to be properly exercised, and you become breathless and strained with any effort.

THE ENERGY BALANCE

Just as a car is fuelled with petrol to produce energy, so the human body is fuelled with food, which is composed of carbohydrates, proteins and fats, our three main nutrients. These foods are converted into energy and their energy value in units of heat is calculated in kilojoules.

Every minute of our lives, sleeping or working, we burn up energy — more or less depending on the degree of effort and our metabolism. Some people are 'fast-burners', using up more energy than they consume, and stay slim no matter how much they eat. Others are 'sleepers', using up fewer kilojoules than they take in, and get fat. What turns you into a fast burner or a sleeper? Scientists now have a theory that it's all to do with the special kind of brown adipose fat found at the base of the neck between the shoulder blades.

It is this special fat which helps to burn up all the surplus energy we consume as food. Fat people, it appears, do not have enough brown fat — and that's one of the reasons why some lucky people can scoff themselves silly on all kinds of fattening foods without putting on a gram while less fortunate people put on weight after eating only an extra piece of bread. Scientists are investigating the means of stimulating the growth of this amazing brown fat and when they succeed — if they succeed — it could be the end of the obesity problem. Until that happens, diet and exercise is the only way to get rid of surplus weight.

The key to maintaining your ideal body weight, as an adult, is to balance the kilojoules you take in against those you expend, rather like a bank account. When you regularly take in more energy than you need to use, your body converts the energy into fat and stores it in fat cells. These lie underneath your skin, and in addition to fat they contain water and other substances. Their number doesn't change, but they shrink or expand according to the amount of fat they contain. Obesity is when your body stockpiles far too much of this fat. When you regularly take in fewer kilojoules than you burn, you lose weight as your body calls on its fat storage for energy.

Exercise and diet is the only way to rid yourself of excess weight. A fad or starvation diet with no exercise is not the answer.

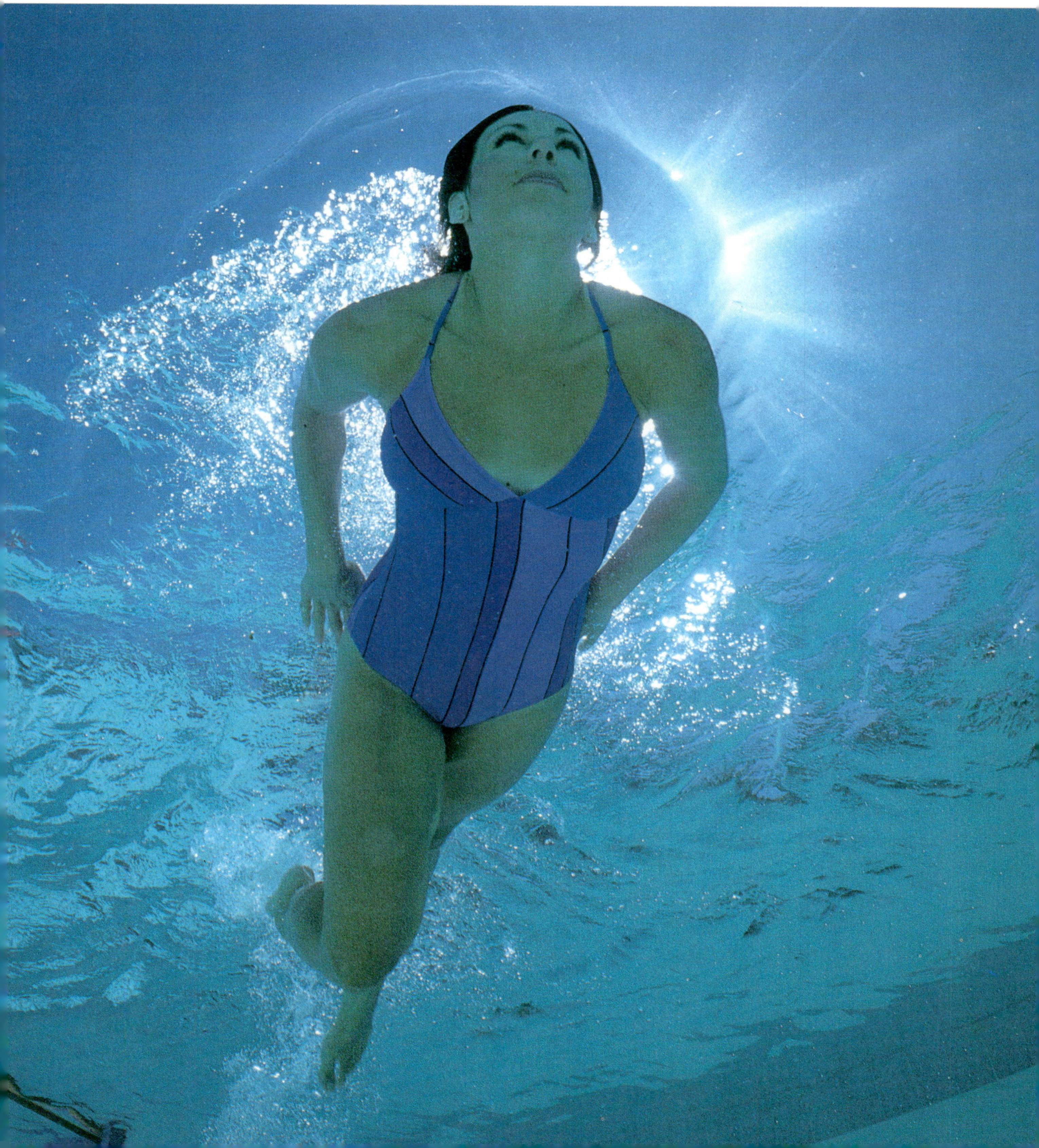

KILOJOULE REQUIREMENTS

Your own daily energy requirement depends on your body size, sex, age, and the degree of phsyical activity you undertake. Women tend to need less energy than men, although needs are increased during pregnancy and breastfeeding. Manual workers use more kilojoules than those who sit at desks all day. Older people tend to need fewer kilojoules than younger ones. The amount of kilojoules you use up in physical activity depends on your weight and how strenuously you work or play. A heavy man will burn up more kilojoules playing a game of tennis than a lighter woman because he is heavier, not necessarily because he runs about more. Cycling up hills and running instead of walking will use up more kilojoules than a gentle stroll or bike ride.

We expend kilojoules in energy even while we are sleeping, sustaining the basic functions of life such as breathing and blood circulation, and we move around quite a lot in our sleep. A woman of 162 centimetres weighing 59 kilograms would use up about 2184 kilojoules during a night's sleep — nearly equivalent to two hours' horseriding or six hours' ironing. It's surprising, though, how much activity is required to work off that little snack which we knew we shouldn't have but didn't really think would matter. In terms of your energy balance, a small packet of peanuts can equal an hour of badminton, a small portion of chips an hour of bowling.

MAXIMUM DAILY KILOJOULE REQUIREMENTS

Age	**Female**
12–15	9660
15–18	9660
18–35	
Sedentary	9240
Quite active	9870
Very active	10 500
35–60	
Sedentary	9240
Quite active	9870
Very active	10 500
60–75	
Sedentary	8610
Quite active	9450
Very active	9870
Over 75	7980

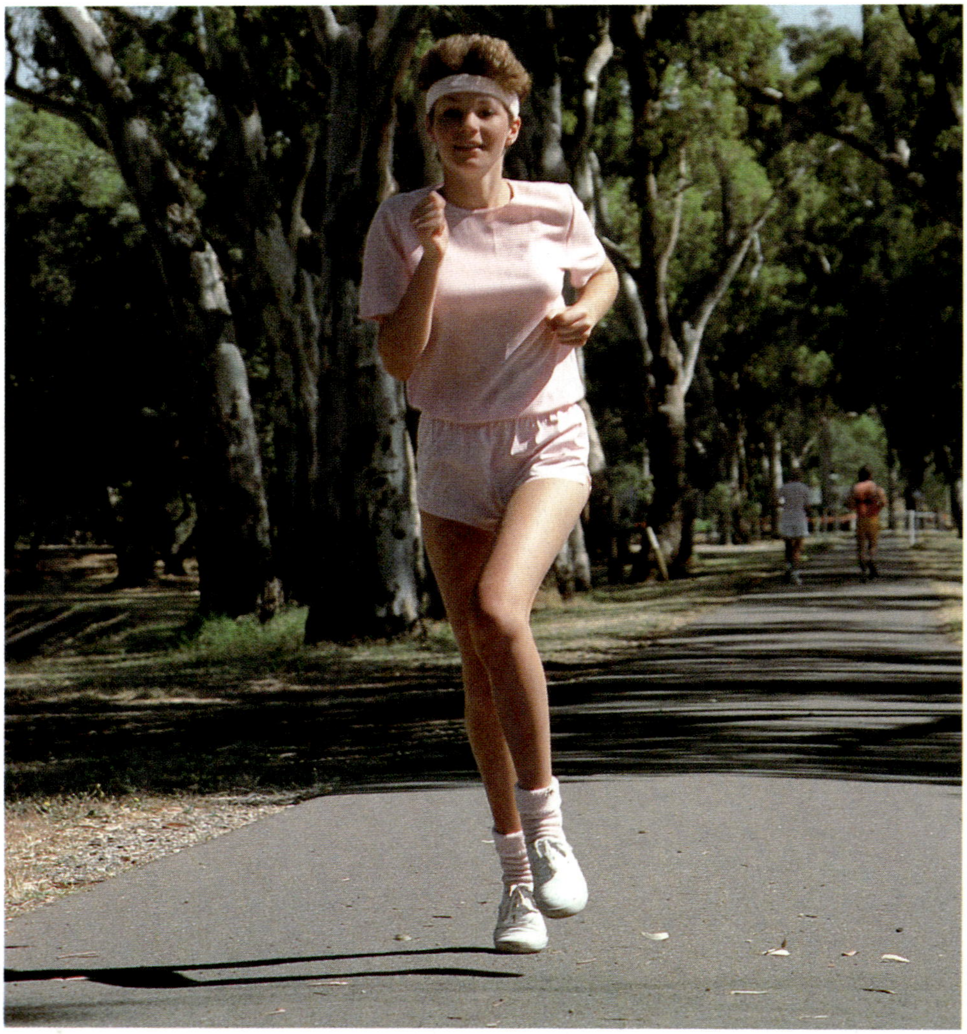

You'd be amazed how much activity is necessary to work off that little 'forbidden' snack. Remember, moments on the lips can mean years on the hips.

taking off

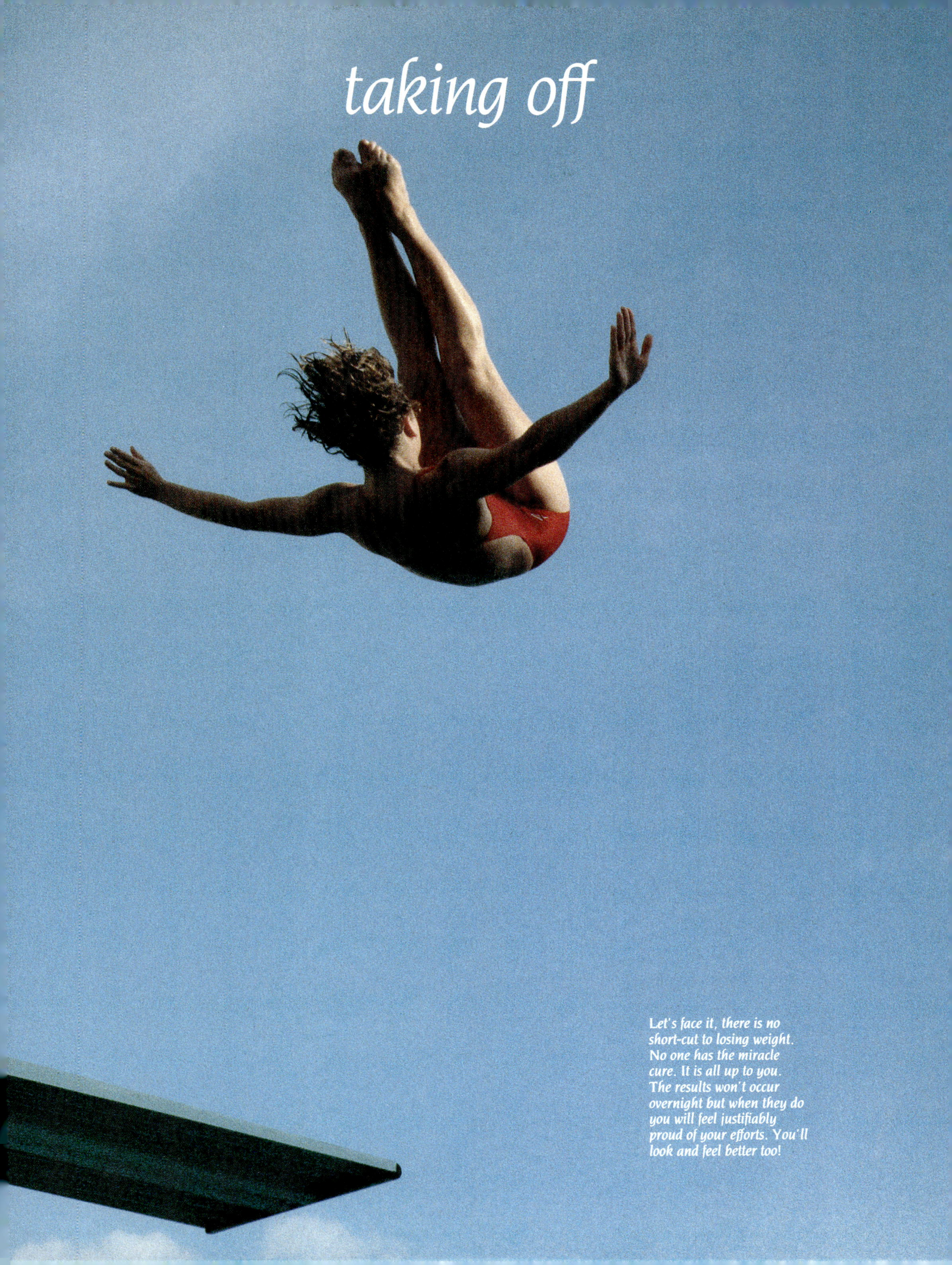

Let's face it, there is no short-cut to losing weight. No one has the miracle cure. It is all up to you. The results won't occur overnight but when they do you will feel justifiably proud of your efforts. You'll look and feel better too!

In order to lose weight, you have to cut down on the kilojoules you eat, but that does not mean cutting down on vital vitamins, minerals and nutrients. If your reduce your food intake from 9240 to 6300 kilojoules your daily kilojoule deficit will be 2940. Over seven days your kilojoule intake/expenditure deficit will be 20 580, and you can expect to lose about half a kilogram of fat. If you reduce your diet to between 4200 and 5250 kilojoules a day, you can expect bigger weight losses. During the first week of any diet you lose water, too. This can be deceptive, when you shed two or three kilograms the first week but much less in subsequent weeks do not be surprised.

Your rate of loss also depends on how active you have been during the week, and whether or not you are a fast burner of energy. Another factor is how overweight you are. If you've been a mighty muncher for years and then go on a 4200 kilojoule-a-day diet, you will drop a great deal very quickly because your body will not have had time to adjust. If, however, you only have a few kilograms to lose, it could take longer than you expect. Don't be too impatient — hopes pitched unrealistically high could lead you to stop dieting altogether because of disappointment.

Your age also affects your rate of weight loss, you need to reduce your kilojoules as you grow older. You may have followed the same kind of diet for all your life, but after 60 your energy expenditure slows down.

DIET PLANNING

When you plan your diet, choose one that is not cranky but which gives you the right balance of nutrients for health and energy. Crash diets which major only in one particular food are flash-in-the-pan diets.

Low-kilojoule diets reduce your kilojoule intake per day by cutting down on foods or portions. A low-carbohydrate diet reduces the amount of sweet and starchy foods you eat. All of these plans involve counting energy units to work out your diet choices. A low-fat diet plan cuts down on foods that contain fat or which are fried in fat, allowing you to eat a sensible amount of carbohydrates such as bread and potatoes. All the diet plans ultimately cut down on kilojoules, reducing your energy intake in order to make your body use up its fat stores.

If you find you dislike counting kilojoules or carbohydrates, and simply want to try to lose weight by cutting down in general and cutting out specific foods, follow the guidelines below. Remember that it isn't just what you eat that counts, but how much, except for fresh vegetables. Also, it's important to include foods from each of the five major food groups — cereals; dairy products; fats; meat, fish and protein; and fruit and vegetables — every day.

Foods to avoid if possible

All alcohol, anything fried, biscuits, butter, cakes, canned fruits in heavy syrup, chocolate, cooking oil, cream, chips, dried fruit, honey, jam, lard, marmalade, mayonnaise, molasses, nuts, pies, puddings, salad dressing, sugar, sweets, syrup, treacle.

Foods to eat in moderation

Beans, bran, bread, cereals, cheese, margarine, meat, milk, oily fish such as salmon, pasta, pork, potatoes, poultry, rice, sardines, thick soups, tuna.

Foods to eat freely

Consomme, cottage cheese, diet drinks, fresh fruit, fresh vegetables, herbs and spices, kidneys, liver, natural yoghurt, seafood, skimmed milk, unsweetened tea or coffee, white fish.

How many kilojoules does it have?

	kj
DAIRY FOODS	
Milk, whole 1 cup (225 mL)	664
skim 1 cup (225 mL)	319
Yoghurt, plain natural 200 g	617
fruit flavoured 200 g	802
non-fat flavoured 200 g	748
Cheese, Cheddar-type, average 30 g	462
Parmesan 30 g	546
Danish Blue, Edam 30 g	420
Mozzarella, Brie 30 g	378
Camembert, Jarlsberg 30 g	357
cream cheese, average 30 g	441
cottage cheese, creamed 30 g	126
FATS, OILS AND CREAM	
Butter 30 g	882
Margarine 30 g	882
Oils (all edible types) 2 tbsp (30 g)	1092
Cream, thickened 2 tbsp (30 g)	399
reduced 2 tbsp (30 g)	252
MEATS	
Beef, lamb, veal, pork, mince (all lean) 30 g	273
Stew (lean meat, vegetables, flour) 240 g	1344
Bacon, fried 35 g strip	399
Sausages 30 g	273
Salami 30 g	420
Chicken, lean, cooked no fat 30 g	231
battered and fried 30 g	315
Turkey, cooked with no fat 30 g	315
Fish, non-oily, light colour, grilled 30 g	168
non-oily, light colour, fried 30 g	273
oily, dark flesh, grilled 30 g	210
tuna or salmon, in brine 30 g	176
in oil, drained 30 g	273
Prawns and crab, cooked, no fat 30 g	155
EGGS	
Whole 45 g	302
Yolk only	252
Egg white	50
Fried egg	454
BREAKFAST CEREALS	
Wheat and corn flakes, toasted, average 30 g	449
Bran cereals, average 30 g	403
Muesli, non-toasted, average 30 g	462
Porridge 120 g	294
Wheatgerm 1 tbsp (7 g)	105
VEGETABLES	
Asparagus, beans (runner), cabbage, bean sprouts, capsicum, chokos, cauliflower, eggplant, garlic, cucumber, lettuce, marrows, parsley, mushrooms, radish, zucchini, tomatoes 90 g	67
Broccoli, onions, spinach, silverbeet, turnips, leeks 90 g	101
Artichokes, beetroot, swedes, carrots, Brussels sprouts, pumpkin, squash 90 g	118
Parsnips 90 g	252
Peas 90 g	252
Potato, boiled, baked in jacket 90 g	286
chips 90 g	958
Corn 90 g	344
SOUPS (1 cup)	
Clear stock, fat free 225 mL	34
Vegetable soup, fat free 225 mL	231
Chicken noodle, packet 225 mL	189
Tomato soup, canned 225 mL	307
Thick soup, e.g. pea and ham 225 mL	588
BREAD	
White, brown, wholemeal, rye (1 slice) 30 g	294
Lebanese (¼ flatbread) 25 g	294
Raisin bread (1 slice) 30 g	357
Rolls, small 30 g	294
average 60 g	588
large hamburger bun 100 g	1050
Crumpets 8 cm diameter 55 g	420
Muffins (½ one muffin) 35 g	294
FLOUR AND GRAINS	
Wheat or rye flour 30 g	433
Rice, boiled 30 g	130
Pasta, boiled 30 g	134
BISCUITS	
Dry, crispbreads, average (1 biscuit)	50–126
Sweet, plain (1 biscuit)	235
Cream-filled (1 biscuit)	378
CAKES AND BUNS	
Bun, sweet, plain (1 bun) 60 g	693
cinnamon, buttered, 120 g	1260
Cake, plain 40 g	567
Fruit cake 40 g	651
Cheesecake, average 120 g	1428
Doughnut, plain (12 average) 40 g	735
Lamington 40 g	693
FRUIT	
Apple (1 small) 120 g	210
Banana (1 medium) 120 g	365
Grapefruit (1 medium) 240 g	370
Grapes (20 average) 120 g	277
Orange (1 medium) 140 g	252
Peach (1 medium) 120 g	189
Pear (1 medium) 130 g	336
Strawberries (7–8 medium) 60 g	101
Watermelon (½ average slice) 210 g	210
Canned or stewed, in syrup (½ cup) 120 g	336
sugar-free (½ cup) 120 g	134
dried fruit, average 30 g	336

THE FILL-UP-WITH-FIBRE DIET

(5040 kilojoules a day)
This is a kind of eating plan that is in line with the latest medical thinking about food and your health. A diet higher in complex carbohydrates and fibre and lower in fat and sugar is one of 'the prudent diets' that doctors recommend. You certainly should not feel hungry or deprived and yet you will lose weight safely and consistently over a period of time.

Remember, fibre fills you up but you also have to make an effort to cut kilojoules. So no fried food, restrict butter, margarine, cheese and pastry. Be sure to drink plenty of water, tea, coffee or any low-kilojoule drink. Try to spread the high-fibre foods throughout the day rather than eating them all at breakfast.

If you are not used to eating a lot of fruit, vegetables and bran cereals, take it easy and increase your fibre gradually. Plunging in to such a changed pattern of eating so suddenly could make you feel uncomfortable.

ALLOWANCES
Each day you are allowed 275 mL skimmed milk for tea and coffee. That is enough for about 7 cups. No sugar in drinks. Grams of fibre are given for each meal.

BREAKFASTS
Choose one each day. If you want to eat it in the evening rather than the morning, do so. But don't eat buns and biscuits at mid-morning because you feel hungry.

1 5 heaped tbsps bran cereal or portion wholewheat cereal
150 mL skimmed milk
1 small chopped apple
2 chopped dried apricots (17 g)

2 2 slices wholemeal toast
2 level tsps butter or magarine
2 level tsps marmalade or jam or honey (7 g)

3 3 dried figs
½ melon filled with grapes
1 slice of wholemeal bread
1 level tsp butter or margarine (15 g)

4 5 chopped dates with 15 g toasted chopped nuts
1 tsp honey
150 g low-fat natural yoghurt (5 g)

5 muesli made by mixing:
3 heaped tbsps oatmeal
1 heaped tbsp bran
1 level tbsp toasted flaked almonds
2 chopped dried apricots
150 mL skimmed milk (11 g)

MAIN MEAL 1
This is a lightish meal, choose one each day.

1 chicken salad made from:
50 g cooked chicken, no skin
shredded white cabbage
½ diced eating apple
4 walnut halves, chopped
2 chopped sticks celery
1 tbsp yoghurt dressing
1 tbsp low-fat natural yoghurt
dessert: 1 orange, 2 apricots (10 g)

2 1 wholemeal muffin split and toasted, topped with 2 sliced tomatoes then 25 g grated cheddar cheese or mozzarella cheese, grill and top with 1 rasher well-grilled bacon
dessert: 1 apple or pear or orange (9 g)

3 salad made by mixing:
50 g cooked butter beans
50 g cooked red kidney beans
110 g cooked cut green beans
chopped celery
4 chopped walnut halves
chopped onion
1 tbsp yoghurt dressing
with 1 slice wholemeal bread (14 g)

4 100 g cod steak (no bone) baked in a foil parcel with sliced onion, stock and 1 sliced tomato
200 g baked jacket potato
1 tbsp sour cream
large portion peas (10 g)

5 open sandwich made with:
1 slice wholemeal bread
lettuce and cucumber slices
50 g peeled prawns mixed with 1 tbsp yoghurt dressing and 1 tsp tomato puree. Serve with lemon wedge
dessert: 150 g fresh or frozen raspberries
4 tbsps low-fat natural yoghurt mixed with 2 tbsps orange juice (15 g)

6 275 mL can any low-kilojoule soup or make your own
1 slice wholemeal bread

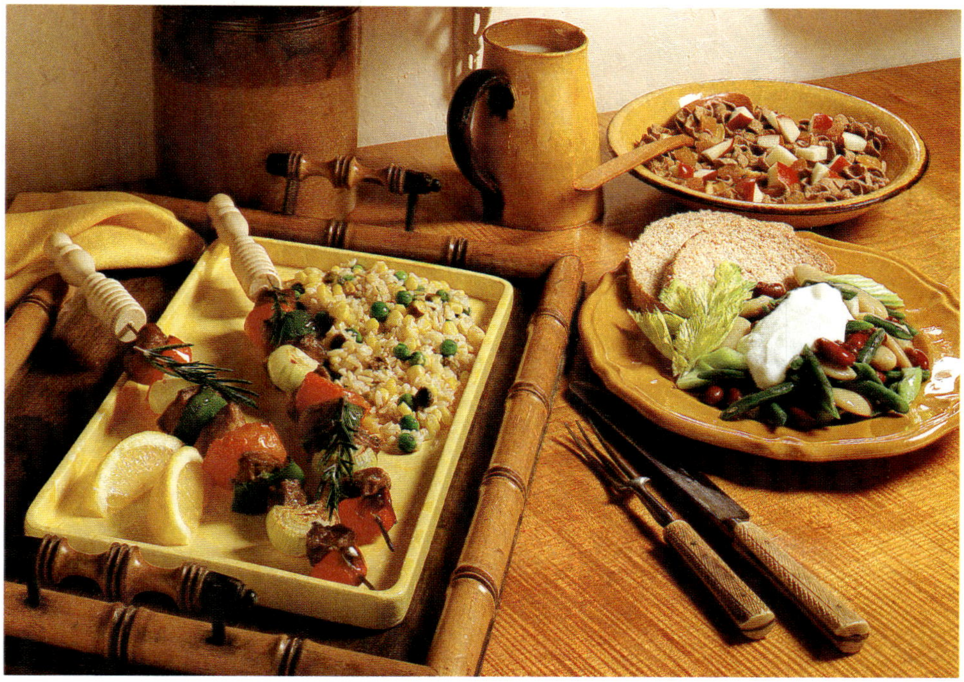

A diet higher in complex carbohydrates and fibre; lower in fat and sugar.

dessert: ½ small melon filled with any soft fruit (10 g)

7 1 poached egg on:
175 g cooked spinach
110 g cooked spaghetti — preferably wholewheat
dessert: 4 dates (15 g)

8 3 sardines on 1 medium-thick slice wholemeal toast
2 grilled tomatoes
dessert: fruit salad made from 1 orange, 1 grapefruit and 6 grapes (9 g)

9 200 g baked jacket potato filled with 3 heaped tbsps cooked sweetcorn
salad of celery, cucumber, onion
dessert: 6 prunes or 3 dried figs (14 g)

10 175 g grilled flounder fillet served with 50 g black grapes
salad of lettuce, sliced cucumber, watercress and 1 sliced orange
1 slice wholemeal bread (6 g)

MAIN MEAL 2

These are rather more substantial meals, choose one each day.

1 2 lamb cutlets, grilled (no fat)
large portion boiled, mashed swede
large portion cauliflower and 2 tbsps white sauce (5 g)

2 110 g pork fillet casseroled with onion, stock, seasoning and 4 dried apricot halves
3 heaped tbsps cooked brown rice
large portion cooked broccoli, sprinkled with 15 g toasted chopped hazelnuts (12 g)

3 200 g trout, grilled and topped with 15 g toasted flaked almonds
large portion spinach
large portion sliced green beens
dessert: 1 peach or pear (13 g)

4 225 g chicken joint, skin removed and casseroled with onion, stock, carrots, tarragon and seasoning
110 g boiled potatoes
large portion peas
large portion broccoli (12 g)

5 75 g roast/boiled lean ham
2 tbsps parsley sauce
75 g broad beans
large portion baby carrots
dessert: 4 fresh plums or 5 prunes
2 tbsps low-fat natural yoghurt (10 g)

6 150 g veal escalope, grilled and topped with 25 g mozzarella cheese and 1 sliced tomato
serve on a large portion spinach
2 grilled tomatoes (12 g)

7 110 g stewing beef casseroled with stock, onion, herbs and seasoning
large portion red cabbage with onion and apple
150 g mashed potato, no butter
dessert: 1 pear or peach or apple (10 g)

8 75 g thinly sliced liver, grilled and topped with orange slices
large portion broccoli
75 g peas or broad beans
dessert: 2 slices fresh pineapple (or canned in water or natural juice, no syrup) and 1 sliced kiwi fruit (11 g)

9 pasta salad made from:
50 g raw weight pasta shells, boiled
75 g poached and diced cod
diced celery and cucumber
75 g peas
dessert: 1 sliced orange (13 g)

10 lamb kebab made with 110 g lean marinaded lamb, tiny tomatoes, red and green capsicum and onion pieces
25 g (raw weight) brown rice, boiled and mixed with 15 g pistachio nuts, 25 g peas and 25 g sweetcorn (6 g)

THE SUIT-YOUR-MOODS DIET

(Strict Days: 3360 kilojoules; Normal Days: 5040 kilojoules; Nibbling Days: 4620 kilojoules)

There are good days, when being sensible about food seems easy, and other times when all you feel you want to do is eat and eat.

This diet allows you to be flexible, both about eating meals and nibbling bits and pieces. There are three basic levels of eating: Strict Days, when you have lots of will-power; Normal Days, when you want to eat just three meals a day; and Nibbling Days, when you feel like eating more frequently.

Whatever the swings and roundabouts, these guidelines should help you cut the kilojoules and lose weight. But aim to have as many Normal Days, where you have three meals a day, as possible. Try to have up to two Strict Days a week, no more; and one or two Nibbling Days at most.

ALLOWANCES

Each day you are allowed 275 mL skimmed milk for tea and coffee, no sugar. Also plenty of low-kilojoule drinks and water.

BREAKFASTS

Choose one of these.

1 3 heaped tbsps bran cereal or portion wholewheat cereal

2 3 pieces fresh fruit

3 1 slice wholemeal bread
1 tsp butter or margarine
1 tsp honey
1 piece fresh fruit

STRICT DAYS
MAIN MEAL 1

Choose one each day.

1 1 apple and 1 banana
110 g cottage cheese

2 huge salad of lettuce, cucumber, celery, 25 g raisins, ½ diced apple, 25 g diced cheddar cheese
1 tbsp yoghurt dressing

3 fruit salad made from:
1 orange, 1 slice pineapple, 1 kiwi fruit, 1 apple, a grapefruit

4 ½ melon, 10 cherries
5 dates or 3 dried figs

5 150 g low-fat natural yoghurt
25 g raisins
1 apple or pear

MAIN MEAL 2

Choose one each day.

1 1 egg boiled, poached or scrambled
1 slice wholemeal bread
either 75 g peas
or 1 portion fresh fruit

2 110 g white fish, grilled or poached
large portions of 2 green vegetables such as green cabbage, broccoli, sliced green beans, whole French beans, spinach, spring greens

3 275 mL any low-kilojoule soup
2 slices wholemeal bread
2 fresh apricots or plums

4 150 g cottage cheese on lettuce surrounded by lots of fresh fruit

5 225 g chicken joint, no skin, casseroled with carrots and onions
green beans or mashed swede and 75 g peas or broad beans

NORMAL DAYS
— when you feel like eating three meals
MAIN MEAL 1

Choose one a day, variations are given in italics.

1 2 frozen fish cakes
2 grilled tomatoes
50 g peas
50 g sweetcorn
1 large apple
omit sweetcorn and add 1 tbsp tartare sauce and lots of sliced green beans

2 100 g cod steak with 75 g white sauce
110 g mashed potato
large portion poached mushrooms
1 large orange
add to the sauce either: 50 g peeled prawns or 15 g grated cheese; omit potato and add 25 g raw weight brown rice

3 75 g any lean roast meat
1 tbsp gravy
75 g roast potato
large portion braised red cabbage
broccoli
make meat into kebabs before cooking; substitute apple, cranberry or horseradish sauce for gravy

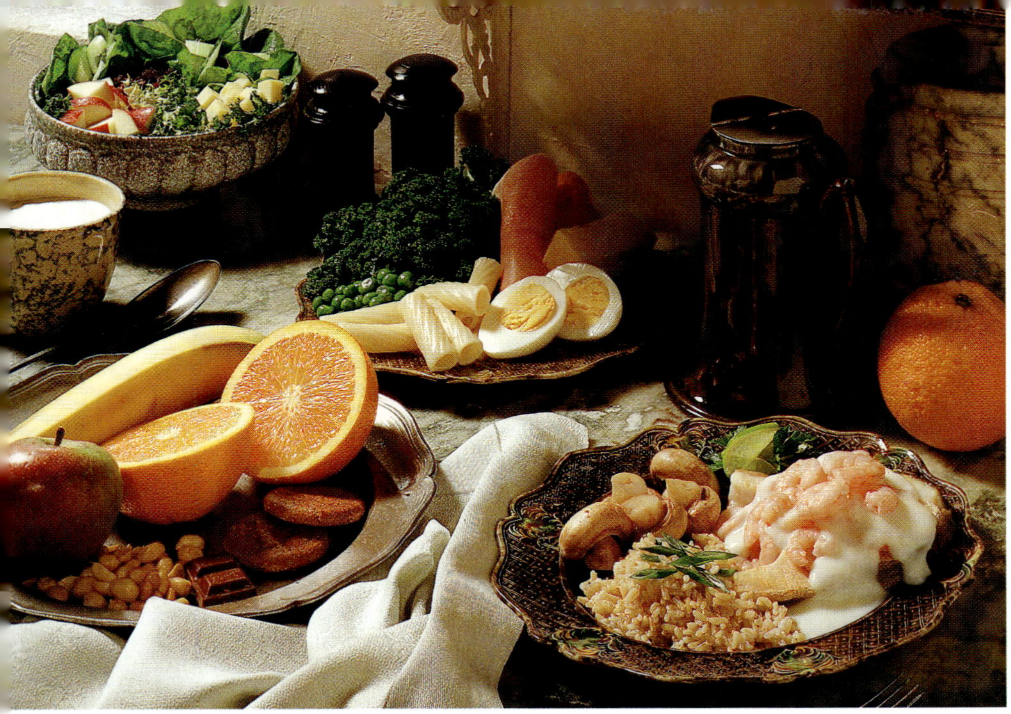

Weidenfeld & Nicolson Ltd/Ken Martin

A flexible diet to suit your mood and changing lifestyle.

4 110 g chicken breast baked in foil with onion, mushrooms and mixed herbs
2 tbsps white sauce
large portion green beans
large portion sliced carrots
use 225 g chicken portion without skin, instead of chicken breast; use any other green vegetable instead of green beans

5 50 g burger, grilled with 50 g bun and
1 tbsp relish
1 sliced tomato
1 portion fresh fruit
use 1 large sausage instead of burger

6 150 g can baked beans
1 slice wholemeal toast
1 tsp butter
1 poached egg
replace toast and butter with 25 g grated cheese on baked beans

7 275 mL can any low-kilojoule soup
2 crispbreads
110 g tub cottage cheese
2 portions fresh fruit
replace crispbreads by ½ slice bread; replace cottage cheese with 25 g hard cheese or 1 hard-boiled egg

MAIN MEAL 2

Follow the guidelines for Main Meal 1 and add any one of these to each meal.

1 110 g boiled or baked potato
2 25 g cheddar cheese
3 1 large glass red or white wine
4 25 g raw weight brown rice or pasta
5 individual tub low-fat natural yoghurt and 1 orange
6 275 mL can any low-kilojoule soup
7 25 g pate and 1 crispbread and salad
8 ½ grapefruit and 1 tsp sugar

NIBBLING DAYS
— when you want to eat all the time

During the day, eat 10 of the following, and try to eat at least 6 different foods.

1 275 mL vegetable soup
2 1 large orange and 1 large apple
3 1 very large banana
4 40 g raisins or sultanas
5 20 g nuts
6 25 g cheddar cheese
7 portion wholewheat cereal
8 2 squares chocolate
9 individual tub frozen mousse
10 1 boiled or poached egg
11 2 beef sausages, well grilled
12 50 g lean cooked meat
13 110 g poached or grilled white fish
14 large portion any leafy vegetable and 50 g peas
15 75 g sweetcorn
16 50 g canned salmon
17 25 g raw weight pasta or rice, boiled
18 10 prunes
19 110 g peeled prawns
20 2 biscuits
21 2 crispbreads and 1 tsp butter
22 1 slice bread, yeast extract
23 110 g cottage cheese
24 150 g tub low-fat natural yoghurt and 1 piece fruit
25 2 grilled fish fingers
plus unlimited lettuce, cucumber, raw carrots and low-kilojoule drinks

THE YOU-DON'T-HAVE-TO-EAT-MEAT DIET

(5040 kilojoules a day)
Vegetarians are usually healthy, rarely overweight and their way of eating generally includes lots of nutritious fruit and vegetables. However, *just* cutting out meat won't make you healthy and slim, unless you remember some of the new guidelines. Don't replace meat with lots of hard cheese because it is high fat and high kilojoule. You can get all the protein you need with fish, pulses, cereals and some dairy foods, and these also provide all the nutrients meat contains.

Although animal protein contains all the nine essential amino acids for your health, vegetable protein is usually missing one or more — but you can balance it all out by combining vegetables with other kinds of vegetables and other foods. For instance, the Mexican dish of corn tortillas and beans does that. Other combinations that work include: leafy vegetables with most grains and cereals; beans with sesame or wheat; peanuts with barley, bran or corn.

Don't forget the value of good wholemeal bread — it contains 9 grams of fibre and 9 grams of protein, as well as 40 grams of starch per 100 grams, and is a rich source of B vitamins.

A diet without meat needs to be well balanced to provide all the essential nutrients.

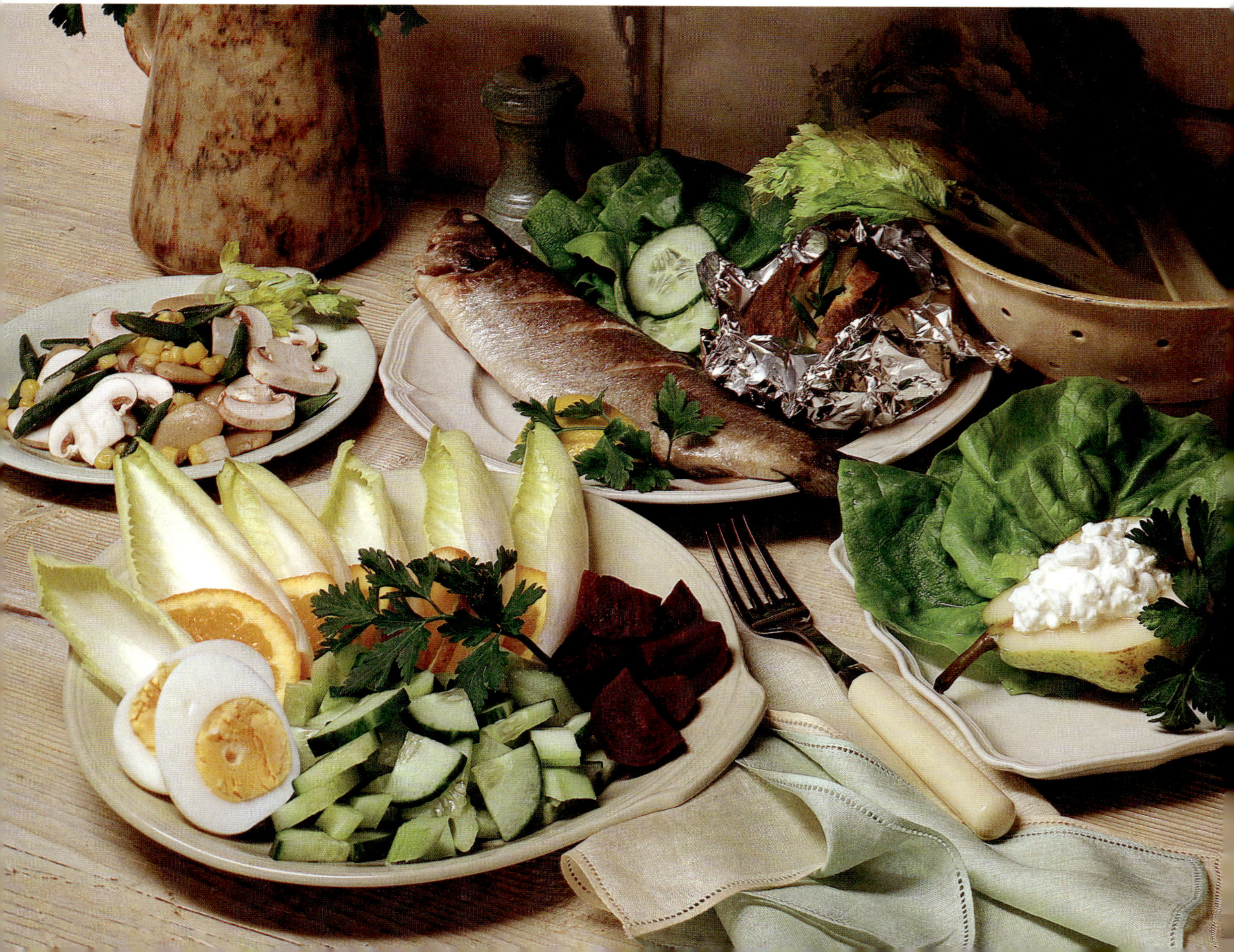

ALLOWANCES

Each day you are allowed 275 mL skimmed milk for tea and coffee. That is enough for about 7 cups. Also drink water and low-kilojoule drinks as often as you like.

BREAKFASTS

Use the same list as The Fill-Up-With-Fibre Diet.

LIGHT MEALS

Choose one each day.

1 Salad
choose one of the following:
3 sardines
75 g canned salmon
75 g tuna in brine
1 hard-boiled egg with 1 tbsp yoghurt dressing
110 g cottage cheese
25 g hard cheese like cheddar
with any 2 salads:
chopped celery, cucumber, 110 g diced beetroot, chicory and slices of orange
onion, 50 g sweetcorn, beans, 75 g butter beans, sliced mushrooms and low-fat natural yoghurt
grated carrot, 25 g raisins and lemon juice

2 Omelette
2 eggs, seasoning, 2 tbsps milk (try a souffle omelette sometimes by separating the egg whites, whipping them and folding into the yolk before cooking)

Fillings
25 g grated cheese and minced onion
75 g cooked sweetcorn
110 g cooked spinach with 15 g chopped peanuts
75 g peeled prawns
75 g peas and sliced poached mushrooms
1 medium-thick slice wholemeal bread
large portion broccoli, cabbage or beans

3 Open sandwich
1 medium-thick slice wholemeal bread with 1 tsp butter or margarine, lettuce and cucumber slices

Toppings
75 g peeled prawns mixed with 1 tbsp yoghurt dressing
50 g smoked or canned salmon with lemon slices
75 g canned tuna in brine and apple slices
75 g cottage cheese and pear slices
2 sardines and 2 slices beetroot

4 White fish
poach or grill 200 g cod, gemfish, flake or ling

Accompaniments
very fine strips of carrot and celery cooked in 15 g butter
25 g wholemeal breadcrumbs, sliced mushrooms and grated onion mixed with 1 tbsp cream
3 tbsps parsley sauce
1 sliced zucchini, tomato and sliced onion, cooked in stock
15 g each of grated cheese and wholemeal breadcrumbs — grill to melt and brown

5 Oily fish
choose one of these:
200 g trout
110 g mackerel fillet

Accompaniments
15 g toasted flaked almonds
3 tbsps mustard sauce
3 tbsps cucumber sauce
serve with 175 g plain boiled rice or baked jacket potato and green salad

6 Baked potato
baked 200 g potato, scoop out some of the flesh and fill
return to the oven to heat filling through

Fillings
75 g sweetcorn and 1 tbsp sour cream
75 g prawns, chopped celery and 15 g chopped walnuts
25 g grated cheese and 1 tbsp sweet pickle
75 g cooked white fish and 1 tbsp tartare sauce
75 g baked beans
50 g cottage cheese and 50 g sweetcorn
dessert: portion of fresh fruit

7 Pasta/rice
50 g raw weight brown rice or wholewheat pasta, boiled, mixed with any one of these:

Accompaniments
1 hard-boiled egg, 2 tbsps curry sauce and 50 g peas
75 g cooked diced white fish, 25 g peas, 25 g butter beans and a chopped tomato
4 tbsps cheese sauce

MAIN MEAL 2

Choose any of the meals indicated for Main Meal 1, and include any one of these starters.

1 275 mL clear soup

2 275 mL home-made vegetable soup

3 ½ melon

4 ½ large grapefruit topped with 1 tsp sugar and grilled

5 segments from 1 small orange and 1 small grapefruit

6 150 mL tomato or orange or grapefruit juice

7 ½ pear filled with 50 g cottage cheese on lettuce

8 1 hard-boiled egg, mix yolk with yoghurt dressing and pipe back into whites
serve with tomato, lettuce

SOCIAL DIET

If there's one thing that's sure to test any slimmer's willpower to the limits, it is eating out socially, or having people round for meals in your own home — although that is at least more controllable.

'Do have another drink,' says one hostess. 'You simply must try my new pudding,' says another, giving your conscience a tweak. And if you have the kind of job that means having business lunches and drinking, you could be faced with delicious choices in smart restaurants. So how can you carry on with your diet, not become a bore, and stay sociable? Here's how to meet some of the challenges.

Drinks

Remember that wines and alcohol are just as full of kilojoules as food. You can't stand around at parties without a drink in your hand, so ask for a spritzer (white wine mixed with soda or mineral water). A long, diluted drink is best, with ice-cubes, because you can sip it slowly and spin it out longer. If you're being very strict, a tonic poured over ice-cubes with a slice of lemon looks convincingly like gin-and-tonic. Low-kilojoule ginger ale on ice looks like Scotch on the rocks. If you think it sounds a bit 'soft' to ask for a diet drink, have one shot of alcohol — and keep on filling up with the mixer. Your glass looks full all the time.

Cocktail and buffet parties

All those chips, dips, nuts and hors d'oeuvres can send your kilojoule-count soaring. Remove yourself from the food corner of any room and keep your hands occupied, with drink and bag, so that you'll find it more difficult to reach for the nuts.

Self-service buffet parties give you the chance to take what you want. Slices of meat or poultry are fine; there's bound to be salad, but go easy on the mayonnaise. Skip the roll and butter. If you cannot bear to miss out on the desserts, have the smallest of helpings to satisfy your taste-buds. But avoid cheesecake at all costs because it is enormously high in kilojoules. A meringue is a better choice, surprisingly.

Dinner parties

These are more difficult when you are at somebody else's house, because you are faced with a meal which the hostess has cooked for you, without alternatives, and it would seem rude to refuse a helping. The only thing you can do is go prepared. Eat the minimal amount beforehand: work out how many kilojoules you think you will eat at dinner, then save them from meals earlier in the day. Don't have second helpings, and don't indulge in both cheese and the pudding. Sip your wine, so your glass doesn't need much replenishing.

Your own dinner parties are easy because you can whip up some fairly low-kilojoule but gourmet-style meals and stock up on slimmers' drinks. There's no reason why your guests have to eat bland, tasteless food because you are on a diet. Home-made soups give plenty of room for invention and make a delicious first course. You don't need to add cream. In casseroles, you can use emulsified vegetables such as onions and carrots as the thickener. Camembert and Edam are lower in kilojoules than other cheeses. Buy yourself a good dieter's cookbook, but test the recipes in advance.

Eating out

When you're in a restaurant the choice is yours, so choose wisely. It is so easy to be seduced by the huge menu, by what the people at the next table

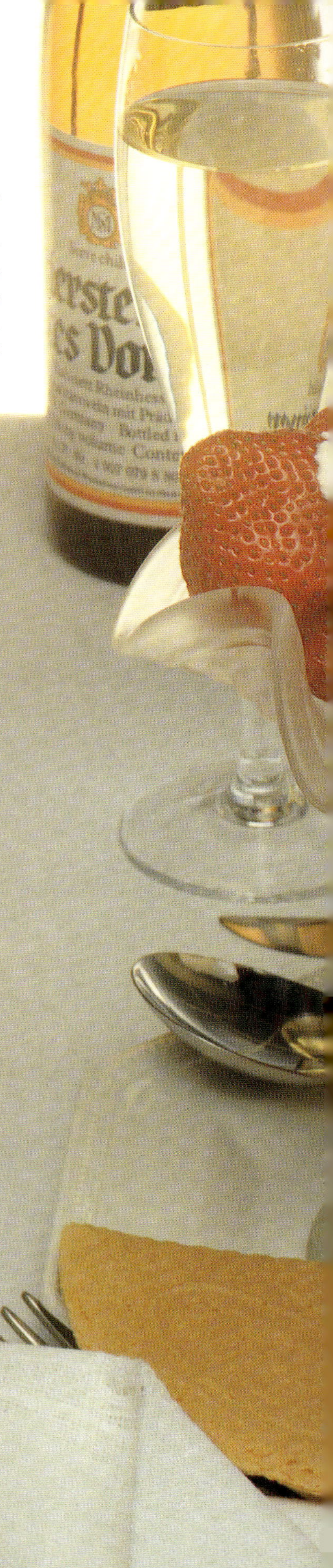
Weidenfeld & Nicolson Ltd

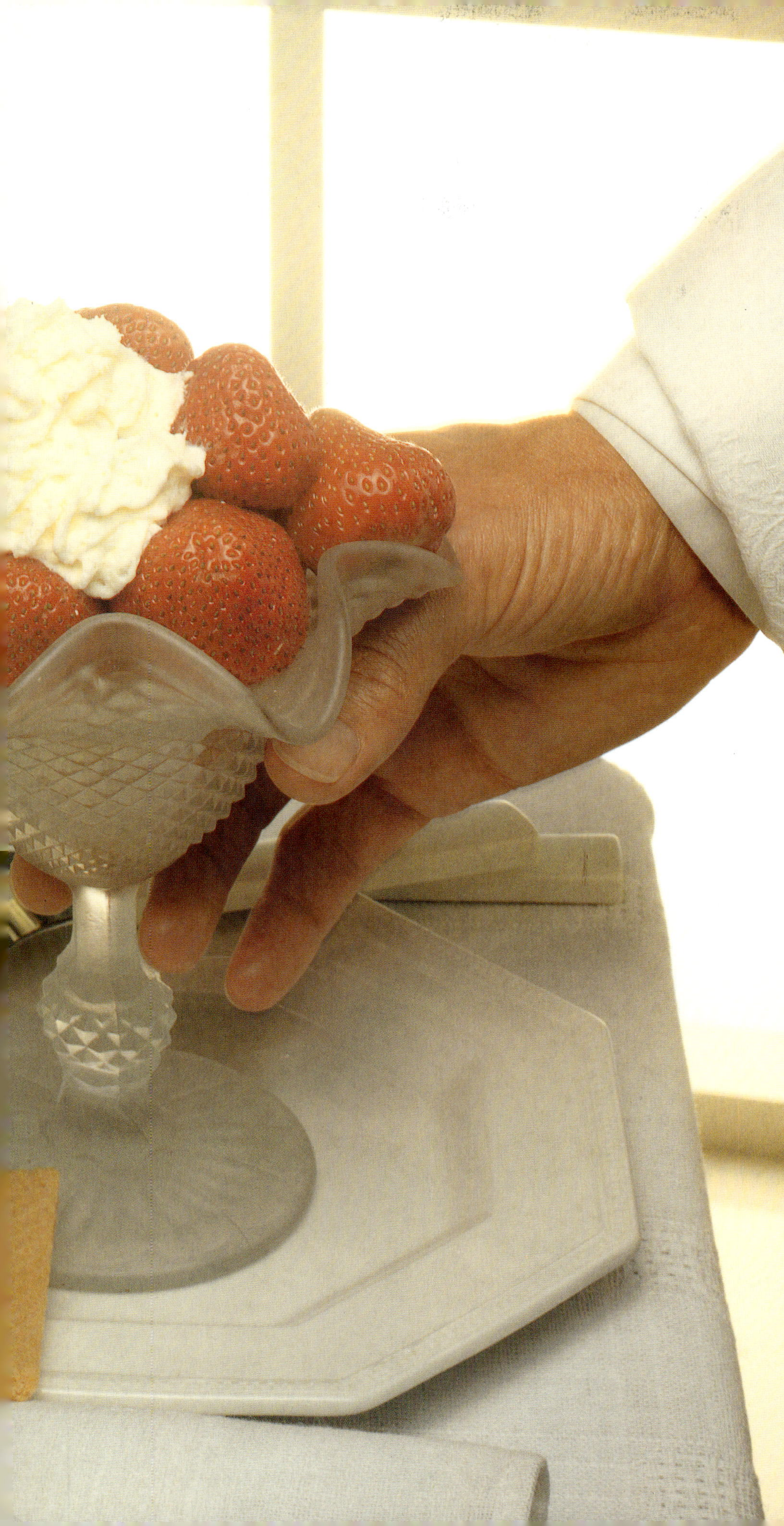

FAST FOODS

These could be your downfall. It is as well to know how many kilojoules you are taking away.

All the quantities are average takeaway portions unless otherwise noted.

Fried chicken

1 piece crispy chicken	945
small portion chips	1134
coleslaw	420
barbecued beans	420

Hamburgers

115 g hamburger	1764
115 g cheeseburger	2184
small french fries	880
chocolate milkshake	1530

Pizzas

whole pizza	2100–3360

Fish and chips

1 piece fish, deep-fried in batter	1365
portion chips	1365

Chinese

3 spare ribs	780
fried rice with pork and shrimps	880
egg fu yong	1660
sweet and sour pork	2184
beef chop suey	1175
chicken chow mein	1095

Kebab house

taramasalata	1325
doner kebab	2730
3 stuffed vine leaves	715
lamb kebabs	1515
Greek salad	420

Indian

beef curry and rice	3675–4200
vegetable curry	1134
chicken vindaloo	2435–2940
1 chapati	500

Sandwich bar

(using sliced white bread)

liver sausage	2015
roast beef	1640
cheese and tomato	1870
chicken salad	1825
ham	1725

are eating, or by the dessert trolley parked close to your left ear. First ask the waiter to remove the bread and rolls and butter from the table — if your companion doesn't mind! Otherwise, make sure it is not too close to you. It just isn't worth filling yourself up before the meal even begins.

Pick your way through the menu as if through a minefield. As you are paying for service as well as food, have the food as you want it. For instance, you can ask the waiter to serve the vegetables without butter.

For a first course, you could have fruit or tomato juice, grapefruit, melon, consomme, or even oysters. The ones to avoid? Rich creamy soups or soups with cheese and bread, such as French Onion soup. Pate is high in fat and lethal to any diet; with toast and butter it could be as much as 3570 kilojoules. Mayonnaise dishes — prawn cocktail, egg mayonnaise — are not such a good idea; nor are dishes with a pastry or pizza base. Smoked salmon is about 170 kilojoules an ounce and portions are usually wafer thin, so you could be quite safe with it as a starter . . . except for the brown bread and butter which usually accompanies it. Half an avocado with oil and vinegar is a very high-kilojoule choice. Melon and Parma ham, smoked eel, any non-creamy, non-buttery soup, or dish which is not fried, can be considered.

For your main course, a simple grilled dish is probably the best. Avoid pizzas, fatty lamb cutlets, mixed grills, anything fried in batter, chips, pies and puddings made with pastry, pork, lasagne. Salads are fine, so long as they are not dripping in high-kilojoule dressing, fried bread croutons, masses of grated cheese and pieces of bacon. Kebabs are a better bet than moussaka, braised kidneys rather than roast duck. A lean piece of grilled fillet steak, grilled chicken (don't eat the skin), or sweet and sour chicken would be better than big fry-ups.

Fresh fruit without cream, or fresh fruit salad, is a good dessert choice for dieters. Sorbet or ice-cream are better than rum baba and chocolate cherry cake, at least in kilojoules. Avoid cheesecake, baked sponge puddings, rich chocolate-cream concoctions, apple strudel, fritters fried in batter, or fruit with crumble topping. Creme caramel, peach melba, oranges sliced in caramel sauce and frothy light zabaglione can be considered. Say no to cheese and biscuits. Irish coffee is about 1470 kilojoules, so don't indulge.

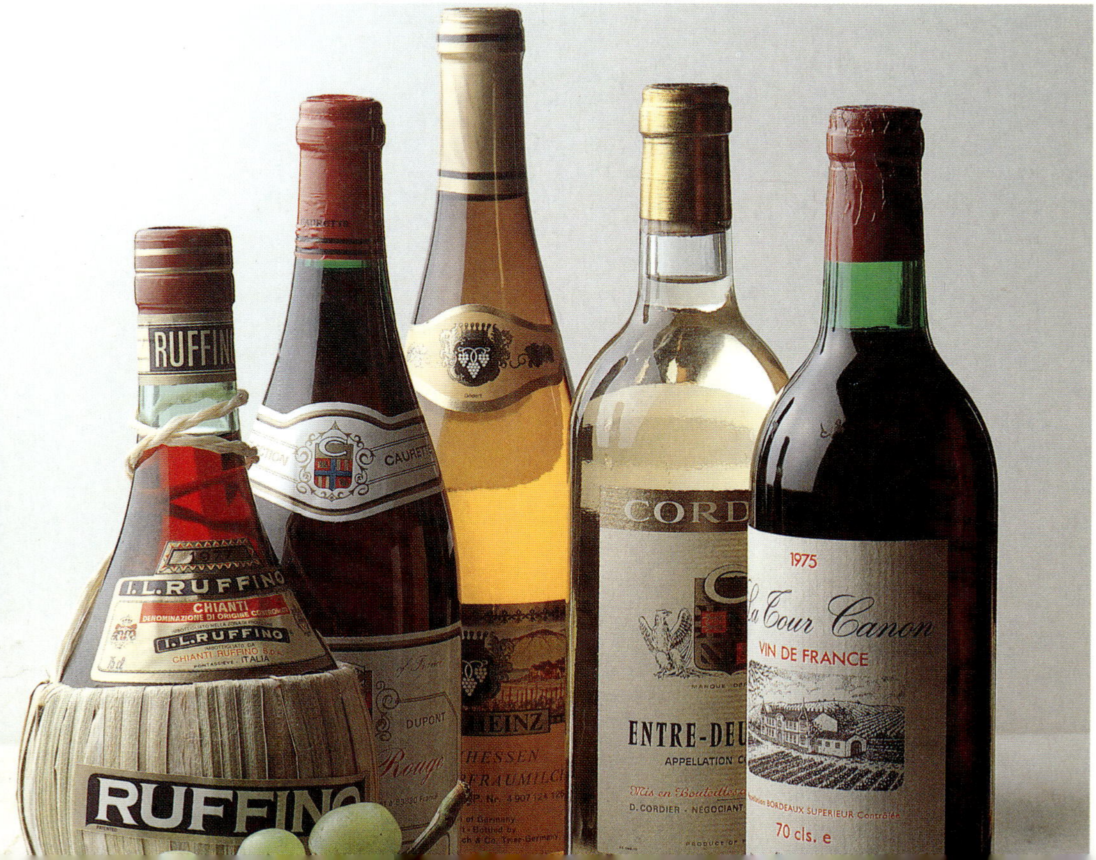

Taking off means learning to say "No"! There are a number of equally refreshing drinks lower in kilojoules.

A kilojoule-counted drinks guide

Counting the kilojoules can be a bit deceptive, since different brands have different values. Cider and beer, in particular, vary considerably according to manufacturer. The figures given here are average amounts.

NON-ALCOHOLIC DRINKS		
Drinks	**Kilojoules**	**Amount**
Bottled spring waters, mineral waters (e.g. Perrier), soda water	0	
Black coffee	Negligible	
Lemon tea without sugar	Negligible	
Low-kilojoule diet drinks and juices	Negligible	
Tea or coffee with 30 mL skimmed milk	40	170 mL
Tea or coffee with 30 mL normal milk	85	170 mL
Tomato juice	85	140 mL
Tonic water	100	140 mL
Dry ginger ale	125	140 mL
Tomato and vegetable juice	125	140 mL
Lemonade	125	140 mL
Orange juice (concentrate)	125	30 mL
Lime juice cordial (concentrate)	135	30 mL
Grapefruit juice (unsweetened)	190	140 mL
Orange juice (unsweetened)	190	140 mL
Tea with 30 mL milk and 10 mL sugar	200	170 mL
Coffee with 30 mL milk and 10 mL sugar	200	170 mL
Cola	230	140 mL
Iced black coffee with 40 g ice-cream	300	170 mL
Pineapple juice (unsweetened)	315	140 mL
Skimmed milk	840	560 mL
Milk (normal)	1555	560 mL

ALCOHOLIC DRINKS		
Spirits (gin, whisky, vodka at 70 proof, rum, bourbon, brandy)	265	30 mL
Dry sherry	278	55 mL
Dry vermouth	285	55 mL
Medium sherry	285	55 mL
Vermouth rosso	315	55 mL
Dry white wine	320	110 mL
Dry red wine	320	110 mL
Sweet sherry	328	55 mL
Rose wine	335	110 mL
Vermouth rose	335	55 mL
Liqueurs	335	30 mL
Vermouth bianco	360	55 mL
Sparkling white wine	370	110 mL
Port	378	55 mL
Sweet white wine	455	110 mL
Beer	315–570	280 mL
Cider	420–840	280 mL

COOKING TIPS

However you plan your diet, the way in which you prepare your food is important. You can make many kilojoule economies through sensible cooking.

☐ Grill, do not fry. That way the fat runs off bacon, sausages or chops, instead of congealing around them.
☐ Cut the fat off meat and the skin from poultry after cooking.
☐ Fry mincemeat without extra fat and throw away any fat residue by straining.
☐ When you cook casseroles, allow time for them to cool — preferably in the fridge overnight. It will then be easy to remove the top layer of fat that forms, before reheating.
☐ Sauces — instead of using traditional fat and flour for the roux, use cornflour or arrowroot as a thickener.
☐ Use skimmed milk instead of ordinary milk.
☐ Use a low-fat spread instead of butter, yoghurt instead of cream.
☐ Make your own low-kilojoule salad dressings to spice up your salads and marinades.

MYTHS AND PITFALLS

Popular theories about dieting seem to be in endless supply, and have been encouraged in recent years by all the fad diets that have come and — in most instances — just as quickly gone. Many of these seem appealing at first glance because they promise rapid weight loss — what you might not realise is that they are often nutritionally imbalanced and rarely offer you the chance to change your eating habits over the long term. The result? You regain all those kilograms just as rapidly as you lost them. Let's look at a few of the more common fallacies.

Grapefruit

Diets which insist that you eat half a grapefruit to start every meal because it 'helps to burn off more fat' are misleading. Grapefruit are low in kilojoules, high in vitamin C and therefore a good, convenient food for slimmers. But there is no evidence to substantiate the claim that a grapefruit can speed up your fat/energy conversion rate. The only way you can make your body 'burn' its stores of fat is to take in fewer kilojoules than you expend.

Fat diets

Diets which allow you to eat as much fat and protein as you like, but have you cut out carbohydrates completely, are now being discredited by expert opinion throughout the world. This fad diet is unsafe for your health. Fat can only be broken down completely in the body when carbohydrates are present. Otherwise ketone substances accumulate, producing giddiness and nausea, and giving your breath the smell of rotten apples. (Acetone, sometimes used as a nail varnish remover, is a member of the ketone family.) The ketosis that results is similar to what happens to diabetics if they have a disruption in supplies of insulin. Such a diet is high in saturated fats and cholesterol and, as described by the American Medical Association, 'unscientific and potentially dangerous to health'.

Water

Drinking an excessive amount of water every day will not help your body to get rid of its fat deposits; your kidneys will simply get rid of the fluid normally. Starting the day with a glass of lemon juice in hot water to 'cleanse your system' is about as effective as grapefruit 'burning up fat'. The vitamin C in the lemon juice is affected by heat, so whatever vitamin is left will not be contributing much to your daily requirements. There's no harm in drinking water of course; in fact, you should never restrict your intake of water when trying to lose weight.

Deceptive foods

Many foods are obviously loaded with kilojoules, but there are a number of others which are deceptive. Beware of concealed fat in avocado pears, Cheddar, coconuts, cream cheese, french dressing, liver sausage, meat, Parmesan, salami, sausages and Stilton. Concealed sugar lurks in some breakfast cereals, canned soups, dried dates and ginger root.

It may seem that a lush diet of oysters and steak, cold soups and smoked salmon is better, nutritionally, than a staple fare of meat and potatoes. In the case of watches and motor cars it may be true that an expensive item is of better value than a cheaper one, but it is not necessarily true of foods. You can diet cheaply, simply and well — and still eat foods prepared with taste and imagination.

SLIMMING CLUBS

Group therapy has a good record of success in helping obese people to lose weight. You get support, encouragement and advice, but you have to pay for it. Clubs say that by paying you have a further incentive to stay the course. If you can slim by yourself or with the help of your family, it would seem budget-wise to do so. But if you have weak willpower and a hard time sticking to any diet, then a commercial or local voluntary group could prove helpful.

The advantages are that you can discuss your slimming problems, be weighed and measured, learn new slimming tips and make friends with people who have similar problems. Some drawbacks are that you may feel like a schoolgirl when you do not achieve an adequate weight loss, grow bored, distrust the lecturers because they do not look slim enough or do not know enough about nutrition.

Some groups are fairly liberal in what diets you follow. Others are very strict and insist that you adhere to a special eating programme. Incentives can vary from small badges to vouchers and scarves. Some groups do exercise sessions at the meeting. All normally have a lecture after your weigh-in.

AIDS TO SLIMMING

A big slimming-food business has grown up in recent years, aiming to capitalise on the millions of people who are too fat. Some products may be useful as substitutes for higher kilojoule foods — slimmers' drinks, for instance — but nothing you can buy will take the place of your own self-control. Nothing you eat can be 'slimming' because all foods contain kilojoules. The best kind of balanced diet helps to re-educate your food habits, so you not only lose unwanted weight, but keep it off, too. Here's a guide to some of the many aids available.

Substitutes

Sweeteners Saccharin tablets are a slimmer's standby, invaluable for adding to hot drinks if you cannot re-educate your palate to do without a tinge of sweetness. Liquid sweeteners, which contain 98 per cent fewer kilojoules than sugar, are useful for cooking. Add them to foods away from the cooker, when they are cooling or cold, to stop any bitter taste. Powder and granulated sweeteners aim to look as much as possible like sugar; some are actual sugar granules coated with saccharin to give extra sweetness; others are concentrated saccharin powders which must be used sparingly. Newer low-kilojoule, granulated, sugar-free sweeteners have 90 per cent fewer kilojoules than sugar, but can be used spoon-for-spoon like sugar, which makes them easier to cope with.

Diet drinks Canned fizzy drinks have almost no calories and are good thirst-quenchers. Low-kilojoule mixers allow slimmers to have the occasional alcoholic drink and half the normal calories. Low-kilojoule squashes are also very useful.

Low-kilojoule dressings These are a useful aid to more interesting diets. Low-kilojoule tomato sauce is another saving.

Low-kilojoule spreads A good replacement for butter, giving you more spread on your bread in a kilojoule-controlled diet. Some taste better than others, so shop around. Processed cheese spreads also give a kilojoule saving.

Bread Slimmers' breads are lighter, weight for weight, than normal bread, but are usually no different in terms of nutrients. Because they weigh less, their energy value is about half that of ordinary bread. They are worth considering, but not if you eat twice as many slices in an attempt to fill yourself up.

Crispbread Made from wholewheat grains of rye or wheat, usually baked with just a little salt, vegetable oil or water, these are good slimming standbys. As crispbread normally retains the husks of grain, they provide fibre and roughage.

Preserves Low-kilojoule jams usually have to be kept in the fridge and have about half the kilojoules of ordinary jam.

Canned fruit Unsweetened, natural juice or water instead of syrup means a kilojoule-saving. A useful substitute, when fresh fruit is not plentiful or available.

Milk Skimmed milk and milk with the cream removed are both great slimming aids.

Soups Tins of kilojoule-conscious soup may prove time-saving, but you can easily make your own diet soups for even fewer kilojoules per serving.

Vegetable cooking spray This provides a less greasy way to pan fry, bake or grill. Since frying is normally forbidden on any slimming diet, this could open up new cooking choices. Spray it onto a cold pan and let the pan warm before adding food; don't be tempted to spray more than the recommended amount.

Meal replacements

Instead of a proper meal, you can have a bar of chocolate, a milkshake, a bowl of soup, a couple of biscuits. They provide you with anything from 525–1533 kilojoules and claim to contain added vitamins, minerals, and/or protein. If you do not have time to eat properly then these can make a quick snack, but they should only be used temporarily. Not only are they unsatisfying, but they do not help to re-educate your eating habits into the balanced, healthy eating pattern which will solve your weight problem for life.

'Medical' aids

Appetite reducers Nowadays doctors are less likely to prescribe pills to

A selection of low kilojoule foods: a crispbread, preferably with no butter or margarine, lettuce and tomato. It need not be a bland snack either; try some freshly chopped herbs such as basil or freshly ground black pepper sprinkled on the tomato and lettuce.

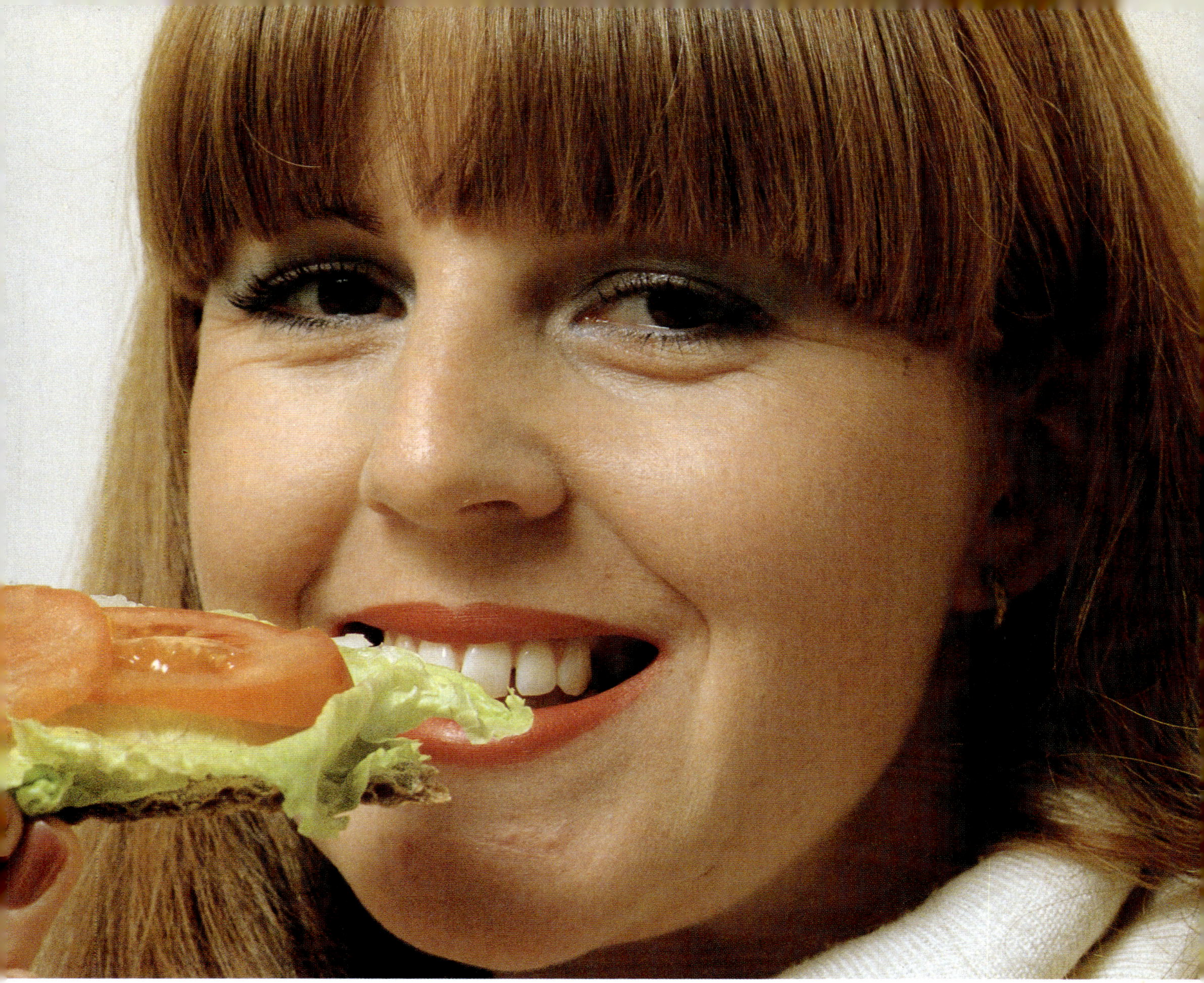

reduce your appetite unless you are grossly overweight, because of the possibility of dependence and addiction. And taking anything with methyl cellulose in it to make you feel fuller is a waste of time.

Diuretics These make you lose water. Unless you have an illness, which has the effect of making you retain water, you will not help your slimming cause by trying to lose more of it with diuretic pills. And it can be dangerous to lose too much water. The body has its own water-regulating system. You can lose water by sweating — and therefore lose weight — if you go to a Turkish bath or sauna. But you will put it back as soon as you have anything to drink.

Injections Some doctors may give injections of HCG (Human Chorionic Gonadotropin) as a treatment for obesity, together with a very strict diet, but it is not generally accepted by the medical profession.

Body treatments

Slimming garments — from a whole suit to ankle bands — wax treatments and plastic treatments are all sold on the theory that you lose weight as you sweat. But you don't lose fat. You only lose water, which you replace at your very next meal. Slimming 'baths' and slimming 'creams' are equally ineffective.

work-out

When was the last time you woke up in the morning feeling really terrific? How often do you pause during the day and realise how happy, healthy and fully in command you are? If you are anything like the average Australian woman, that rush of fulfilment and well-being is a rare moment of joy.

With a little bit of effort and persistence you can feel on top of the world just about every day of your life. The key to feeling terrific is physical fitness. The benefits of a healthy, fit body are numerous — from making your heart and lungs more efficient to increasing your feelings of self-esteem.

Note: Do not undertake any of the following tests and exercises if you are very overweight, or have a history of illness or back trouble, without first checking with your doctor.

TEST YOUR FITNESS

Stamina . . . how long can you last out?

The Step Test This test was first devised by Harvard University during the Second World War, and involves stepping up on to a stool, bench or the stairs (preferably about 40 centimetres high) and down again for a period of 3 minutes. Step up with one foot, bring up the other, then step down again, one after the other, repeating the sequence in a steady rhythm about 21 times per minute (women) and 24 times per minute (men).

After 3 minutes of 'step ups', remain standing and count your pulse over 15 seconds, beginning your count 5 seconds after the completion of the tests. The lower your heart rate over the 15 seconds, the better your physical condition.

Number of heartbeats counted in 15 seconds . . . and your rating

WOMEN

Under 45	Over 45	Fitness rating
Below 20	Below 21	EXCELLENT
20–22	21–23	GOOD
23–28	24–29	AVERAGE
Above 28	Above 29	POOR

MEN

Under 45	Over 45	Fitness rating
Below 18	Below 19	EXCELLENT
18–20	19–21	GOOD
21–25	22–26	AVERAGE
Above 25	Above 26	POOR

Simple Stamina Tests 1 Walk steadily, without stopping, up three flights of stairs (try it the next time you go to a big store and don't take the lift). Each flight should comprise about 15 to 20 steps. Can you climb and still carry on a normal conversation? **Fit**

Are you so breathless when you reach the top you cannot talk without panting? **Average**

Are you too breathless to continue after only one flight? **Unfit**

2 Can you run for a bus — say a distance of about 45 metres — without gasping for breath? **Fit**

Or do you wheeze and gasp? **Unfit**

3 Run on the spot lifting your feet at least 15 centimetres off the ground. If you are over 50, you should manage 2 minutes comfortably. Younger women should find 3 minutes easy. If you are fit, of course!

4 Try this running test only if you are fit enough to do the step test without problems. Jog for a kilometre. You should be able to talk comfortably without being over breathless during and after the test if you are really fit.

If the run takes . . .

More than 22 minutes: You are very sedentary

17–22 minutes: You are inactive

Less than 17 minutes: You are moderately active

12–14 minutes: You are an active person — probably you go jogging

Less than 12 minutes: You sound like an athlete.

As a simple rule of thumb, if you are under 45, you are fit if you can do it in about 12 minutes. Over 45? Add a minute for every 5 years. Men checking

It makes you feel terrific, fully in command of yourself, your self-esteem rises, your fitness and stamina levels increase; so with all these advantages why don't more of us do more exercise?

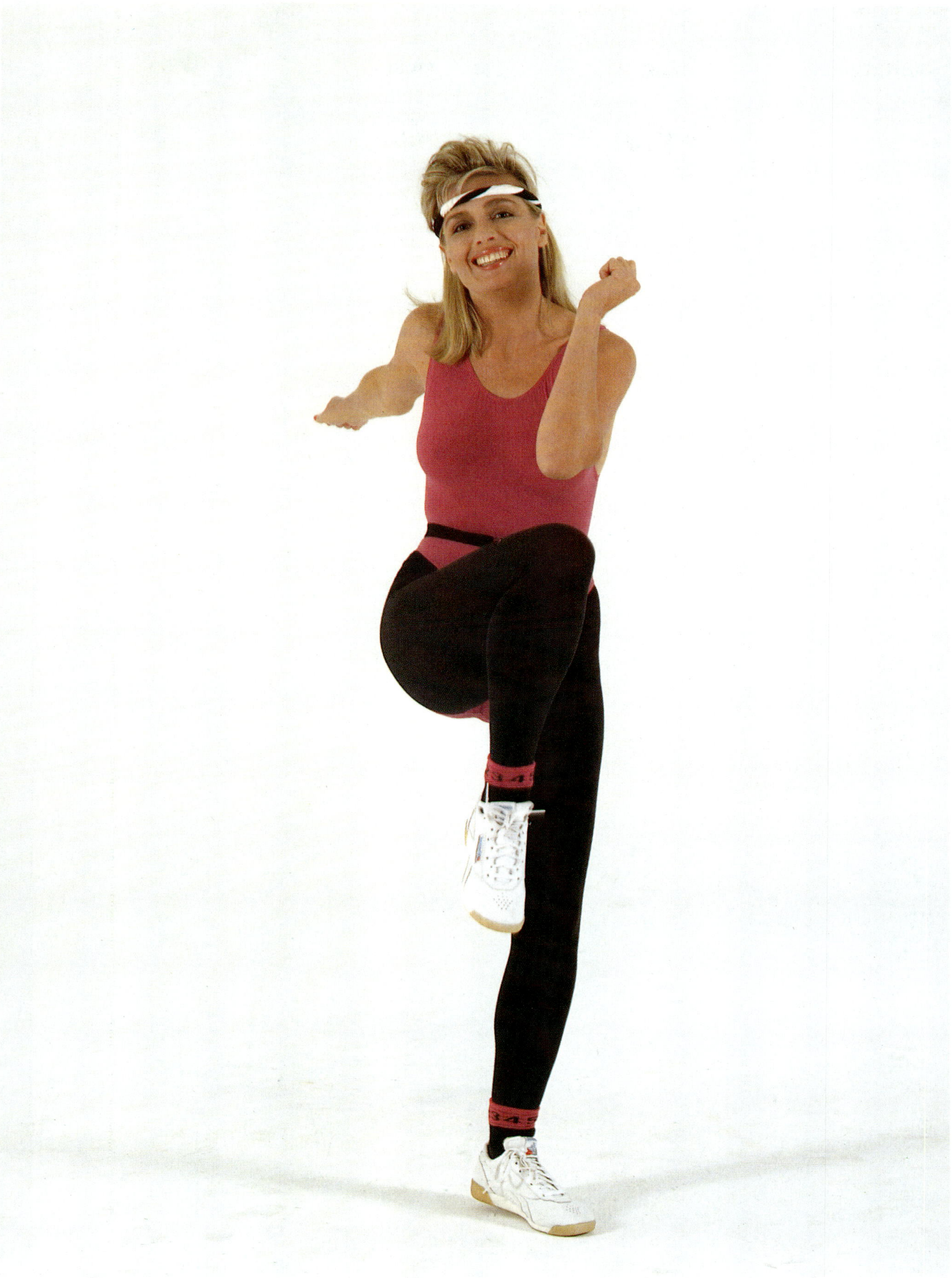

their fitness levels with this stamina test should subtract 2 minutes in each age group.

Strength test

Lie face down on the floor, elbows bent, hands resting on the floor. Now do push-ups. Extend your arms and push yourself up off the floor, keeping the body in a straight line. Lower gently back. Do this as many times as possible in 2 minutes. But *don't* push yourself to do more than you can — be honest.

FEMALE					
Age	**Excellent**	**Good**	**Average**	**Fair**	**Poor**
20–29	49+	34–48	17–33	6–16	0–5
30–39	40+	25–39	12–24	4–11	0–3
40–49	35+	20–34	8–19	3–7	0–2
50–59	30+	15–29	6–14	2–5	0–1
60–69	20+	5–19	3–4	1–2	0
MALE					
Age	**Excellent**	**Good**	**Average**	**Fair**	**Poor**
20–29	55+	45–54	35–44	20–34	0–19
30–39	45+	35–44	25–34	15–24	0–14
40–49	40+	30–39	20–29	12–19	0–11
50–59	35+	25–34	15–24	8–14	0–7
60–69	30+	20–29	10–19	5–9	0–4

Suppleness . . . how flexible are you?

1. Stand with legs together and try to clasp your hands behind your back, with one hand over your shoulder. (Repeat on the other side.) If you can do a full handclasp, score 2 points. Fingers touching: 1 point. Fingers cannot touch at all: 0 points.

Score
11–14 points You are very flexible. You haven't allowed yourself to become stiff or inactive. You probably have an active life.
7-10 points You are quite active, keep up the good work.
3–6 points You are not *too* bad, but you need to exercise before you stiffen up.
0–2 points Not so good. You must be very stiff. Ageing isn't the problem so much as inactivity. You need to start a gentle programme of flexibility exercises.

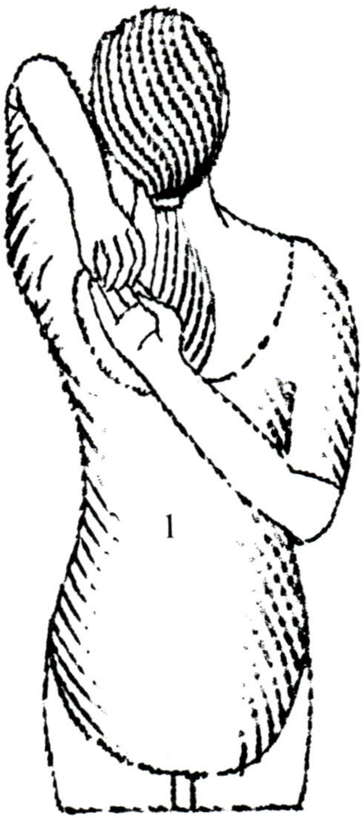

2. Stand straight, with legs together and arms at your sides. Keeping your hips and shoulders to the front, tilt the top part of your body over to one side as far as you can. Then bend to the other side. If you can bend 45° from the upright, score 3 points. Less than 45°: 2 points. Head tilt only: 1 point.

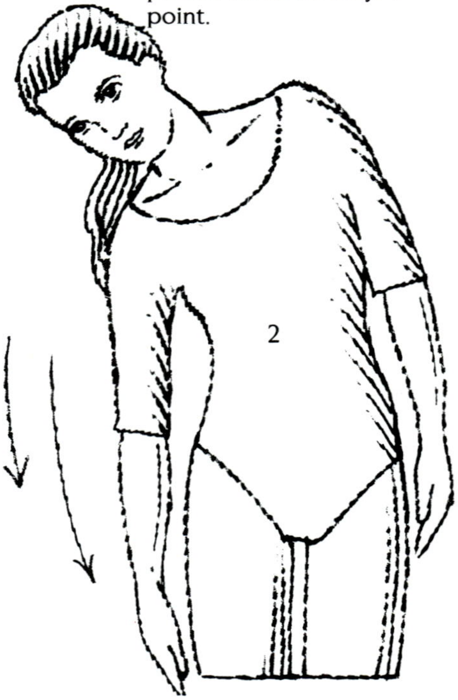

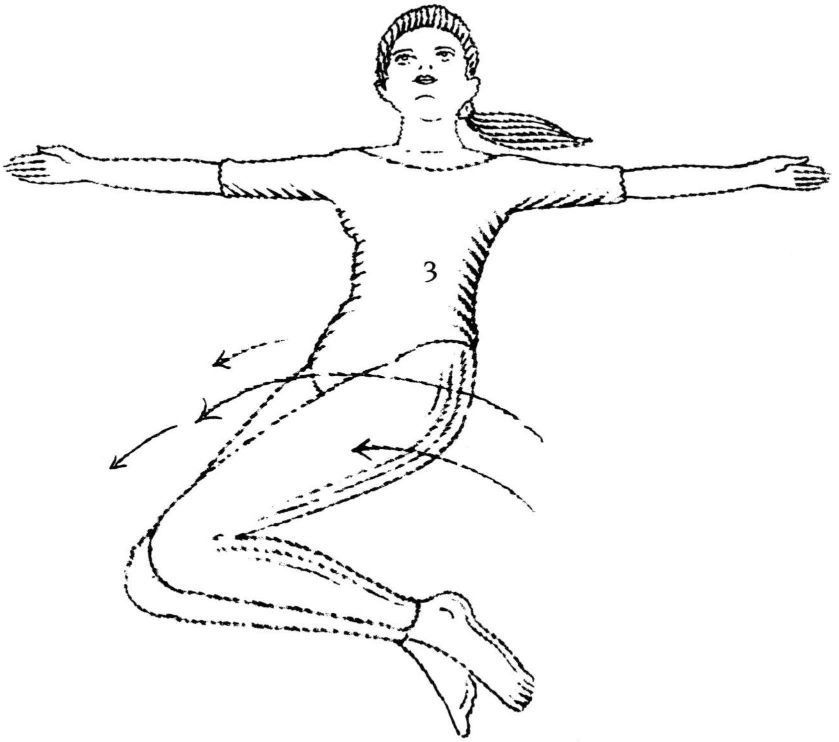

3. Lie on the floor on your back, arms outstretched at shoulder level, knees bent, shoulders flat on the floor. Drop both knees over to one side and then to the other. If you can touch the floor with your knees and keep your shoulders flat, score 3 points. If either shoulders or knees are 8 centimetres from the floor: 2 points. More than 8 centimetres from the floor: 1 point.

4. Sit on the floor with legs straight out in front and bend over to try to touch your toes (feet flexed up) with straight arms. Don't bend your knees! If you can touch your toes or beyond them, score 3 points. If you can reach your ankles: 2 points. If you can only reach your calves: 0 points.

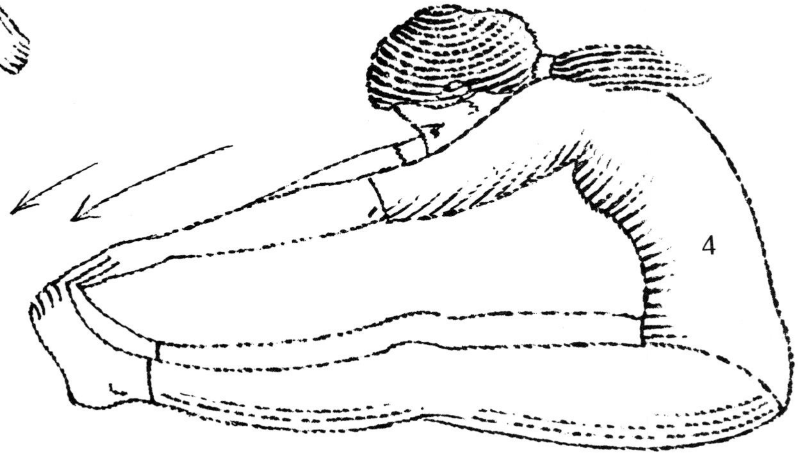

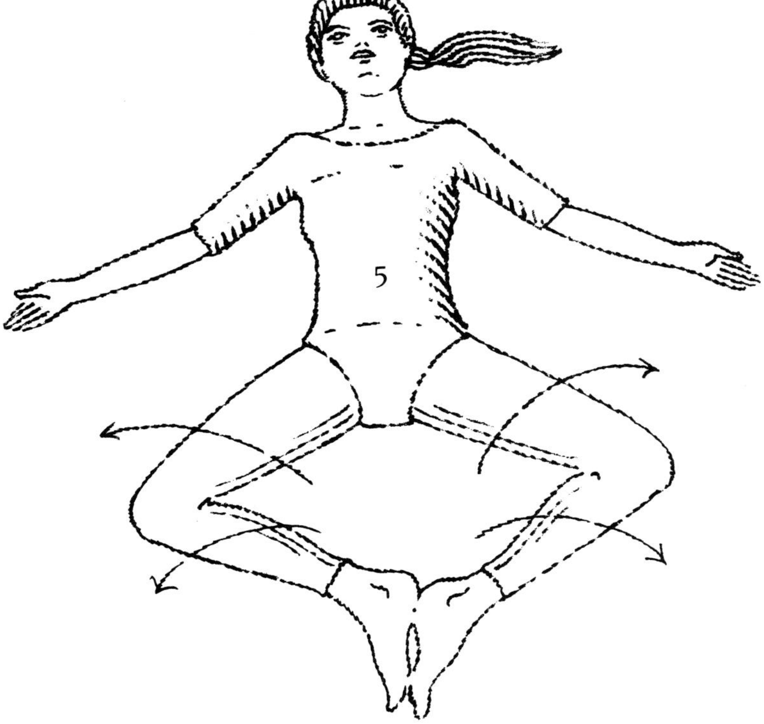

5. Lie on your back, with knees bent up and feet flat on the floor, and arms resting slightly away from your sides. Allow your knees to drop open, keeping the soles of your feet together and your spine in contact with the floor. This tests the flexibility of your hips without straining your back. If your knees are near the floor, score 3 points. If half-way between the vertical position and the floor: 2 points. Less than half-way: 0 points.

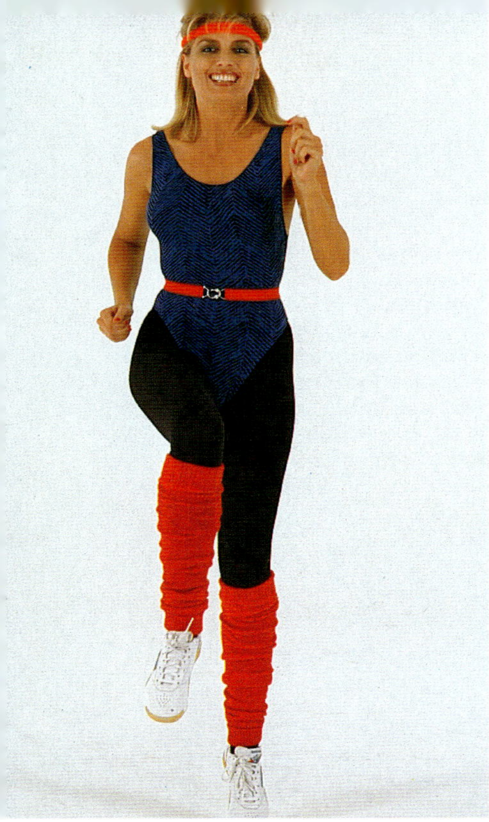

Aerobic exercise stimulates the whole body.

A BALANCED FITNESS PROGRAMME

A balanced fitness programme combines warm-up and cool-down exercises and muscle strengtheners. This fitness programme has been specifically designed to include all the necessary categories in the correct order. It is essential that you follow the exercises correctly so that you avoid injury and gain the maximum amount of benefit in the minimum time.

Programme One involves routines which improve your body's flexibility, suppleness and muscle tone. The exercises are also excellent in helping to reduce stress caused by the demands of modern living. Many of the positions are based on traditional yoga practices.

Programme Two combines flexibility and stretching routines with more strenuous aerobic activity. Aerobic activity stimulates the entire body and improves the health of your heart, lungs and circulatory system. These programmes also include muscle strengtheners designed to give your body endurance and power.

Both programmes begin and end with gentle warm-ups and cool-downs. These exercises may seem easy, and therefore of no benefit, but do not neglect them as they are essential to avoid injury, especially painful muscle strains. When your body is properly warmed-up, the ligaments and tissues are more flexible, lessening the chance of damage.

Cool-downs are equally important. Never rush away from a vigorous aerobic routine, no matter how busy you are. Relaxing exercises at the end of each programme gently stretch your tired muscles and help reduce stiffness and soreness. To neglect cool-downs can lead to light-headedness, dizziness, nausea or even fainting.

On reaching 35 or 40, most women become concerned about the slackening muscle tone in their face which inevitably leads to wrinkles. Nothing will stop you becoming older, but you can slow down the rate at which your face ages by doing simple facial exercises. There are four exercises for you to do each day which help to prevent lines on your face and neck.

The fitness programme also includes a special section on back exercises. Millions of Australians suffer from back pain, often in the lower back. Prevention is the best medicine when it comes to back problems. Learn to lift things properly, bending from the knees, keeping your back straight and using your powerful leg muscles to bear the weight. But 80 per cent of all back pain can be traced to lack of exercise. Do the prescribed back exercises every day to strengthen muscles and ease back pain.

Sleep

As people get older they find it more difficult to sleep. The amount of sleep you need is determined by a variety of factors including age, personality, heredity, health, lifestyle and occupational stress. Try not to worry about sleep — that will only make the problem worse. Here are a few tips to help you make the most of sleep.

☐ Go to sleep and wake up at the same time each day. Your body functions best on a regular schedule. Don't go without sleep during the week and then try to make up for it on the weekend.

☐ Avoid strenuous exercise just before bed. Fit people sleep better, but your body needs a couple of hours after exercise to wind down.

☐ Don't drink caffeinated or alcoholic drinks in the evening. Try some warm skim milk or herb tea instead.

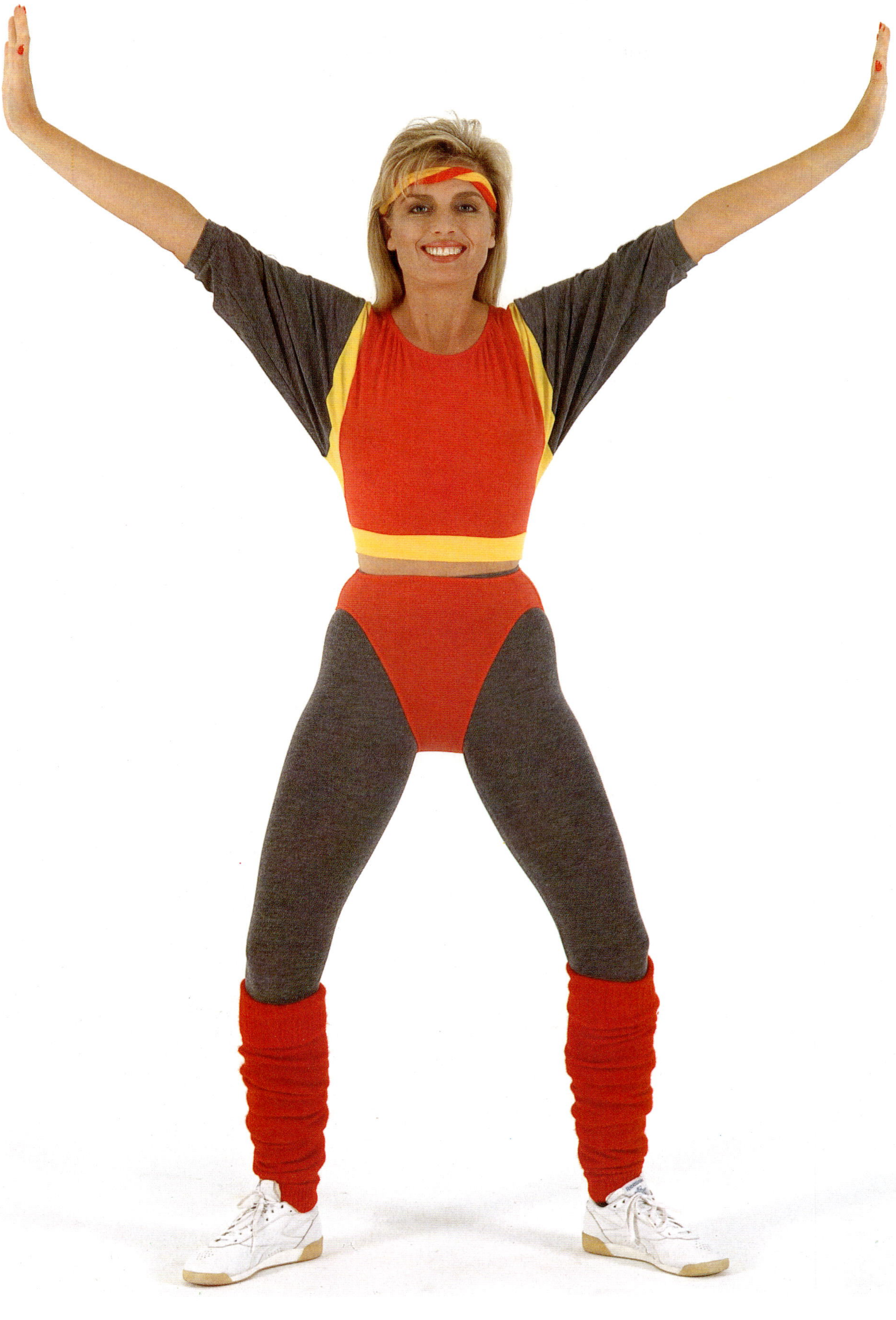

PROGRAMME ONE

FLEXIBILITY, BREATHING, TENSION-REDUCERS

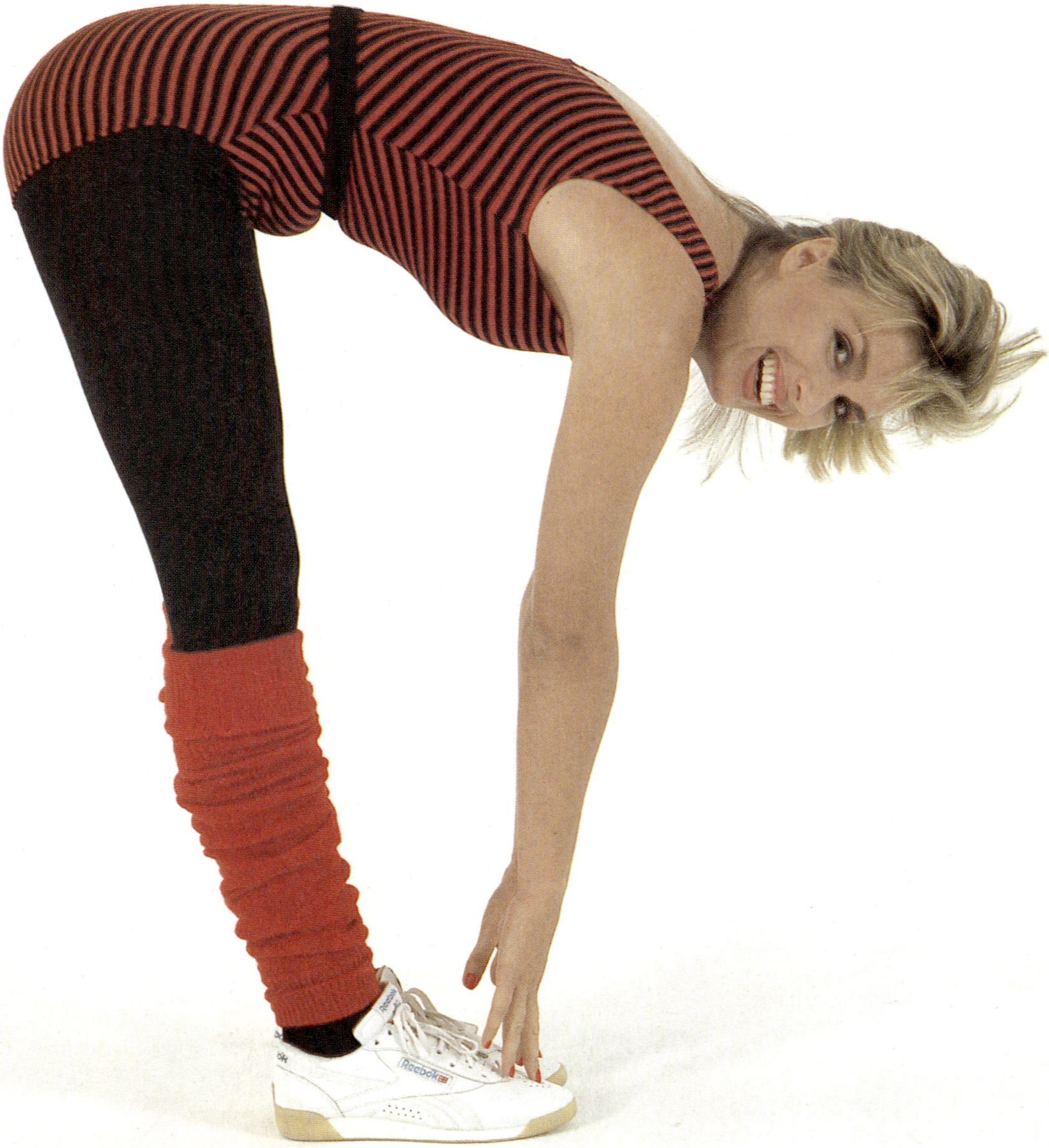

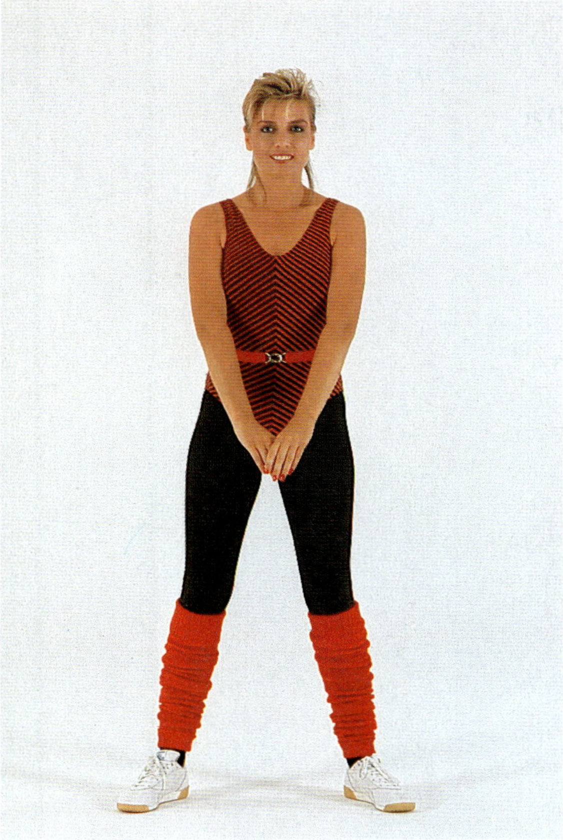

1

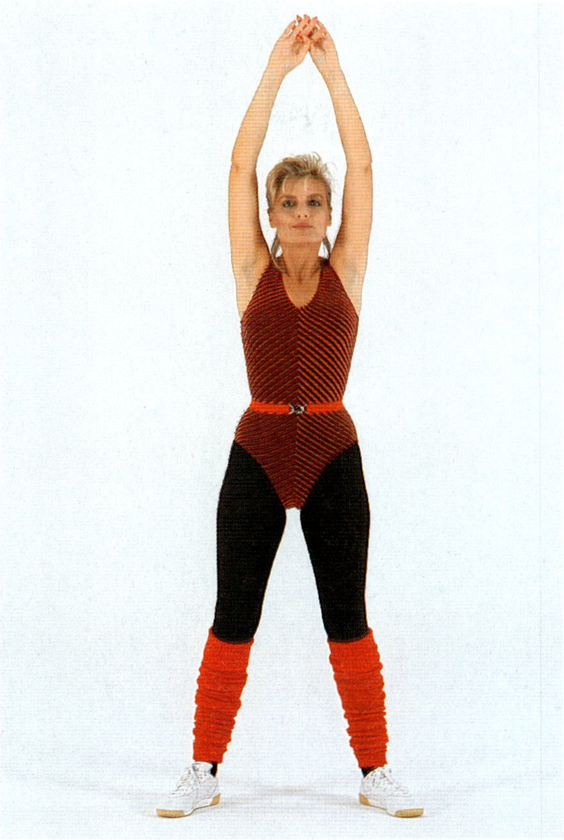

2

THE AXE

1. Starting position.

2. Breathe out slowly until the lungs are empty. With hands clasped as though gripping the shaft of an imaginary axe, raise 'the axe' slowly above your head, breathing in as you do so. Swing your arms back as far as you can, bending from the waist. Hold for three seconds.

3. Bring your arms down with full force, through your legs. Breathe out through the mouth as you swing down. Repeat three times.

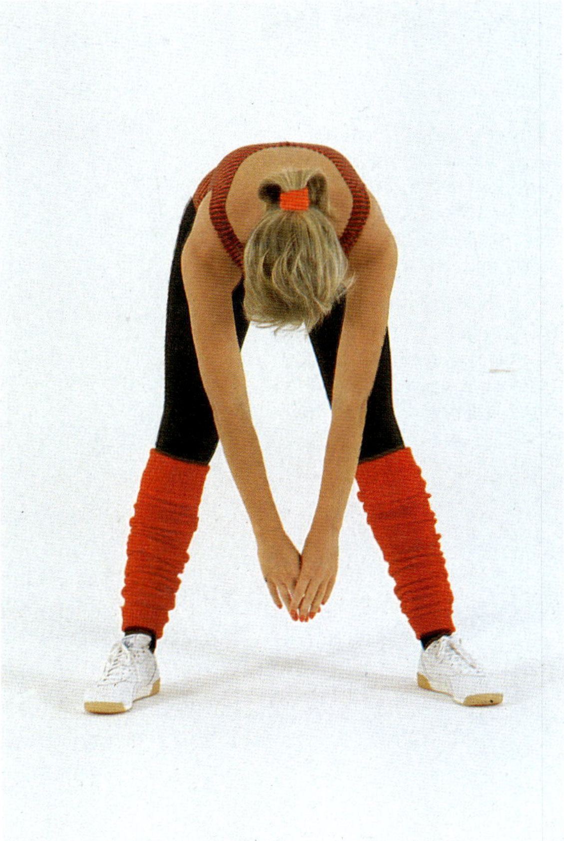

3

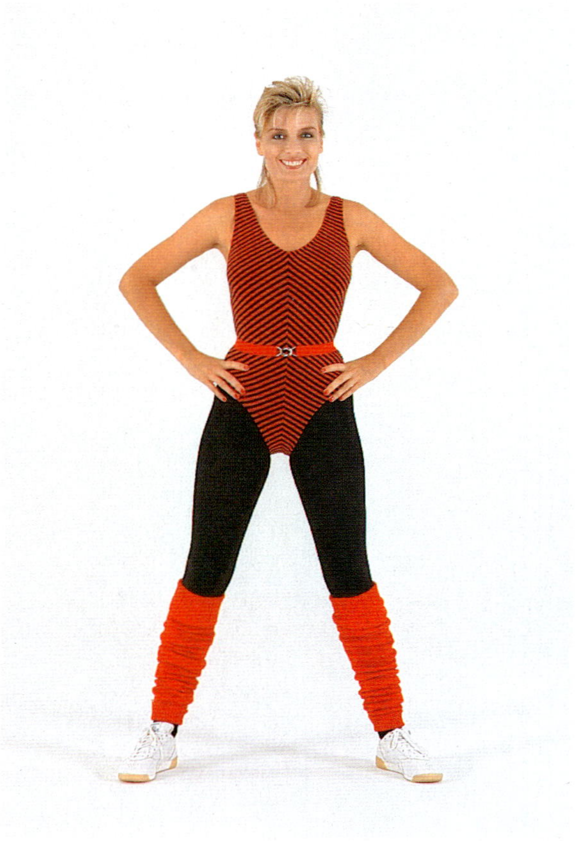

1

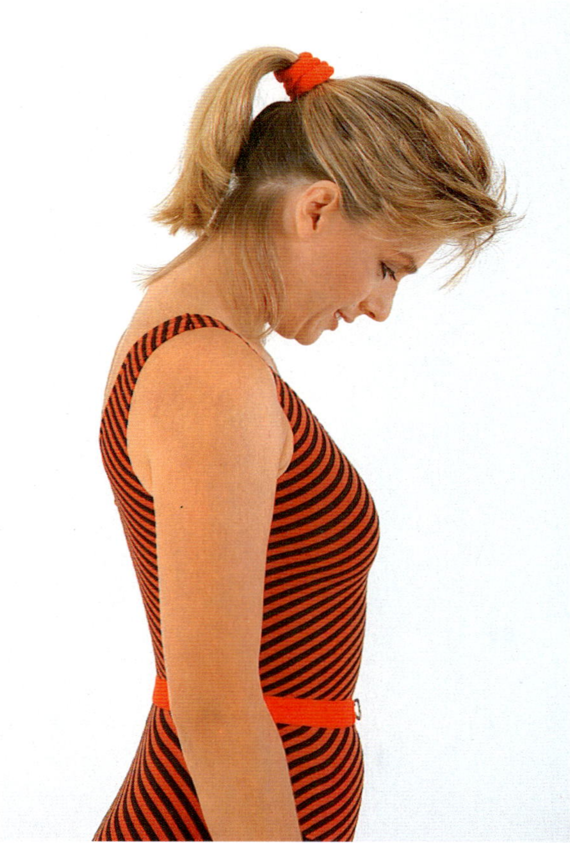

2

FLOP NECK

1. Starting position.

2. Drop your chin down slowly towards your chest, hold, and relax. Slowly bring your head back up. This exercise must be done slowly and gently.

3. Gently and slowly tilt your head backward so that you can see the ceiling. Hold, then bring your head back down. Repeat four times.

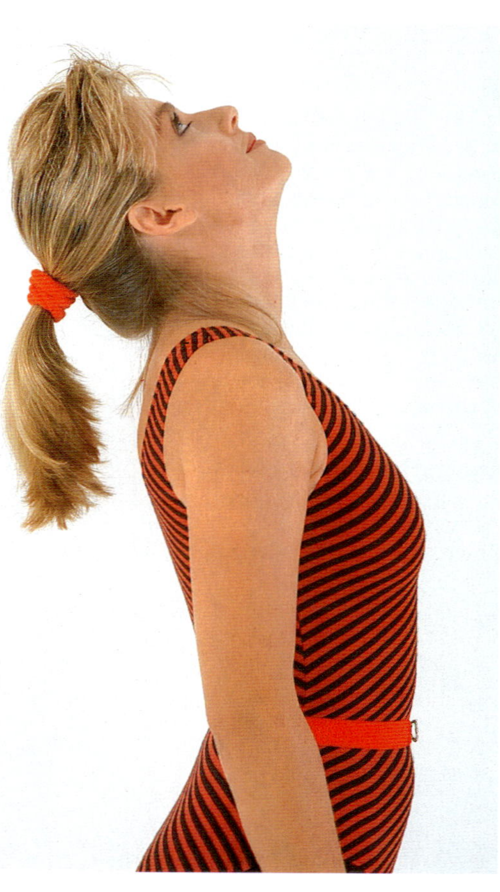

3

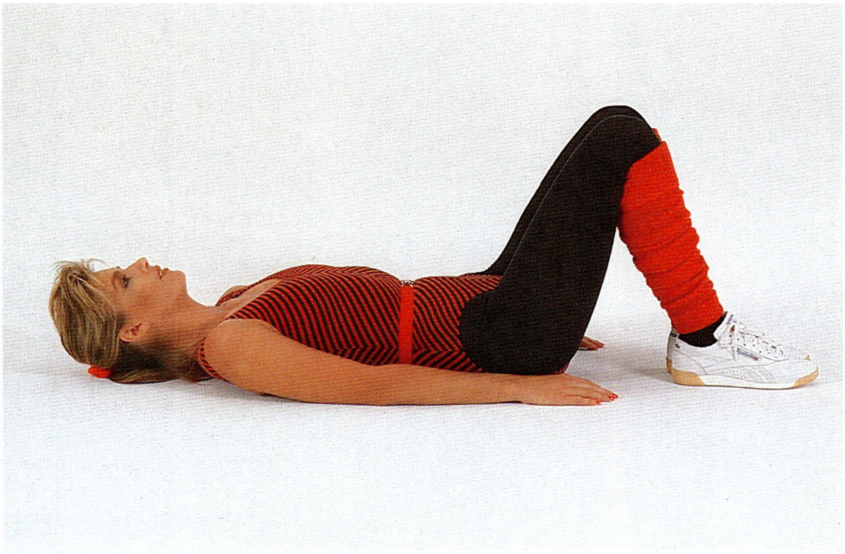

1

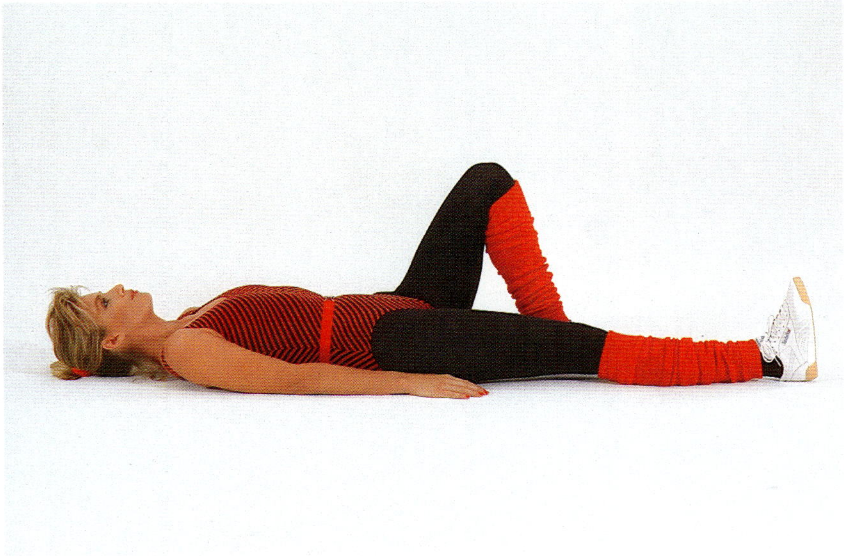

2

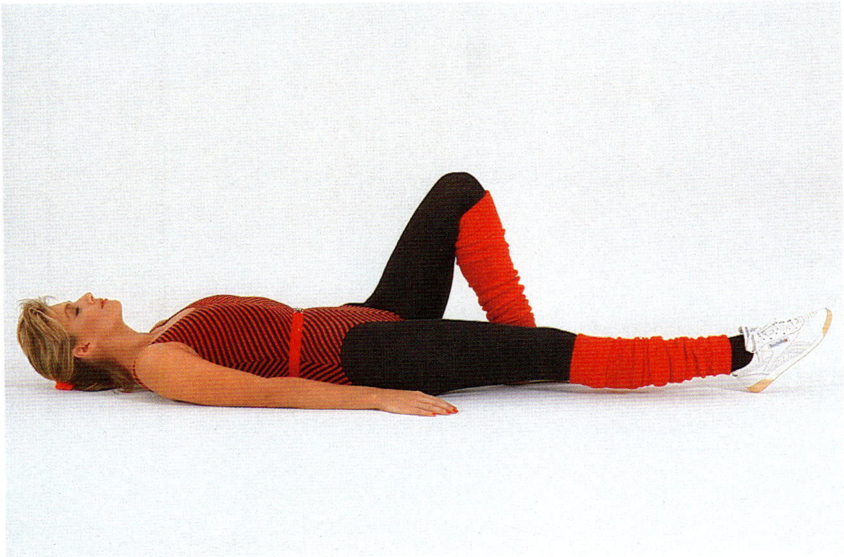

3

QUADRICEPS-HAMSTRING DOUBLE

1. Starting position.

2. Straighten your right leg and tighten your front thigh muscles — the *quadriceps* by trying to push the back of your knee to the floor. Make your leg as stiff as possible. Hold for five seconds, relax for five seconds, then repeat. Do five times.

3. To strengthen your hamstring muscles, with right leg out straight and toes pointed, press to the floor with your heel. Hold for five seconds, relax for five seconds, then repeat. Do five times. Repeat 1 and 2 using your left leg.

BOTTOM TAPPER

1. Starting position.

2. Bend your left leg up, bringing your heel as close as possible to your bottom. Hold for three seconds, then let foot down slowly. Repeat five times. Repeat with your right leg.

3. This time bend both legs together, reaching your heels as close as possible to your bottom. Hold for three seconds, then let your feet down slowly. Repeat five times.

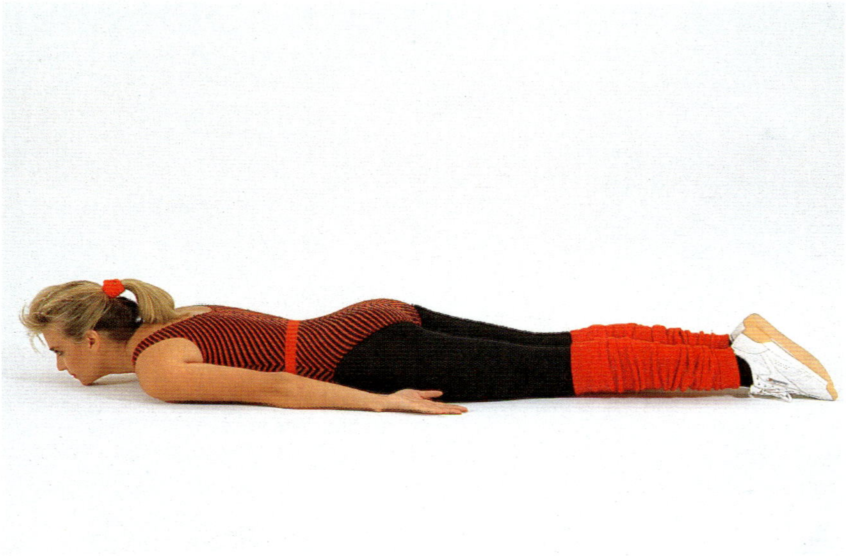

1

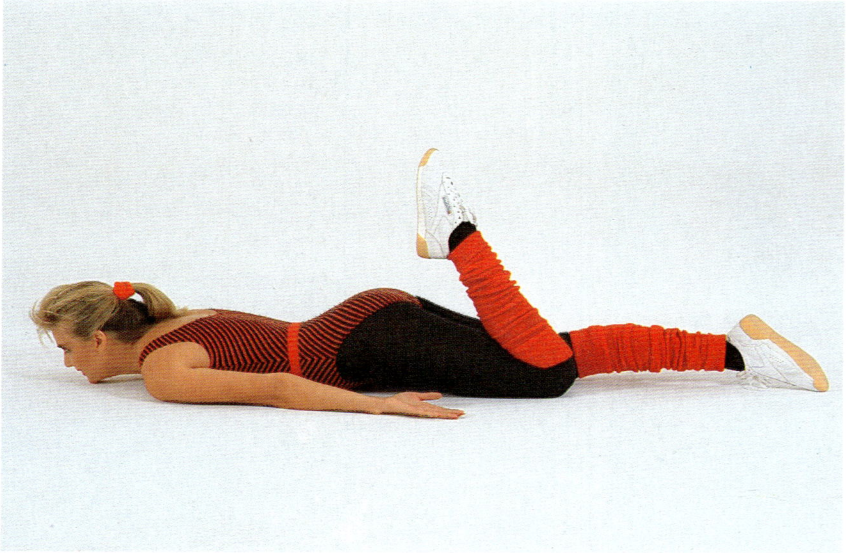

2

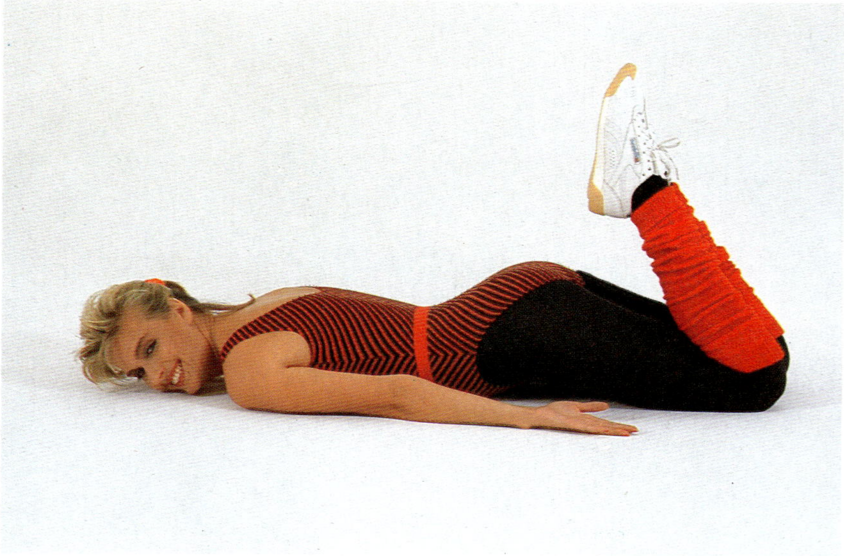

3

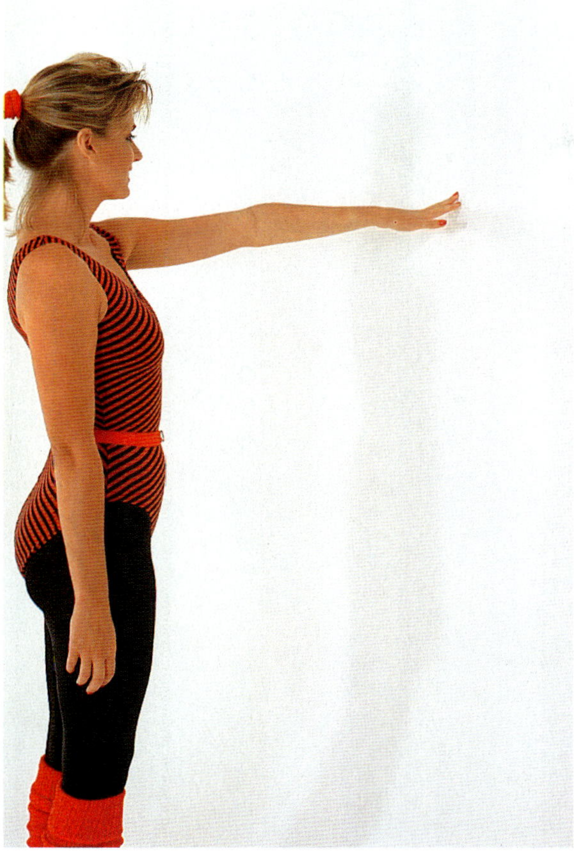

1

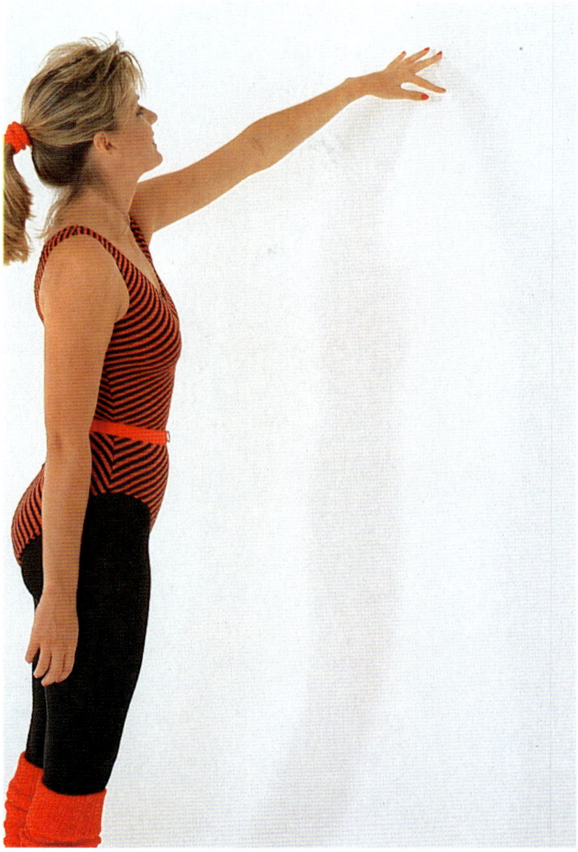

2

THE WALL WALK

1. Starting position.

2. 'Walk' the fingers of your left arm up the wall as far as you can go. Begin at waist level. This exercise is excellent for strengthening the shoulder and working on those fatty deposits in the upper arm. Repeat five times.

3. Repeat five times using the right arm.

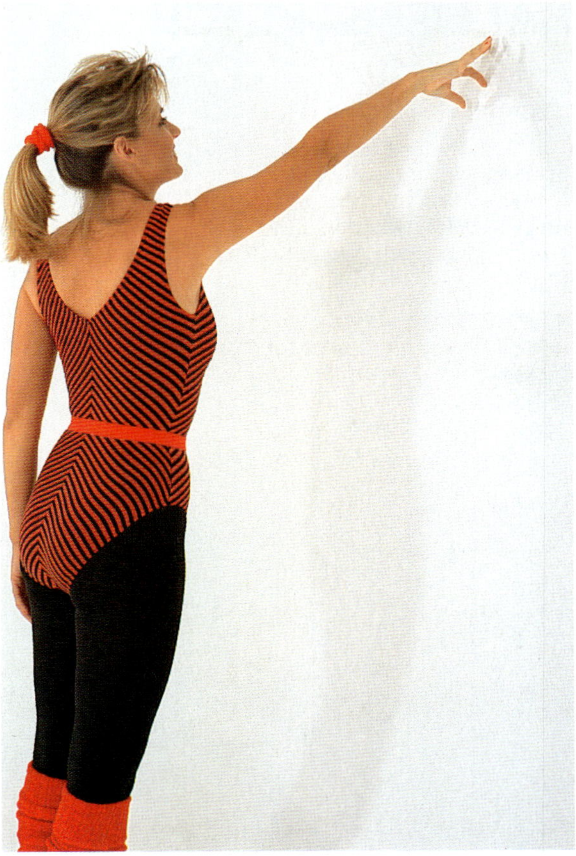

3

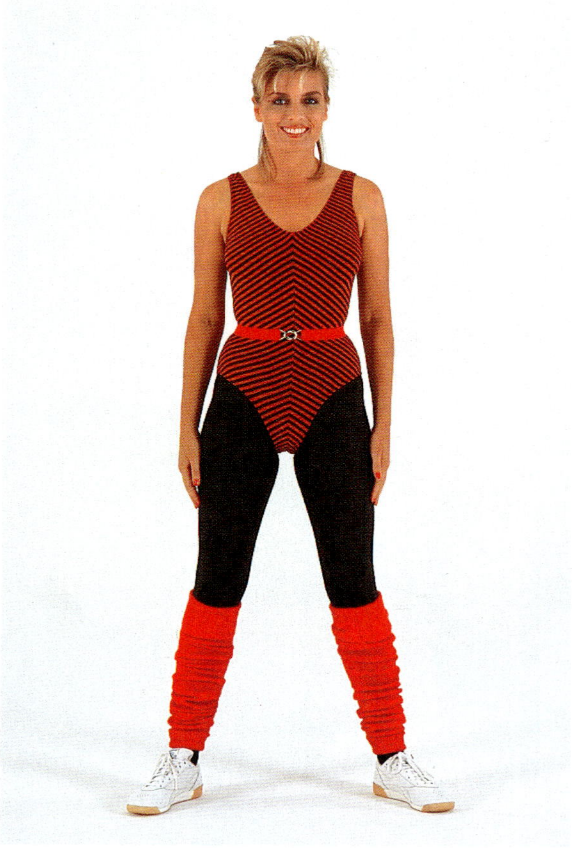

1

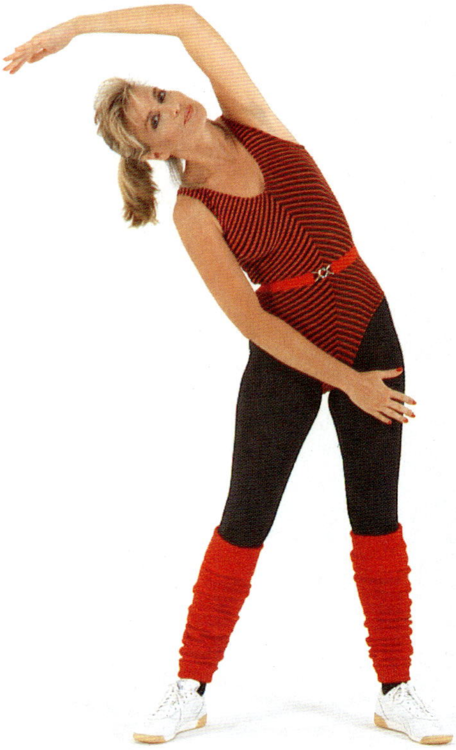

2

BALLET STRETCH

1. Starting position.

2. Keeping your body facing forward, swing your left arm over your head and out to the right. You should feel the stretch right down your left side.

3. Return to the starting position and stretch over to the left. Repeat 10 times each side.

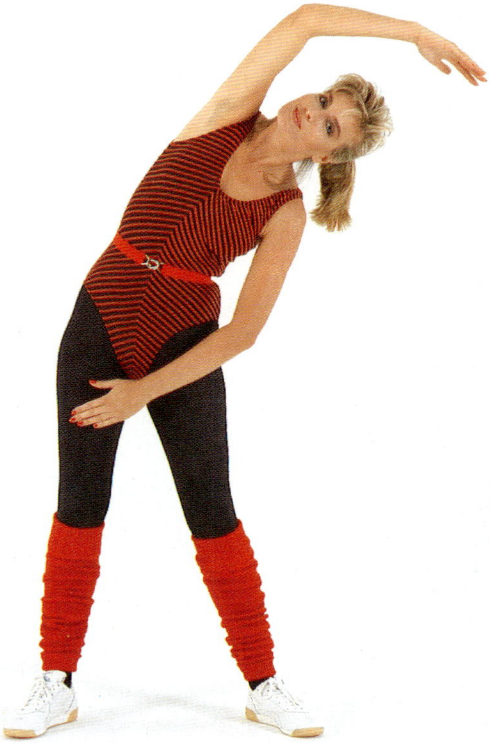

3

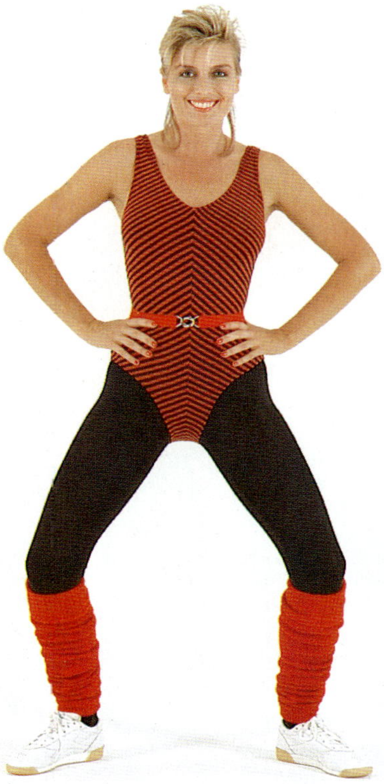

1

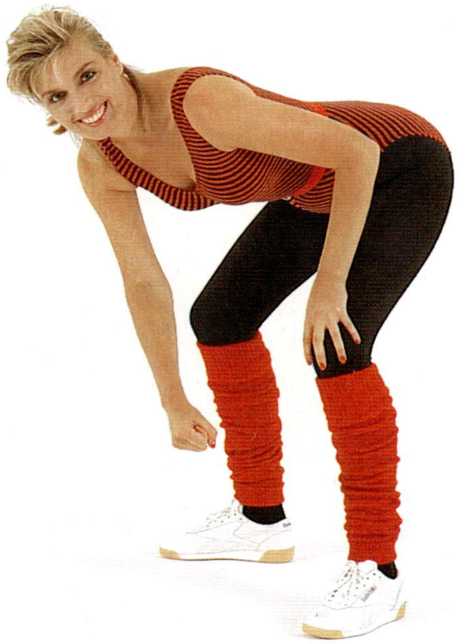

2

SQUATTING PUNCH

1. Starting position.

2. Moving your body weight from side to side in a rocking motion, with knees bent, bend over from the waist until your back is flat and straight. Punch your right arm down towards your left foot, then punch your left arm down towards your right foot. Repeat in rapid succession twice.

3. Continue rocking from side to side. Straighten your body and punch your arms out from side to side. Punch right arm across your body to the left, then left arm across your body to the right. Repeat in rapid succession twice. Alternate 1 and 2, repeating the sequence 10 times.

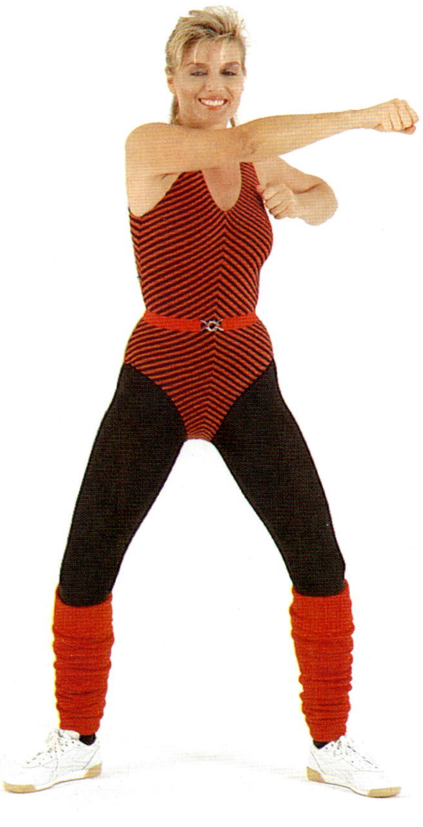

3

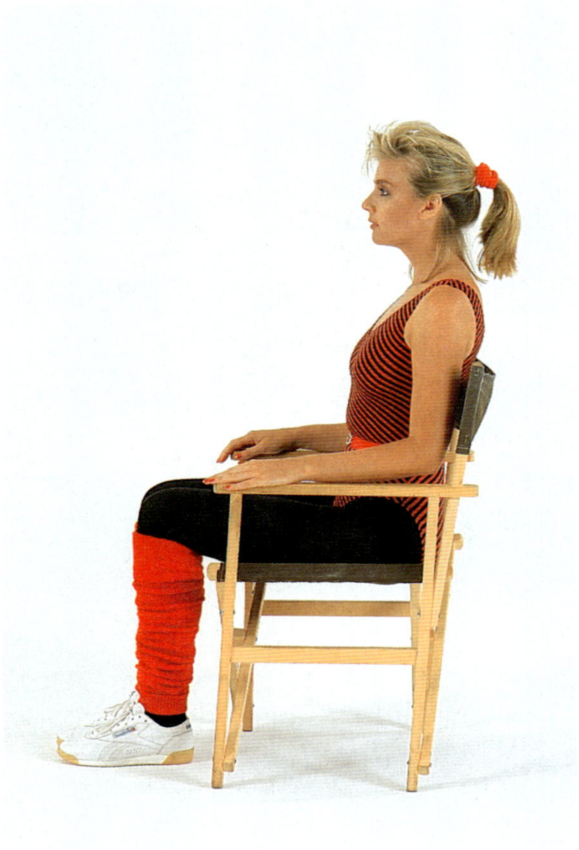

1

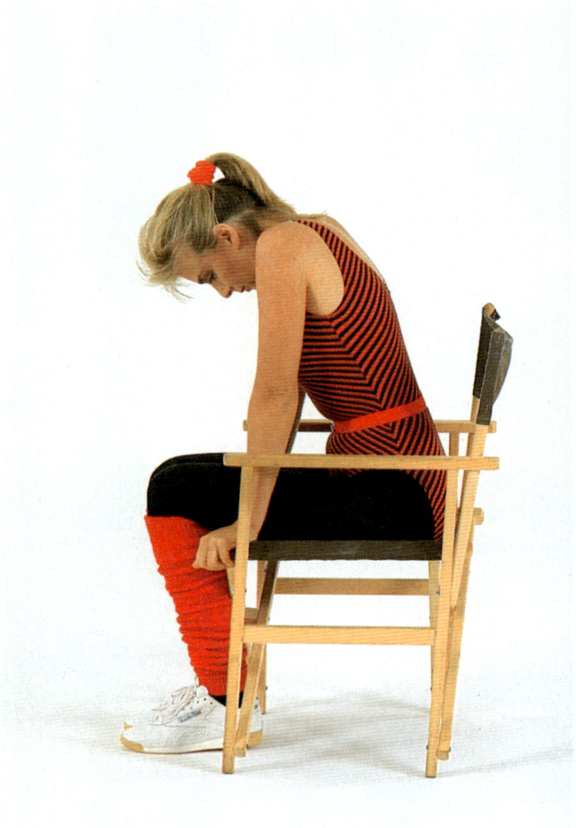

2

TENSION REDUCER

1. Starting position.

2. Grasp the front of the seat with your hands, on either side of your legs. Let your head and shoulders slump forward.

3. Using the chair for leverage and balance, sit up and arch your back. Breathe deeply as you arch and exhale as you slump forward. Repeat five times.

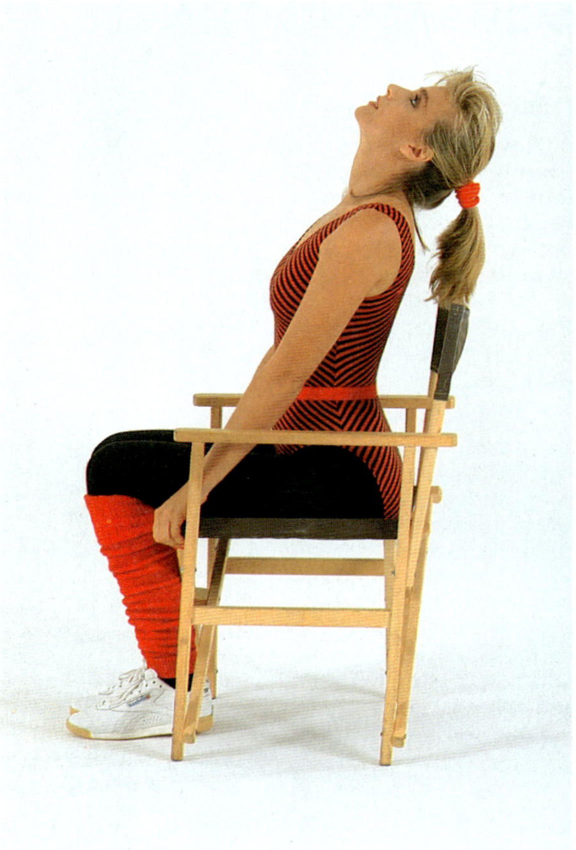

3

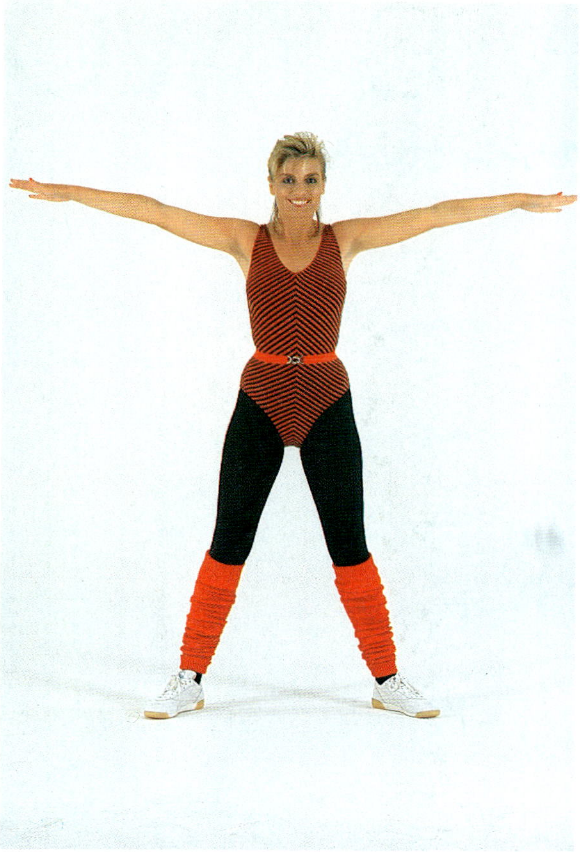
1

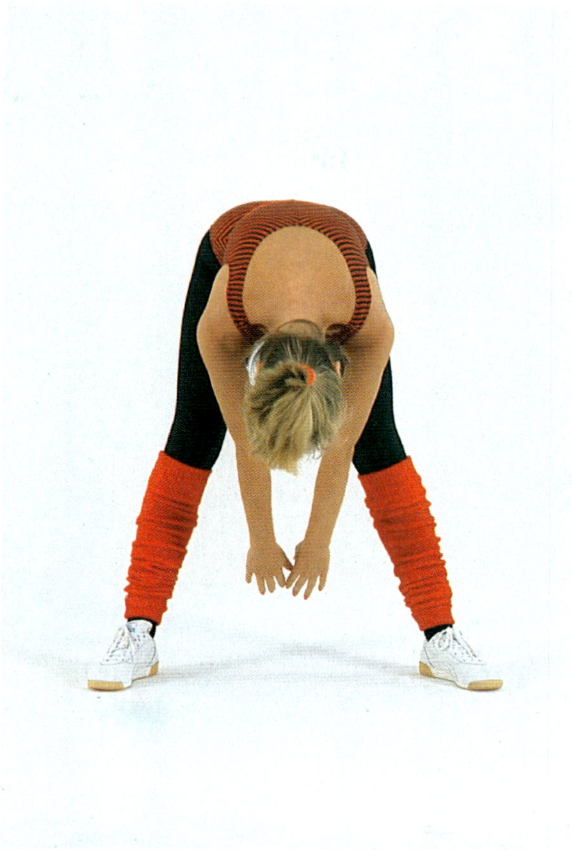
2

FLYING FLOP

1. Starting position.

2. Keeping your legs absolutely straight and your heels on the floor, bend forward from the waist and swing your arms through your legs as far as you can comfortably reach.

3. Roll up one shoulder at a time until you're standing upright.

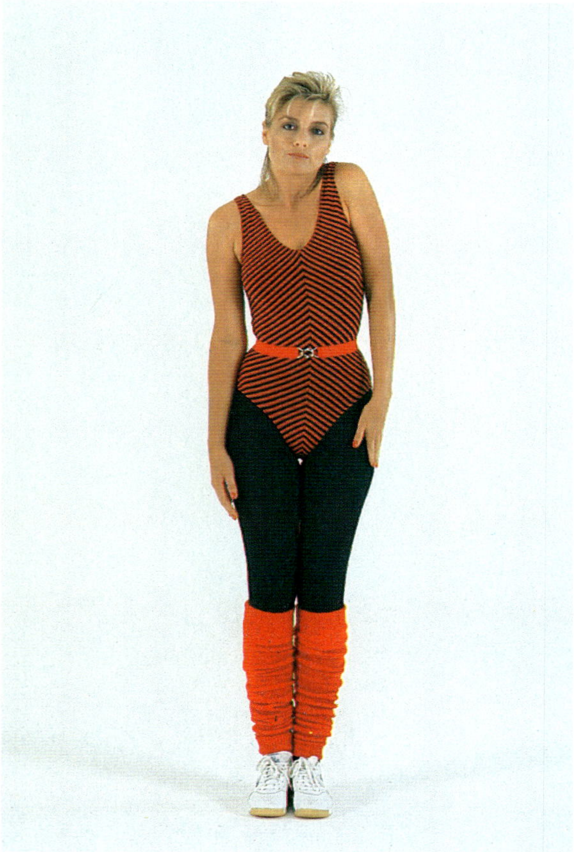
3

PROGRAMME TWO

BREATHING, WARM-UPS, AEROBIC, COOL-DOWNS

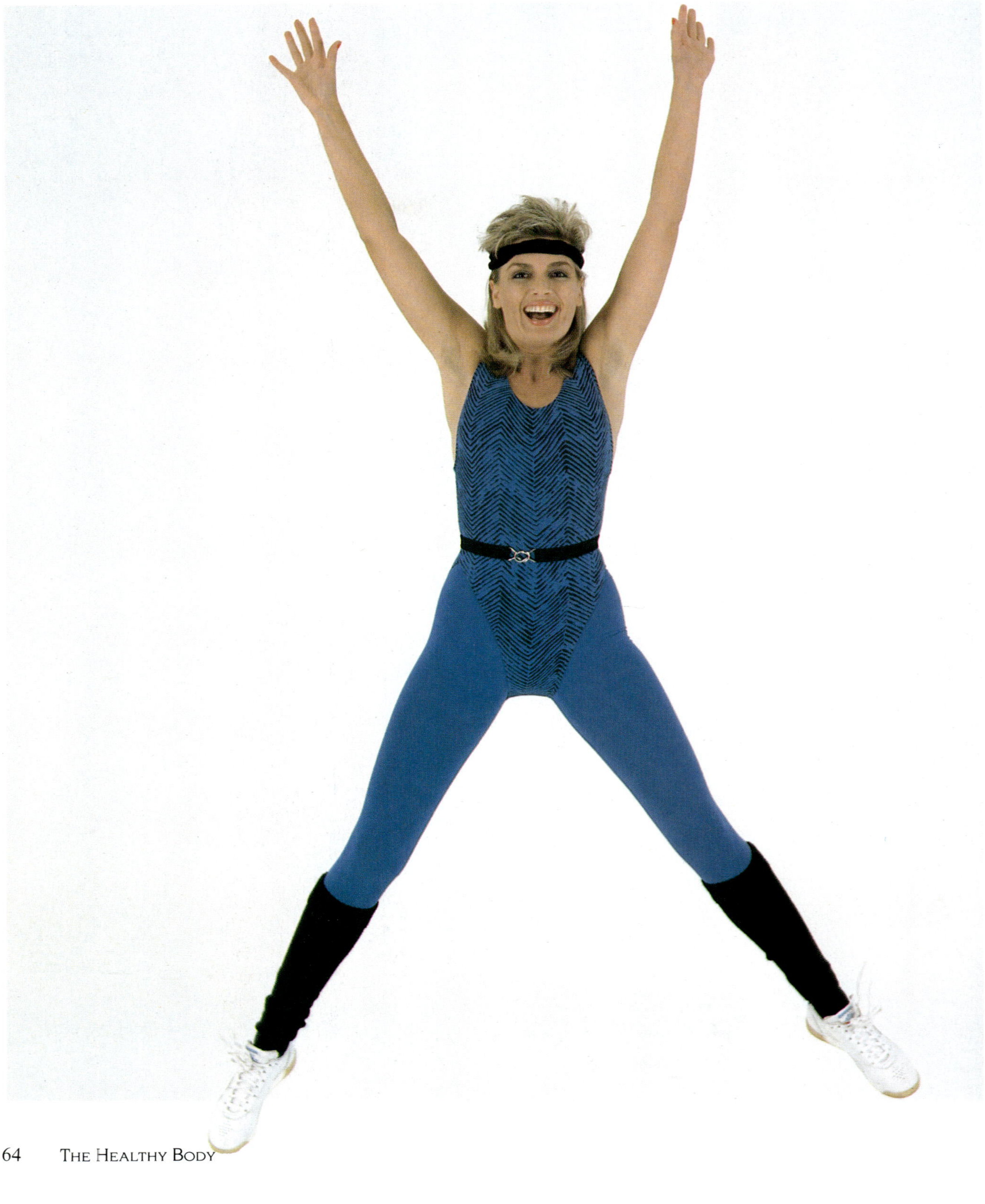

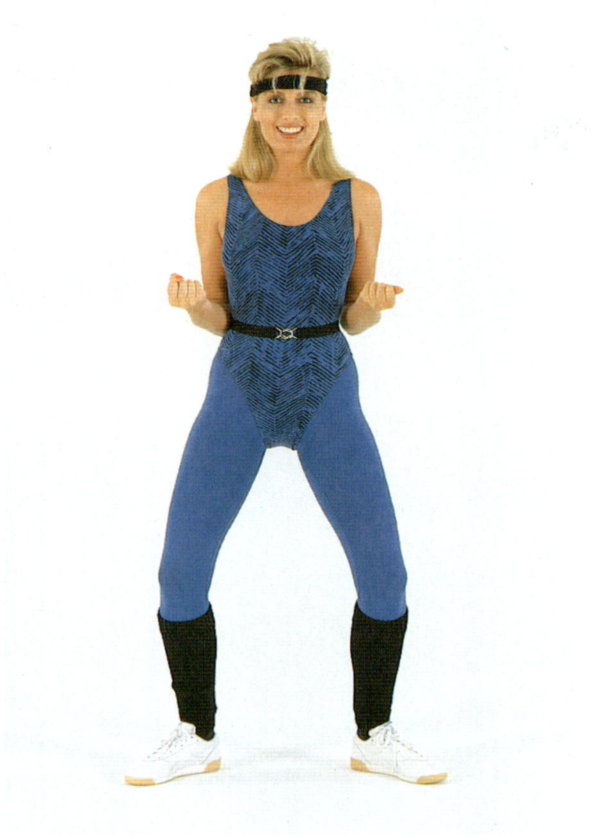

1

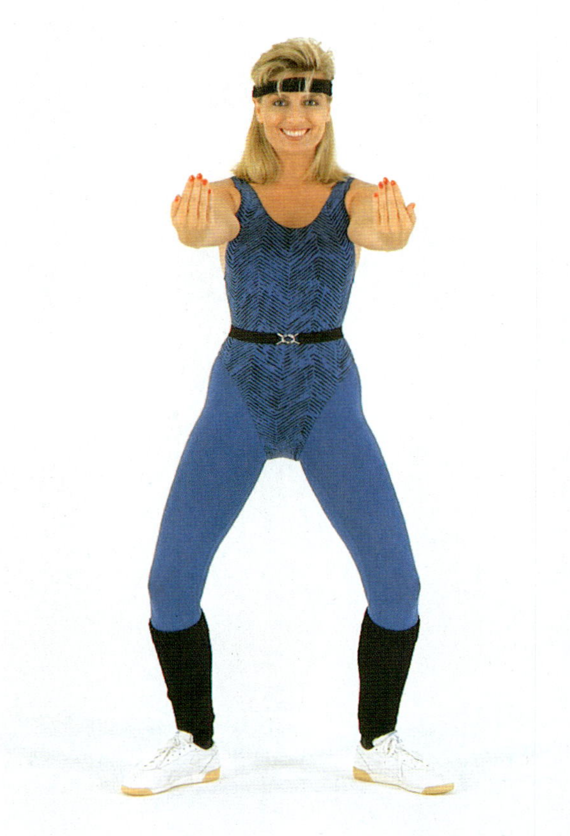

2

FIGHTER'S SQUAT

1. Starting position.

2. Inhale deeply. Exhale slowly as you push your hands forward slowly, palms inward, and bent at the wrist. Hold for three seconds.

3. Inhaling deeply again, push your hands out slowly, until your palms are facing the front. Draw your arms back slowly to the starting position, exhaling slowly. Repeat the sequence five times.

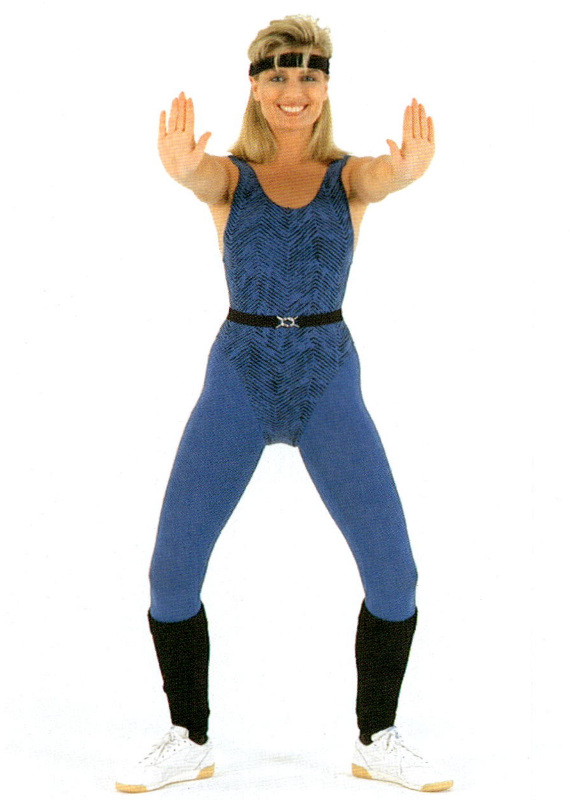

3

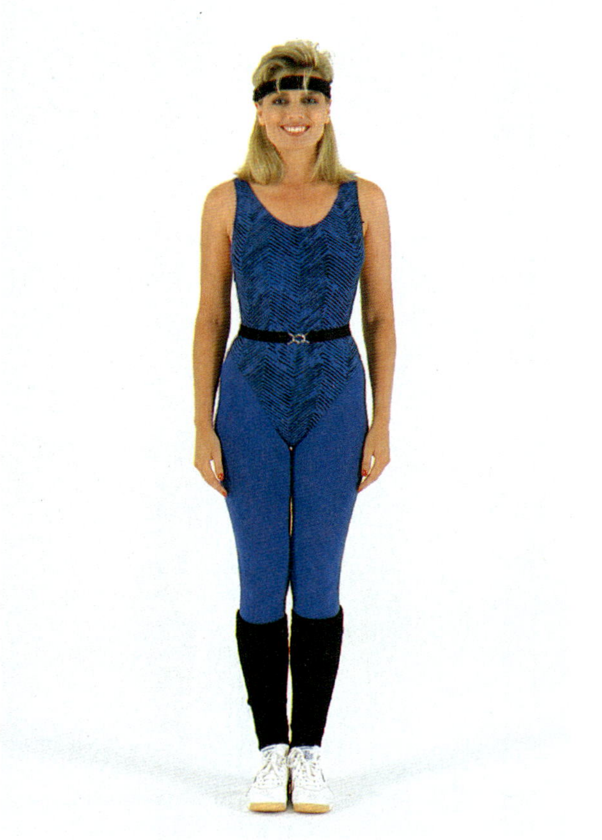

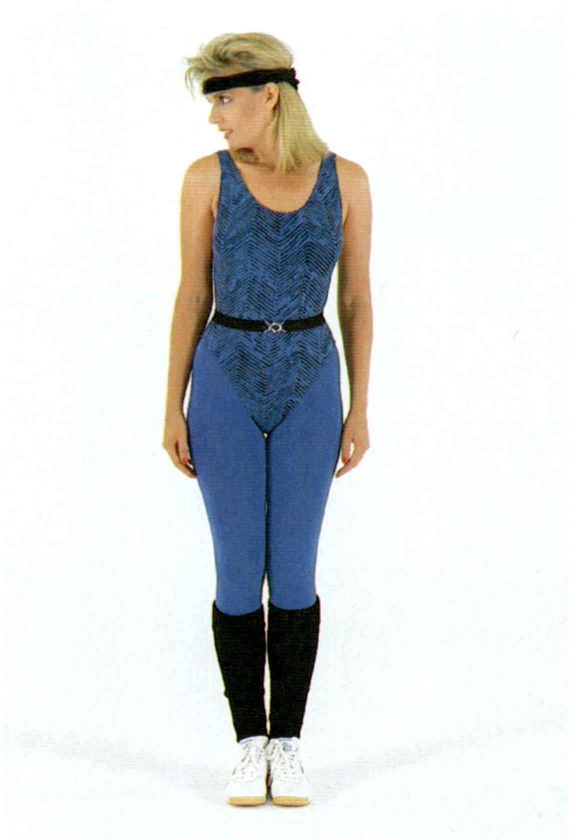

THE RELEASER

1. Starting position.

2. Turn your head slowly to the right, then to the left. Repeat 10 times. Tilt your head to your right shoulder and then to your left 10 times.

3. Slightly bend your knees and roll your shoulders back three times, then forward three times.

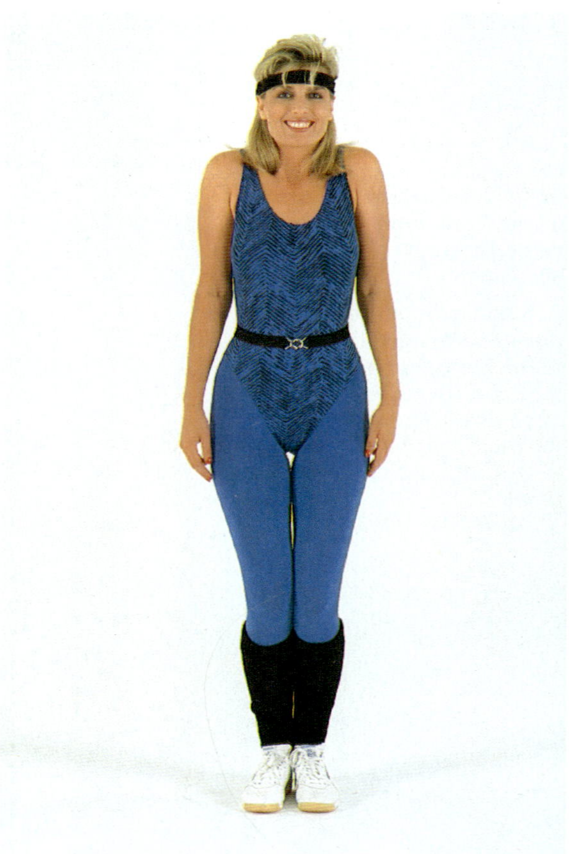

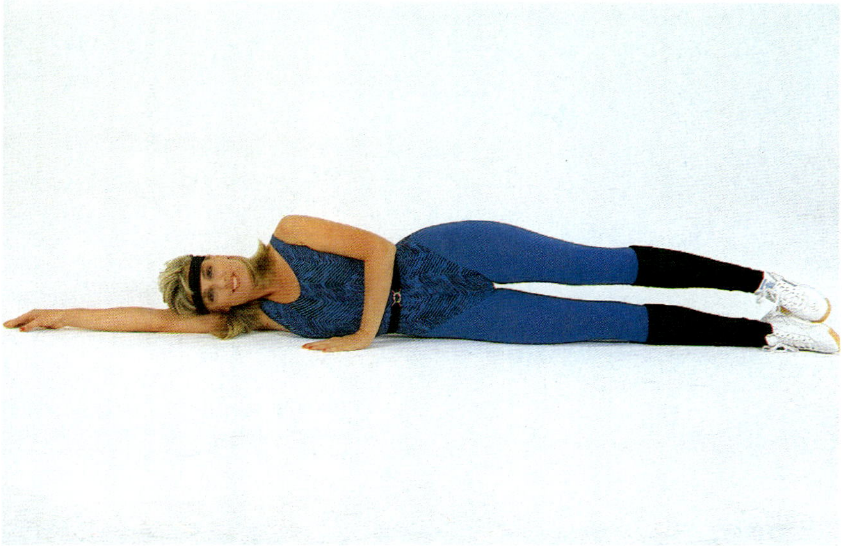

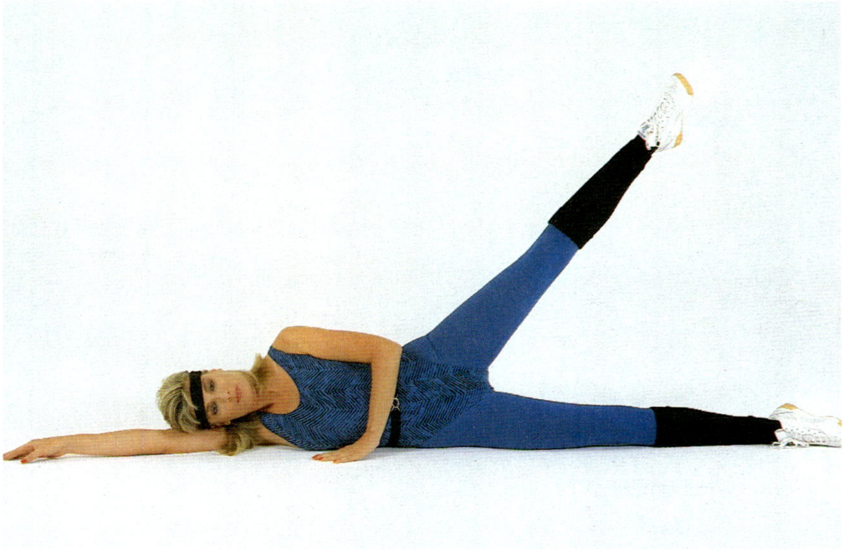

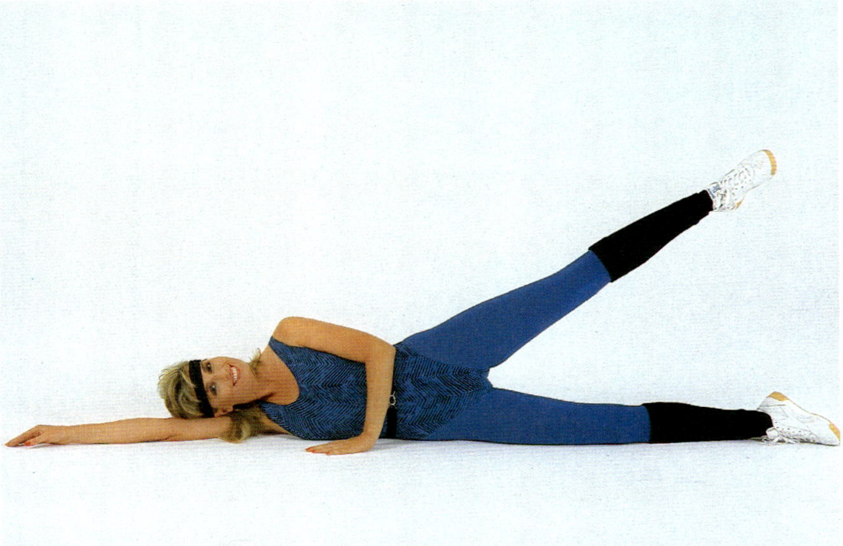

V-LIFTS

1. Starting position.

2. Keeping your left hand on the floor as a lever, slowly raise your left leg as high as you can. Lower your leg without touching it down to your right foot. Repeat, slowly, five times.

3. Quicken the pace and raise and lower your leg half-way six times. Keep your toes pointed down. Finish off with four slow, full leg raises as in 1. Roll to your left side and repeat the sequence raising your right leg.

LEG LIMBERER

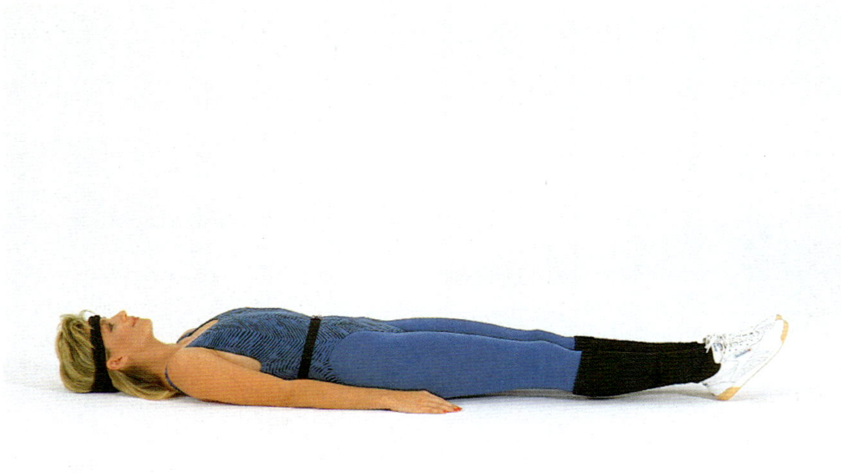

1

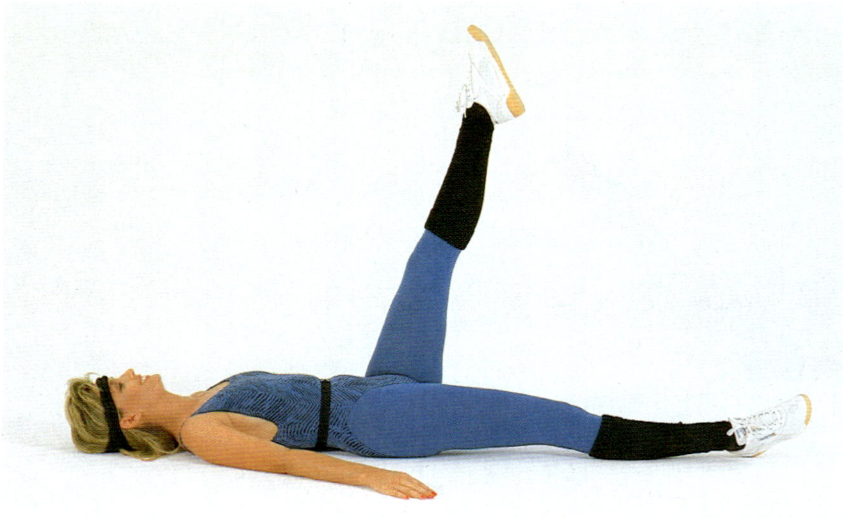

2

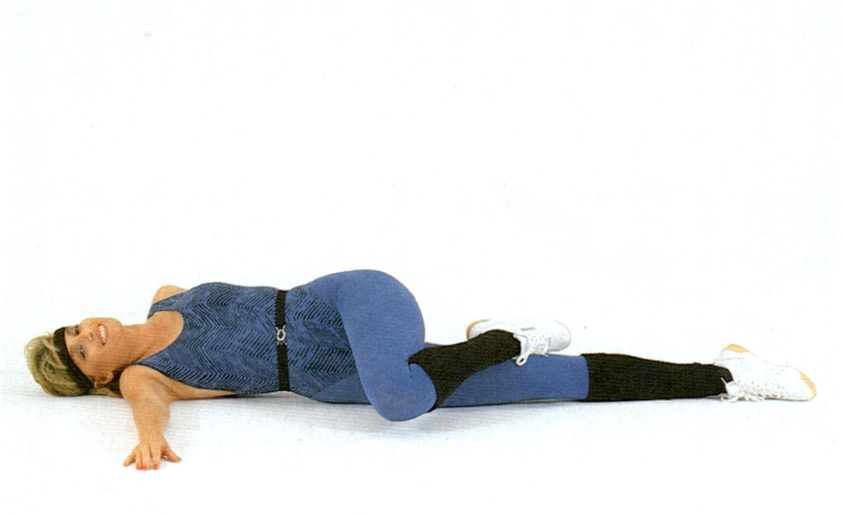

3

1. Starting position.

2. Slowly lift your left leg off the floor. Lift it to about half a metre, keeping it straight all the time. Then, bending your knee slightly, touch your leg down to the floor on the right side of your body.

3. Return to starting position and repeat with the right leg. Do 15 repetitions, alternating legs.

A-FRAME KNEES

1. Starting position.

2. Bend your right leg toward you so that the sole of your right foot touches your left inside knee. Return to starting position. Bend your left leg so your left foot touches your right knee. Alternate rapidly 15 times each leg.

3. Bend legs simultaneously so that the soles of your feet meet in front of your body. Return to starting position and repeat 10 times.

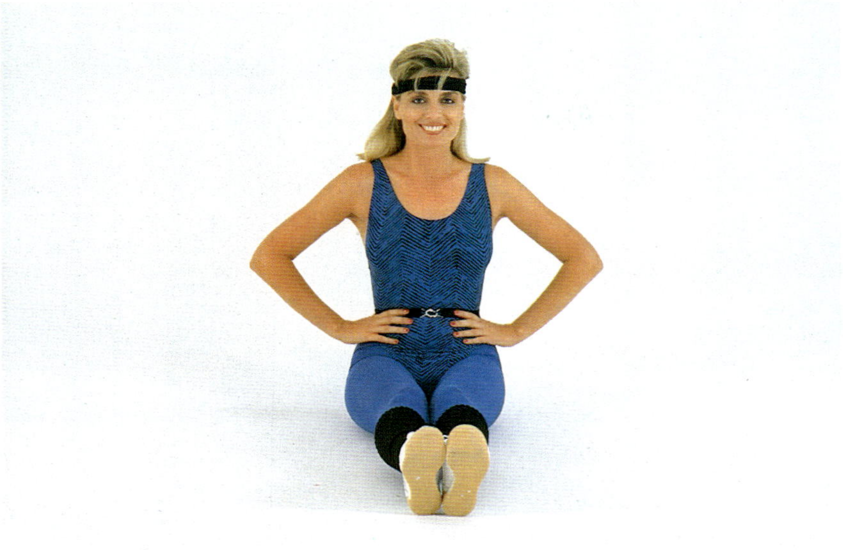

1

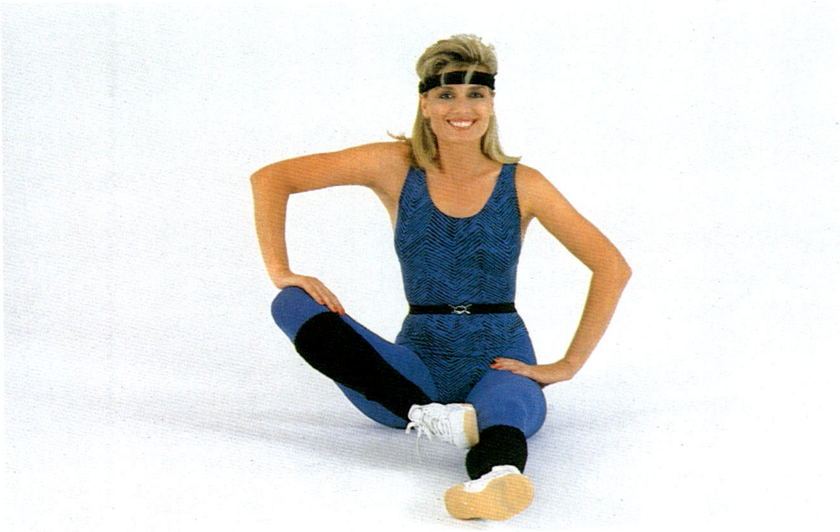

2

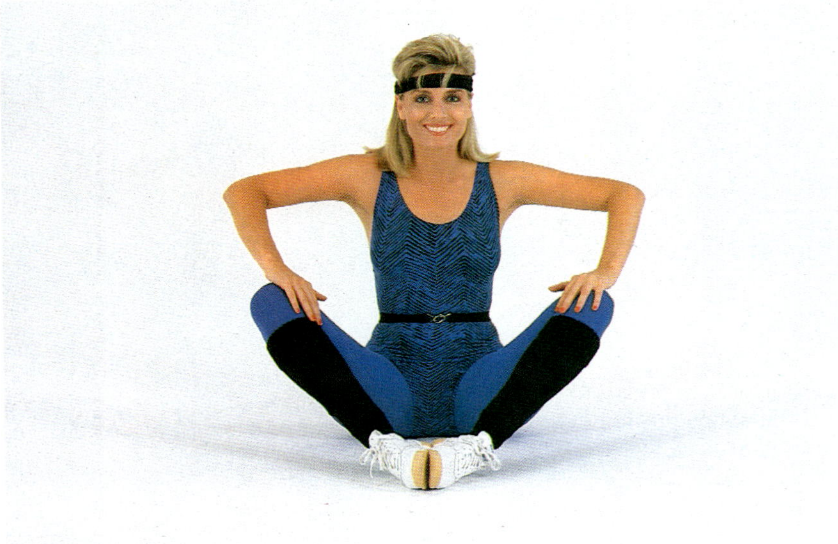

3

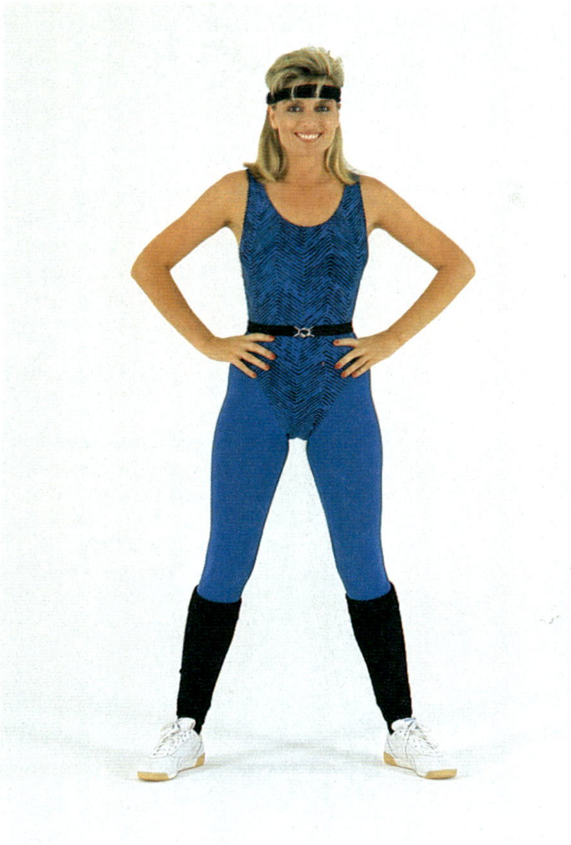

1

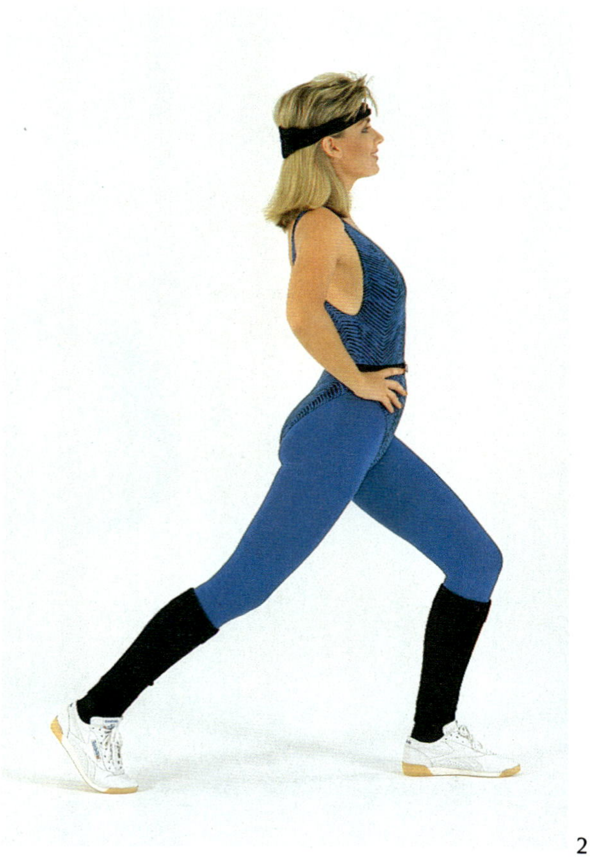

2

FOOTBALLER'S GRIP

1. Starting position.

2. Take a long step forward with your left leg. Your left knee should be bent but your right leg should be straight.

3. Make a circle around your left thigh with both arms. Grasp each arm at the elbow. Hold for a second, then repeat the exercise with your right leg. Do 20 full repetitions, alternating legs.

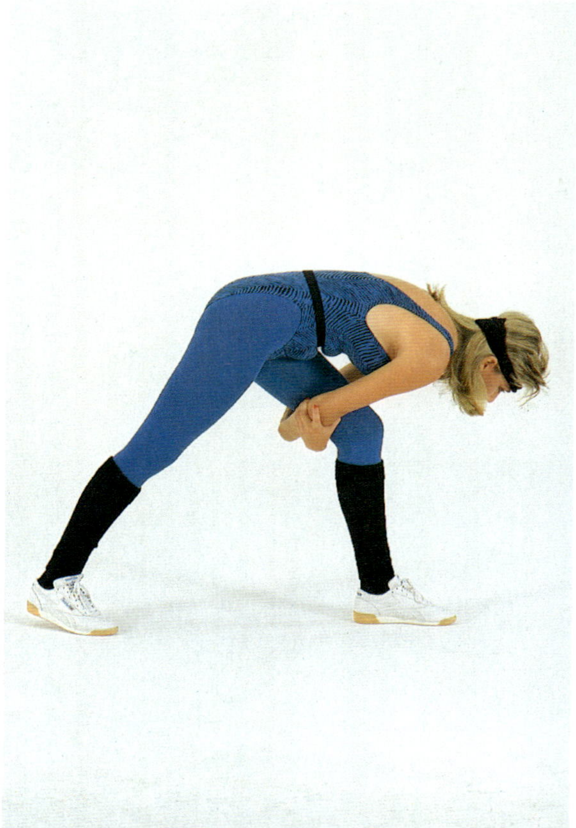

3

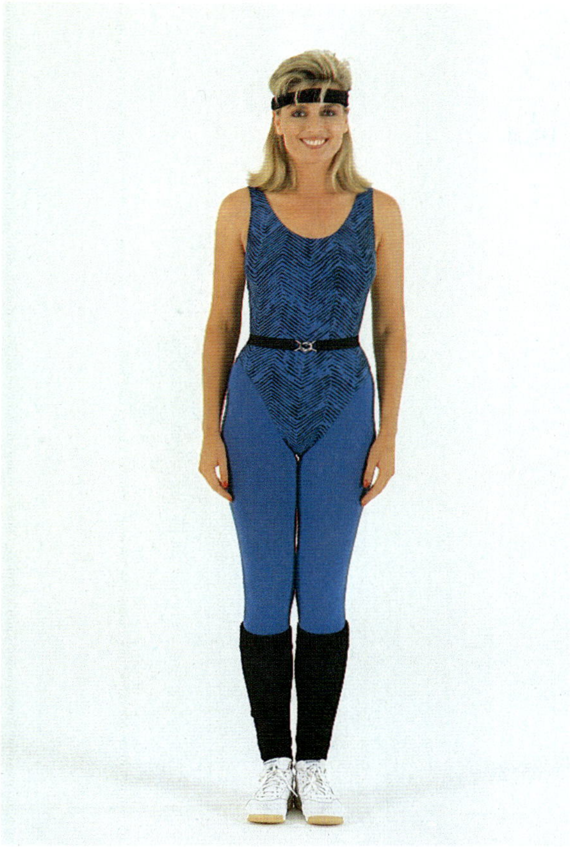

1

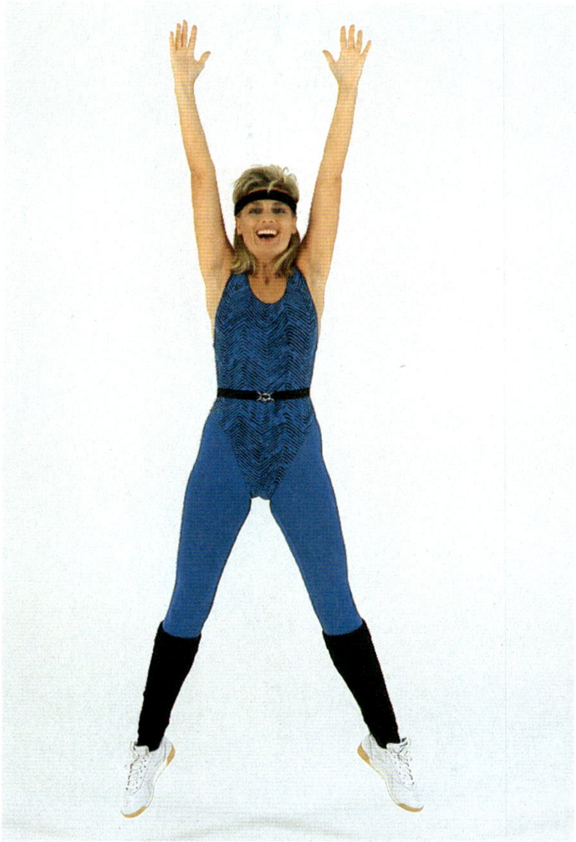

2

JUMPING JACKIES

1. Starting position.

2. Jump to spread your legs apart while touching your hands over your head. Jump back to starting position and repeat rapidly 20 times.

3. Jump, spreading your legs apart, but this time open your arms wide. Then, as you jump back, clap hands together in front of you. Repeat rapidly 20 times.

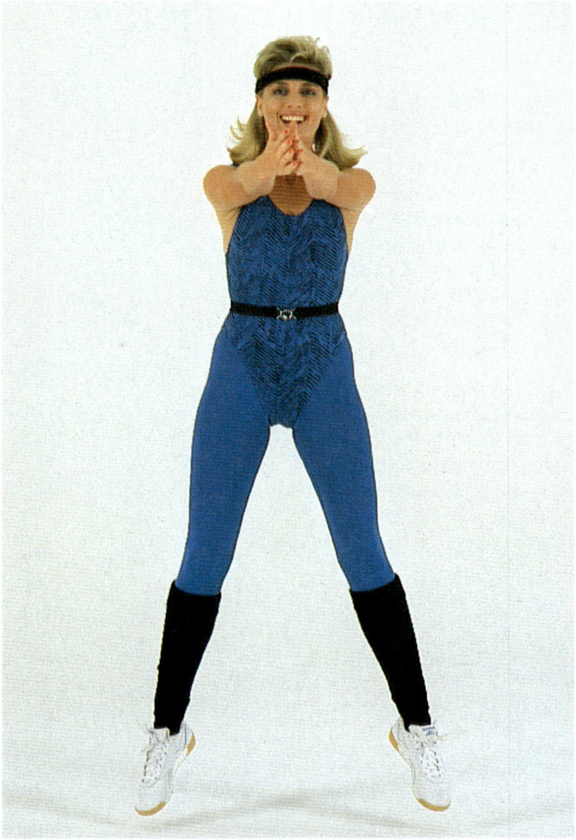

3

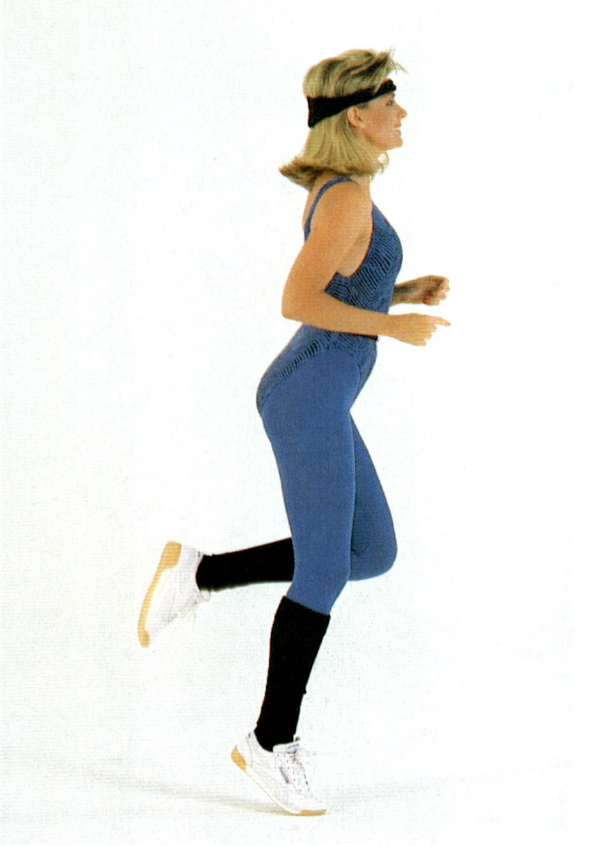

1

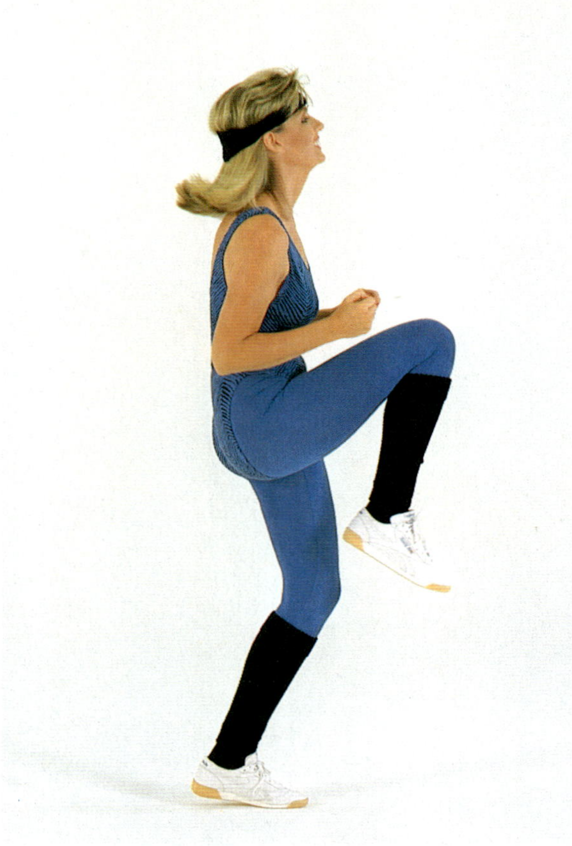

2

JOGGING ROUTINE

1. Starting position, jogging slowly on the spot.

2. Jog slowly on the spot for 20 steps, then get your heart rate pumping by lifting your knees waist-high as you jog for at least another minute. If you are breathing very hard though, slow down and return to a slow jog.

3. Instead of kicking your knees up high, this time jog on the spot kicking your heels up behind you. Try to do this for a minute, but again, if you are over-exerting return to a slow jog.

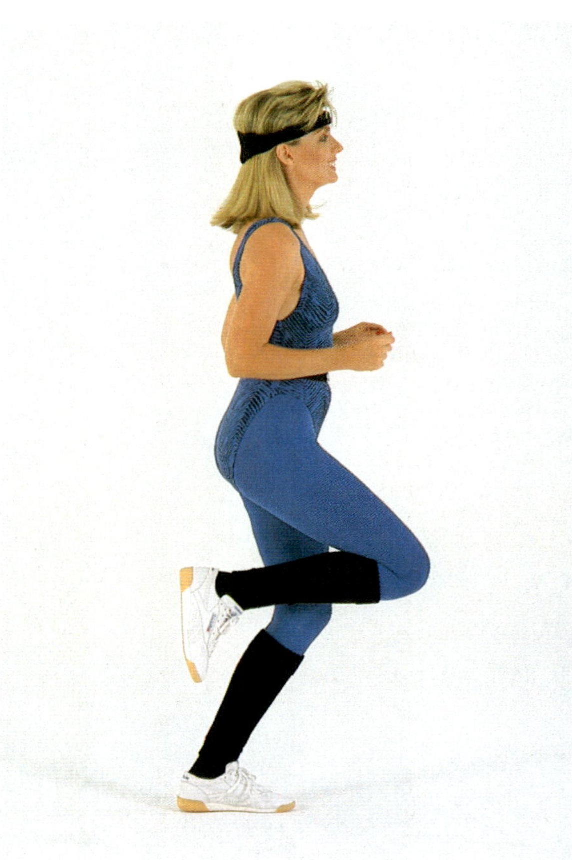

3

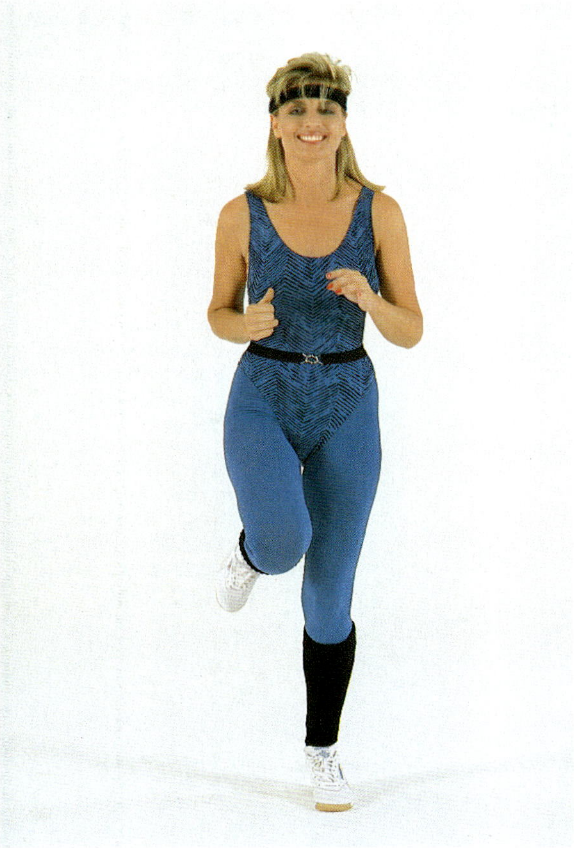

1

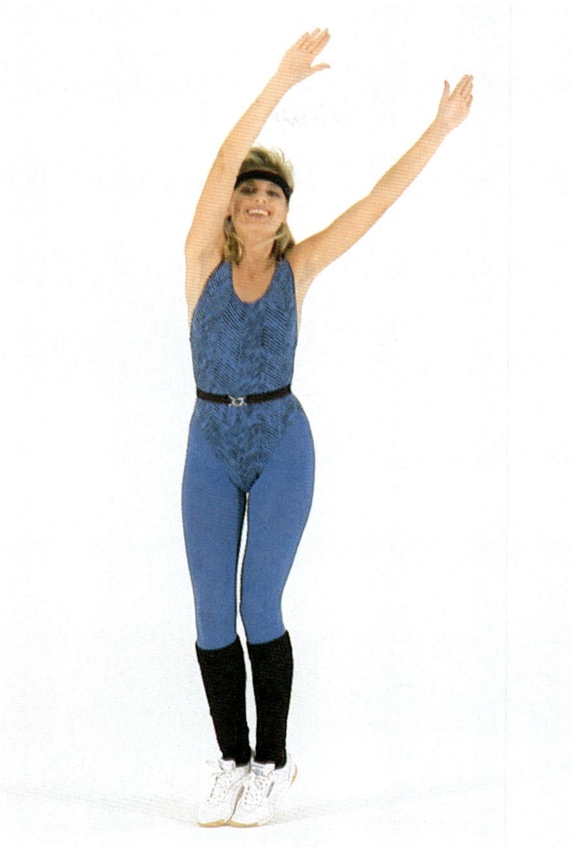

2

TWISTER SHUFFLE

1. Starting position, jogging on the spot.

2. Swing your arms up high in the air. Jump from side to side, twisting your hips in the opposite direction to the jump. Do 20 jumps each side.

3. Lower your arms to chest height. Keep jumping and twisting. Do 10 twists to each side with your feet together. Separate your feet until they are about 30 cm apart. Twist 20 times each side.

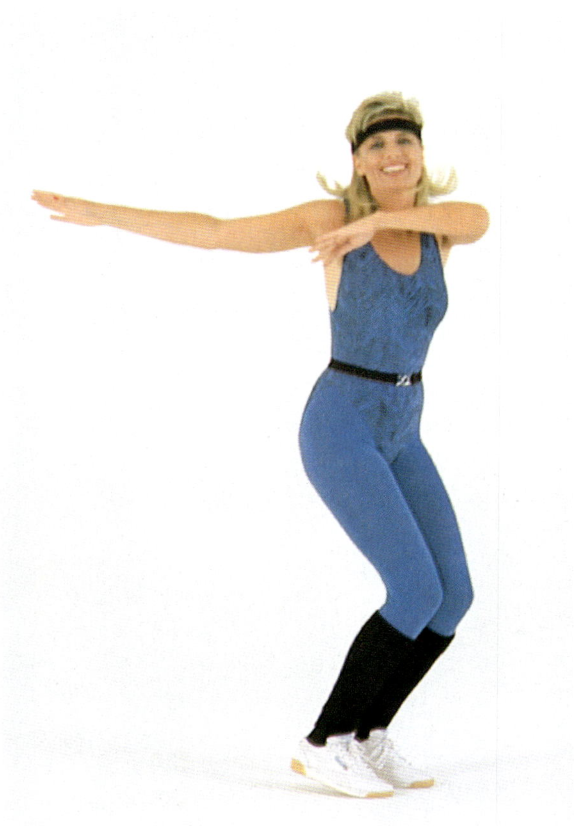

3

CLAPPING SITS

1. Starting position.

2. Keeping your knees bent and your hands touching the sides of your head, curl your shoulders and chest up off the ground. Do not clasp your hands behind your neck. As you come up in a curl, reach your hands out and touch your knees. Repeat 10 times.

3. Now separate your knees slightly. As you come up in a curl, clap your hands between your legs twice. Return to starting position and repeat 10 times.

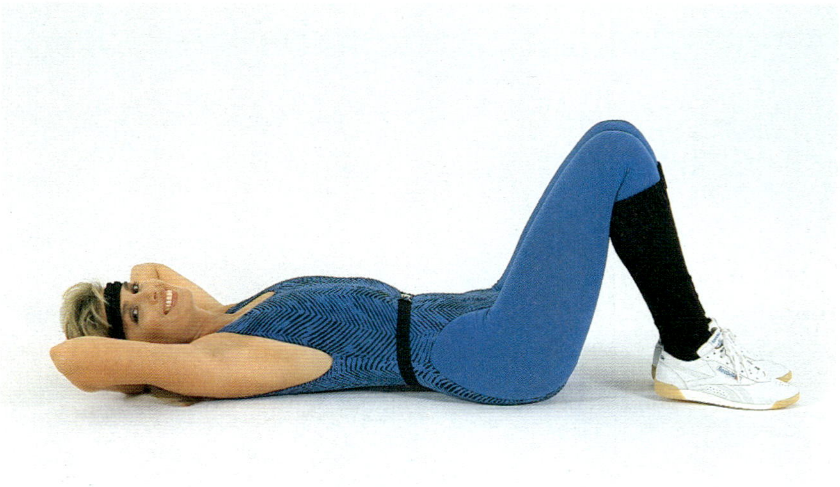

1

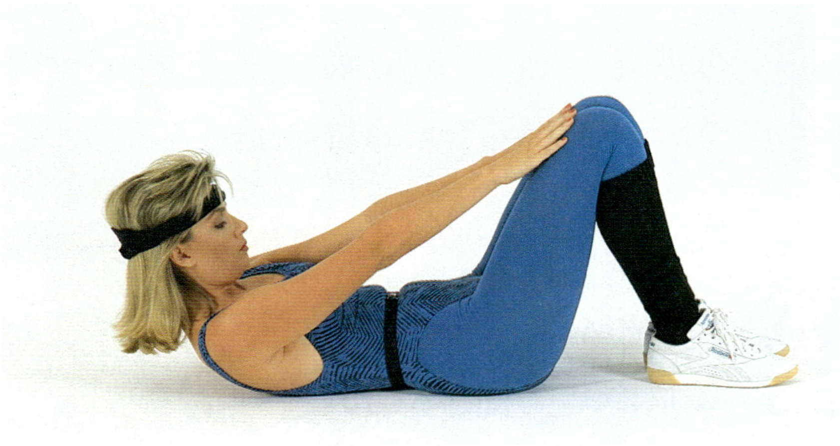

2

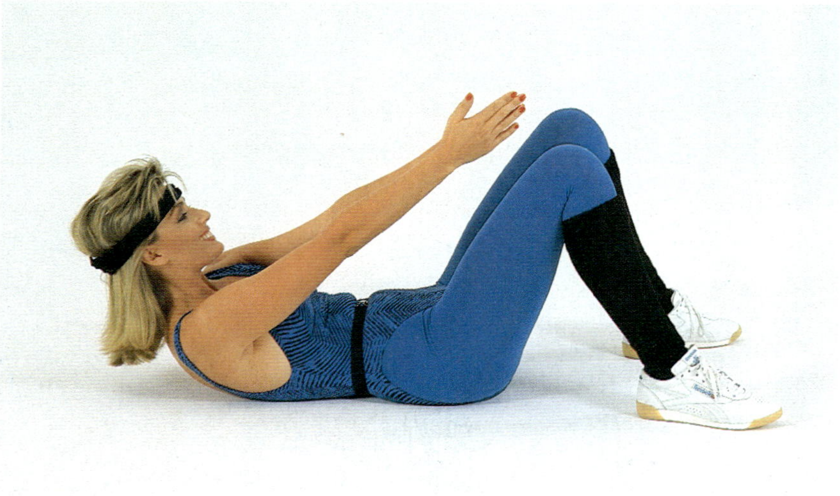

3

BANANA BRIDGE

1. Starting position.

2. Raise your arms up as far as you can behind your back and at the same time lift both your legs up in the air together. Hold for three seconds and relax. Repeat 10 times.

3. Turn over onto your back. Slowly curl your legs up to your chest and pull them close. Hold for five seconds and relax.

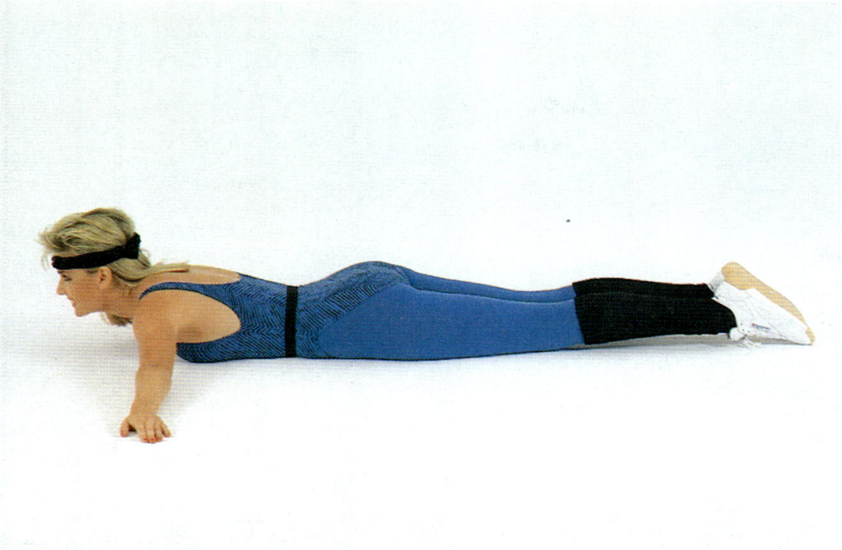
1

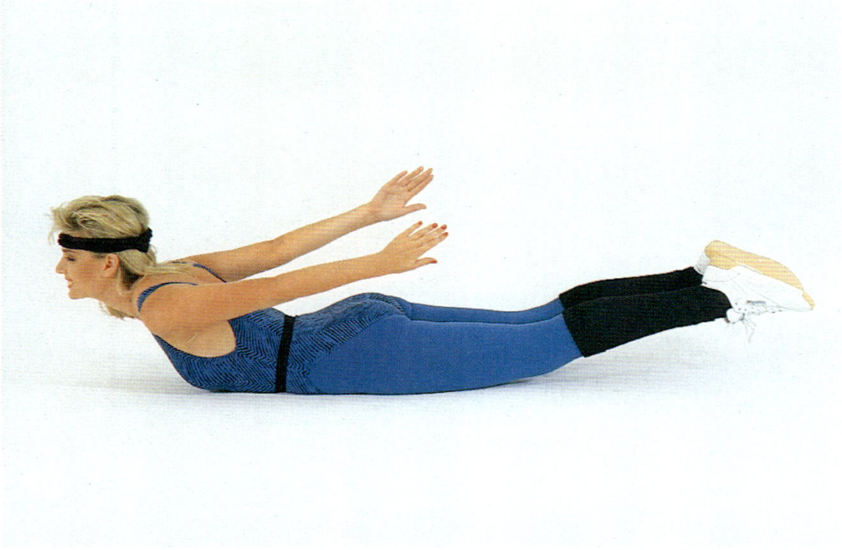
2

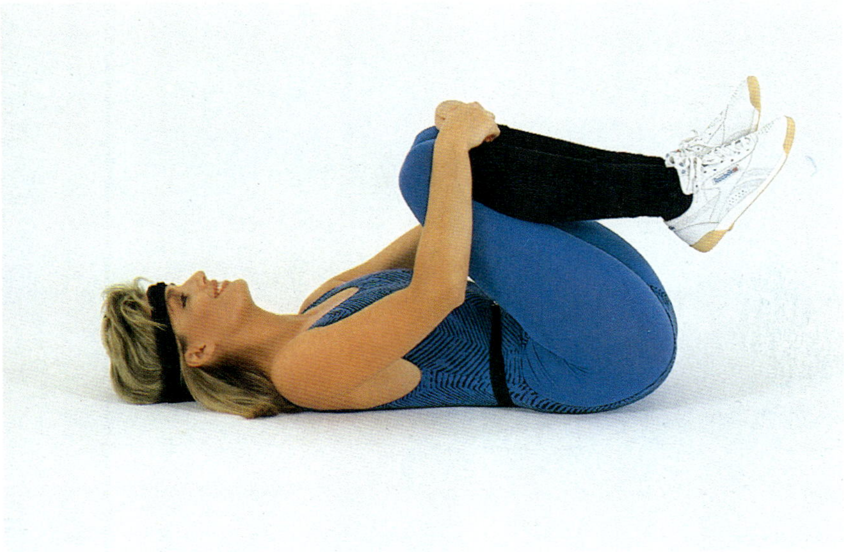
3

SNAKE STRETCH

1. Starting position.

2. Bring your arms level with your chest, palms down. Slowly lift the upper part of your body from the floor, stretching your back in a curve. Look up towards the ceiling. Lower your body to the floor. Repeat 10 times.

3. To relax the body, sit back on your heels. Lean forward with your forehead resting on the floor and with your arms loosely by your sides. Hold for 10 seconds.

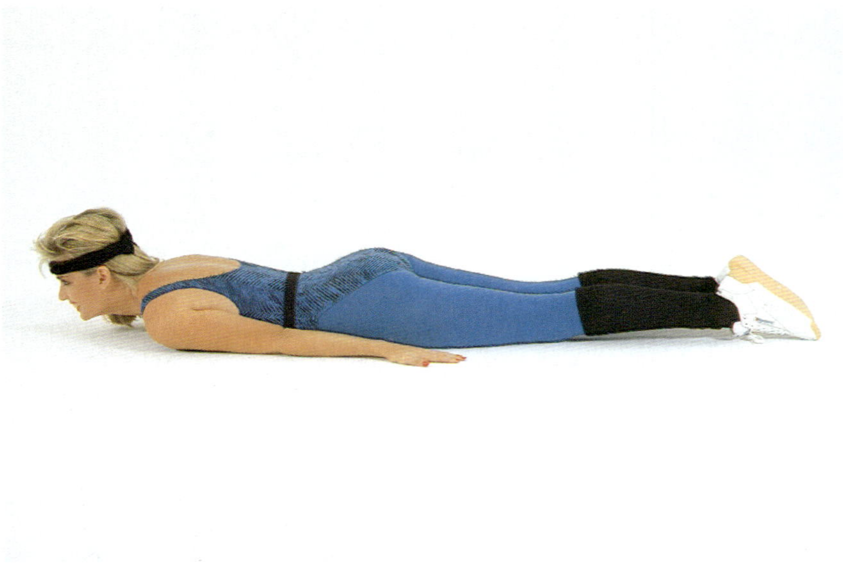

1

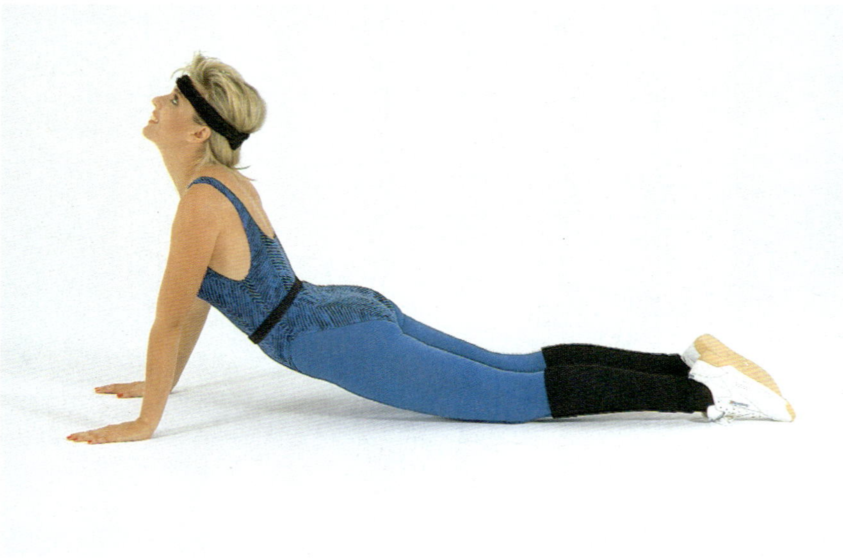

2

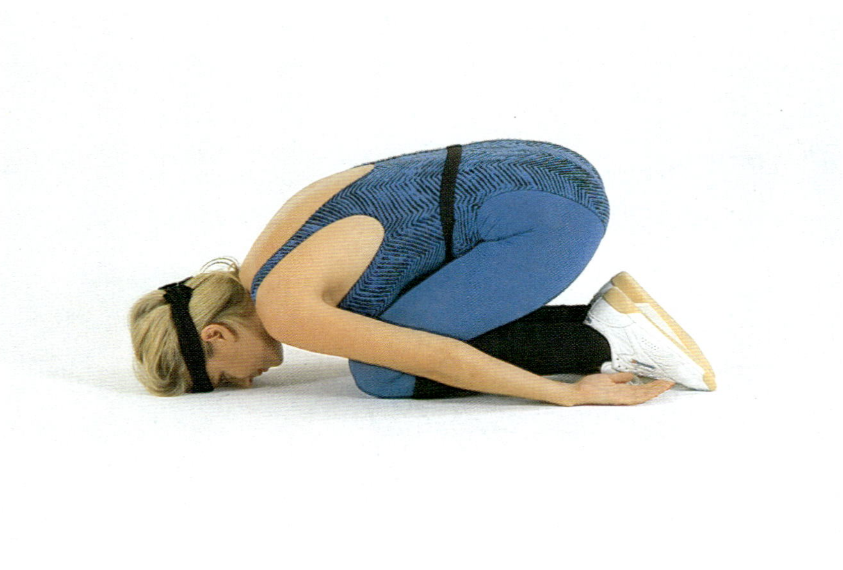

3

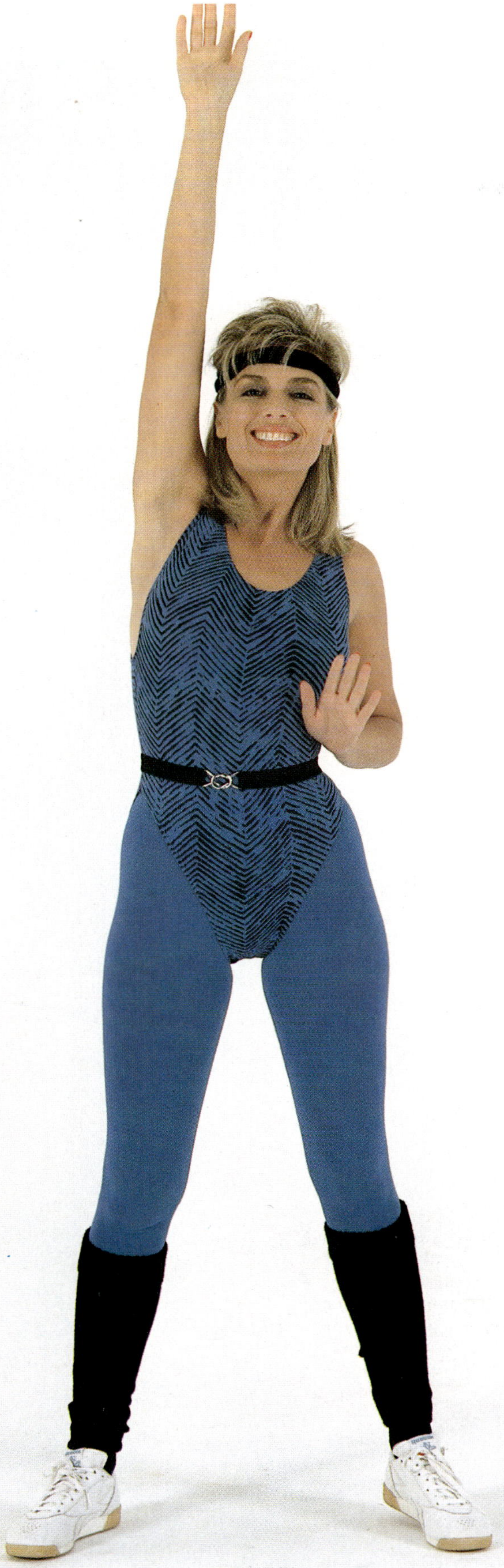

FACE EXERCISE PROGRAMME

DAILY FACE FIRMERS

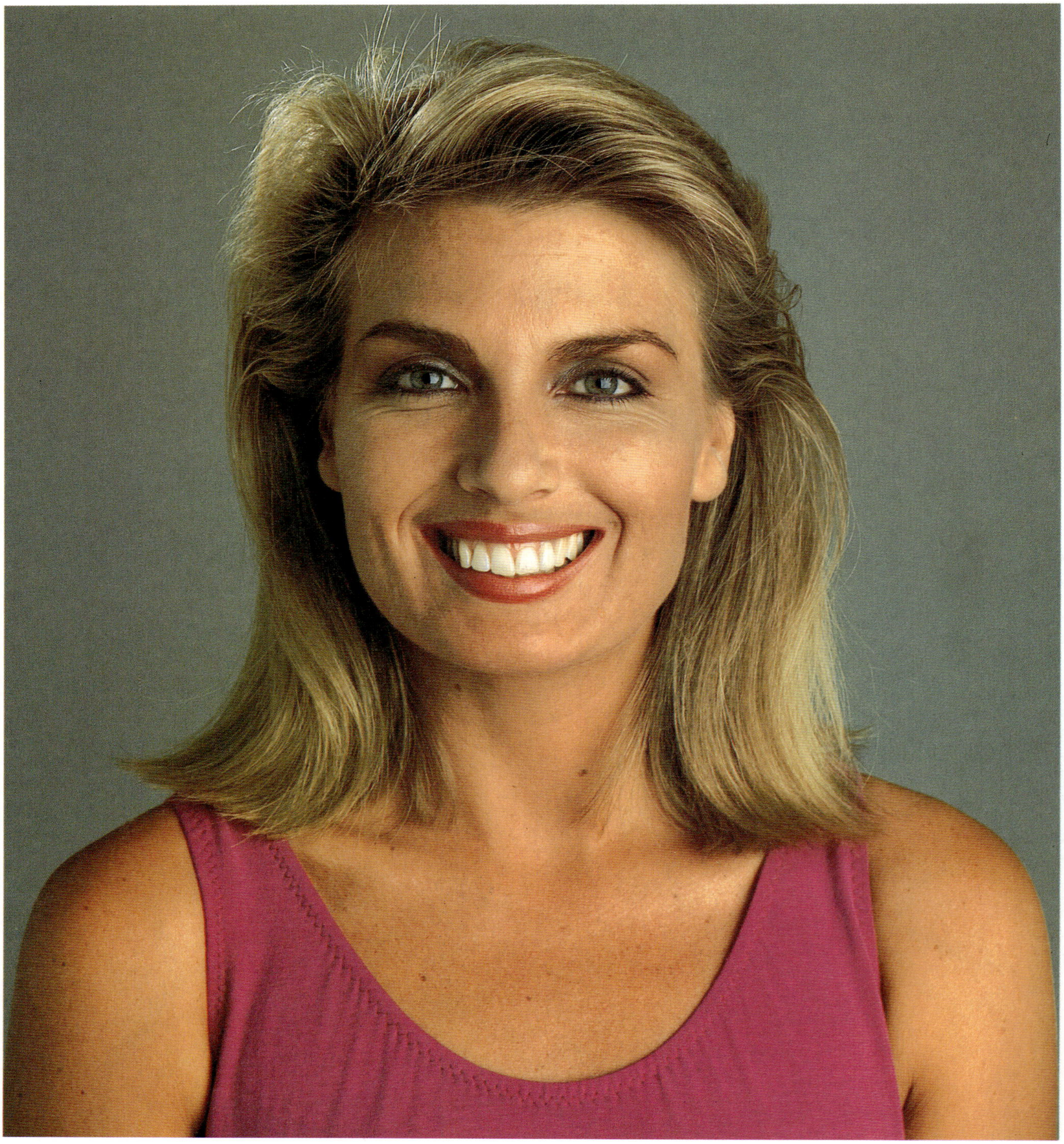

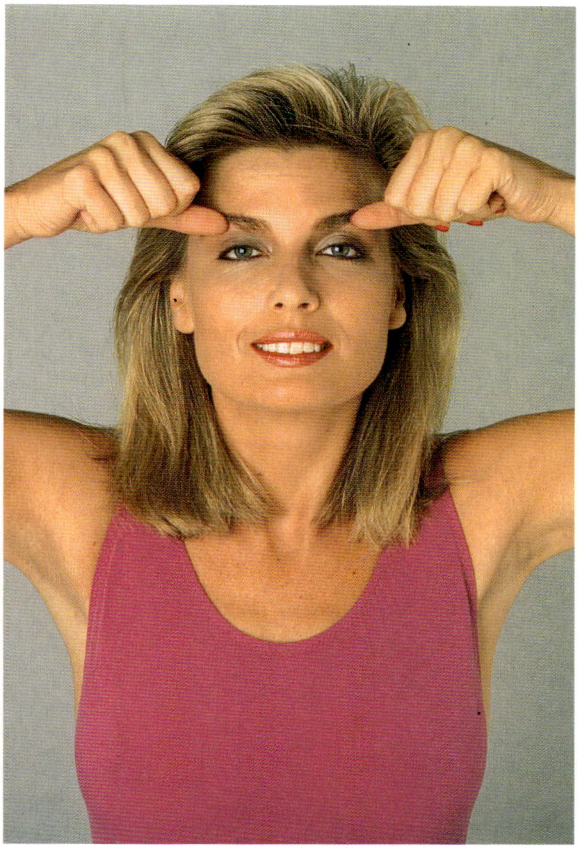

1

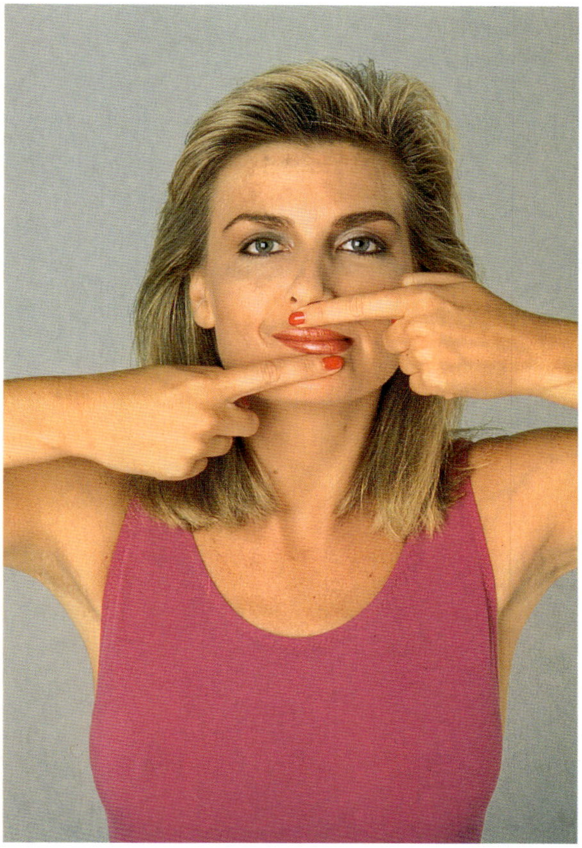

2

EYE AND LIP MASSAGE

1. Using the back of your thumbs, gently stroke your upper and lower eyelids, massaging from the inner corners outwards. Repeat several times with eyes open at first, and then closed.

2. Place your index finger of the left hand between your upper lip and nose and the index finger of your right hand just beneath your lower lip. Push your left finger gently to the right, and your right finger gently to the left. Repeat 10 times.

3. Place your index fingers on either side of your mouth and nose. Slowly draw them down to your mouth, then massage in a circular motion. Repeat 10 times.

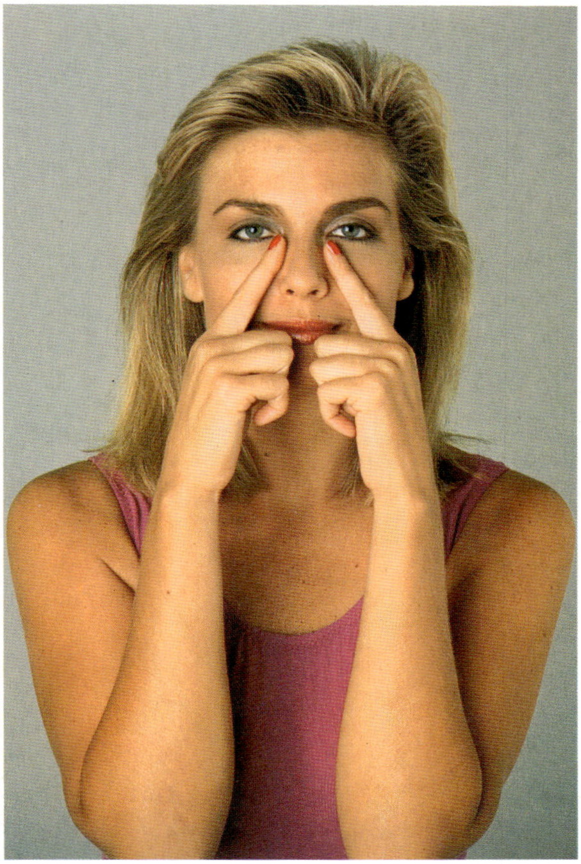

3

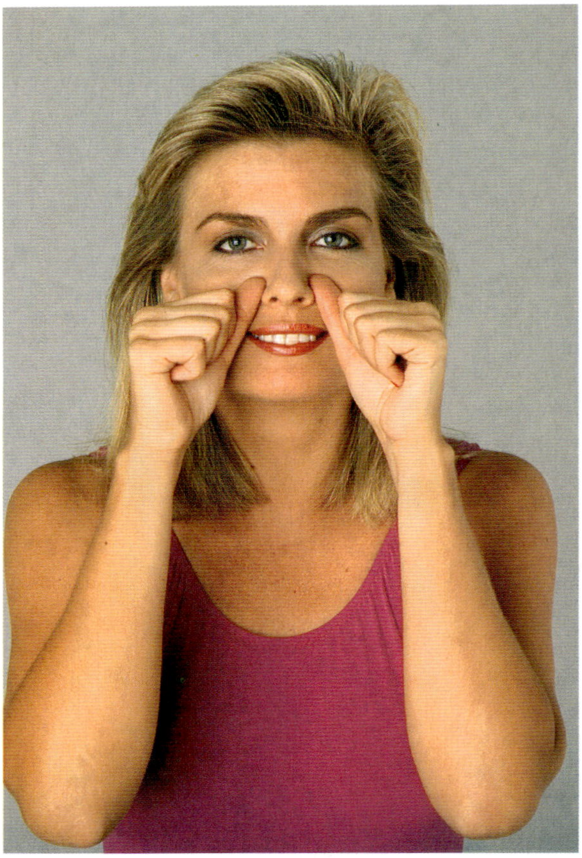

1

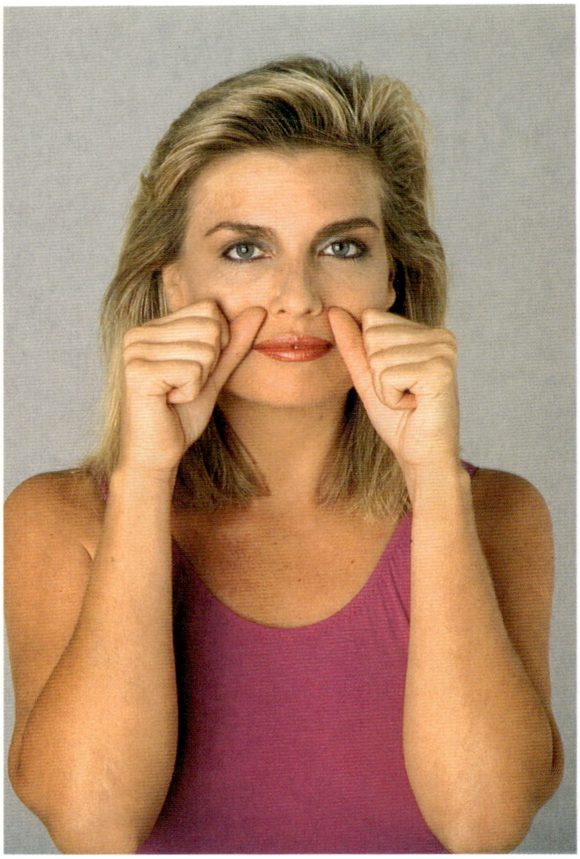

2

NOSE AND NECK SOOTHER

1. Starting position.

2. Using the back of your thumbs, massage down on either side of your nose. Use a little more pressure than you did for the eyes.

3. Place your left hand on the right side of your neck and stroke it firmly downwards 10 times. Repeat the same movement, this time with the right hand down the left side of the throat.

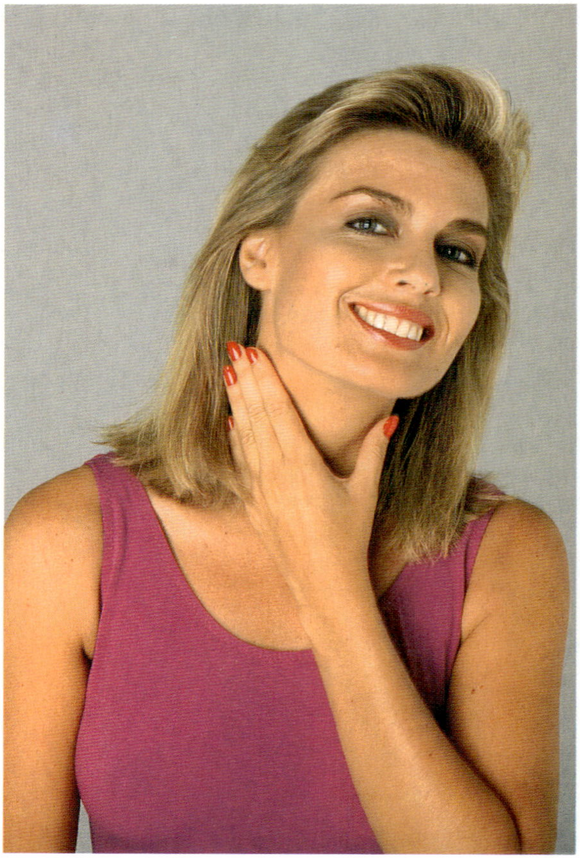

3

1
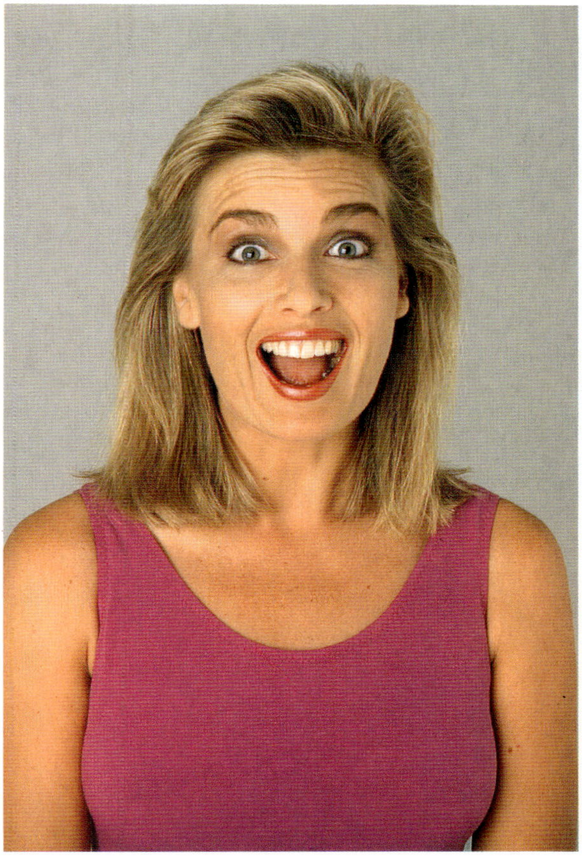

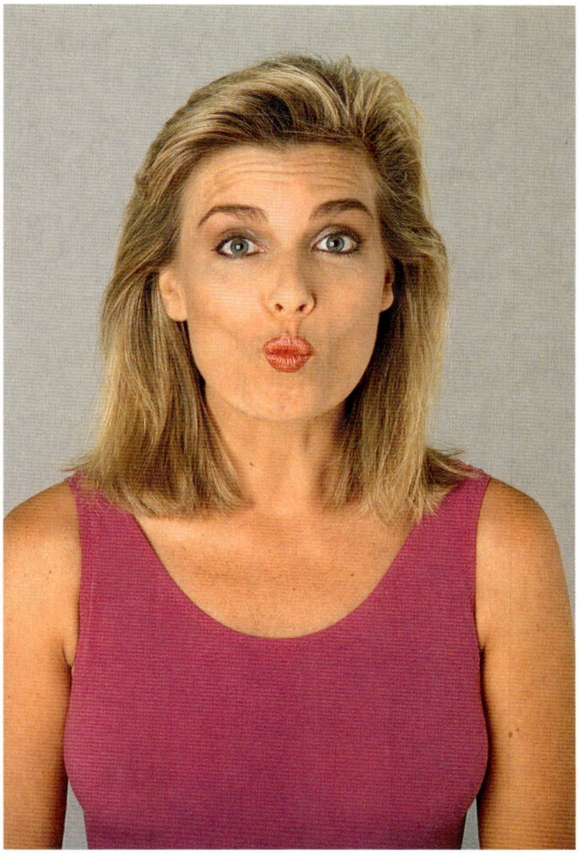
2

FACE CONTORTER

1. Starting position.

2. Close your mouth tight and suck in your cheeks as tightly as you can. At the same time, stretch your eyebrows and forehead skin upwards. Hold for three seconds. Relax and repeat three times.

3. Wrinkle your nose, purse your lips and lower your eyebrows down over your eyes. It doesn't look pretty, but it does work! Hold for five seconds and relax.

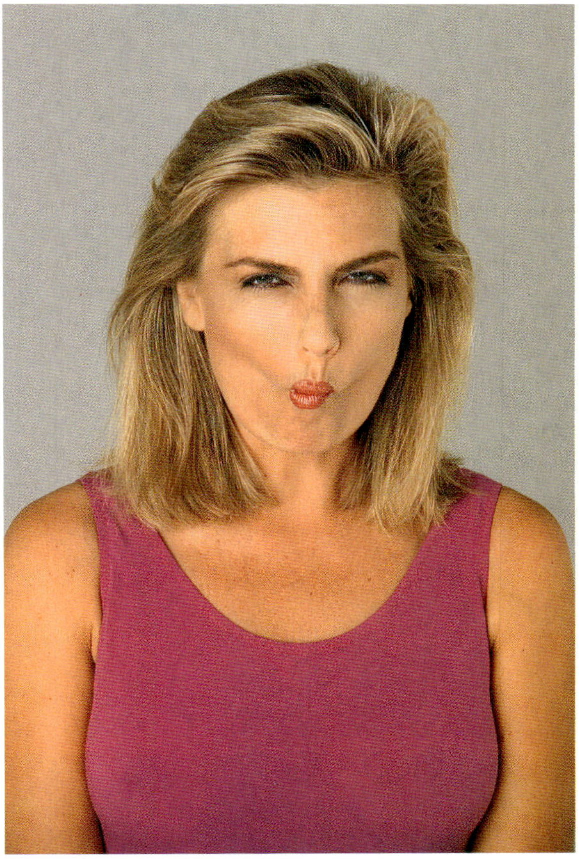
3

BACK EXERCISE PROGRAMME

DAILY BACK STRENGTHENERS

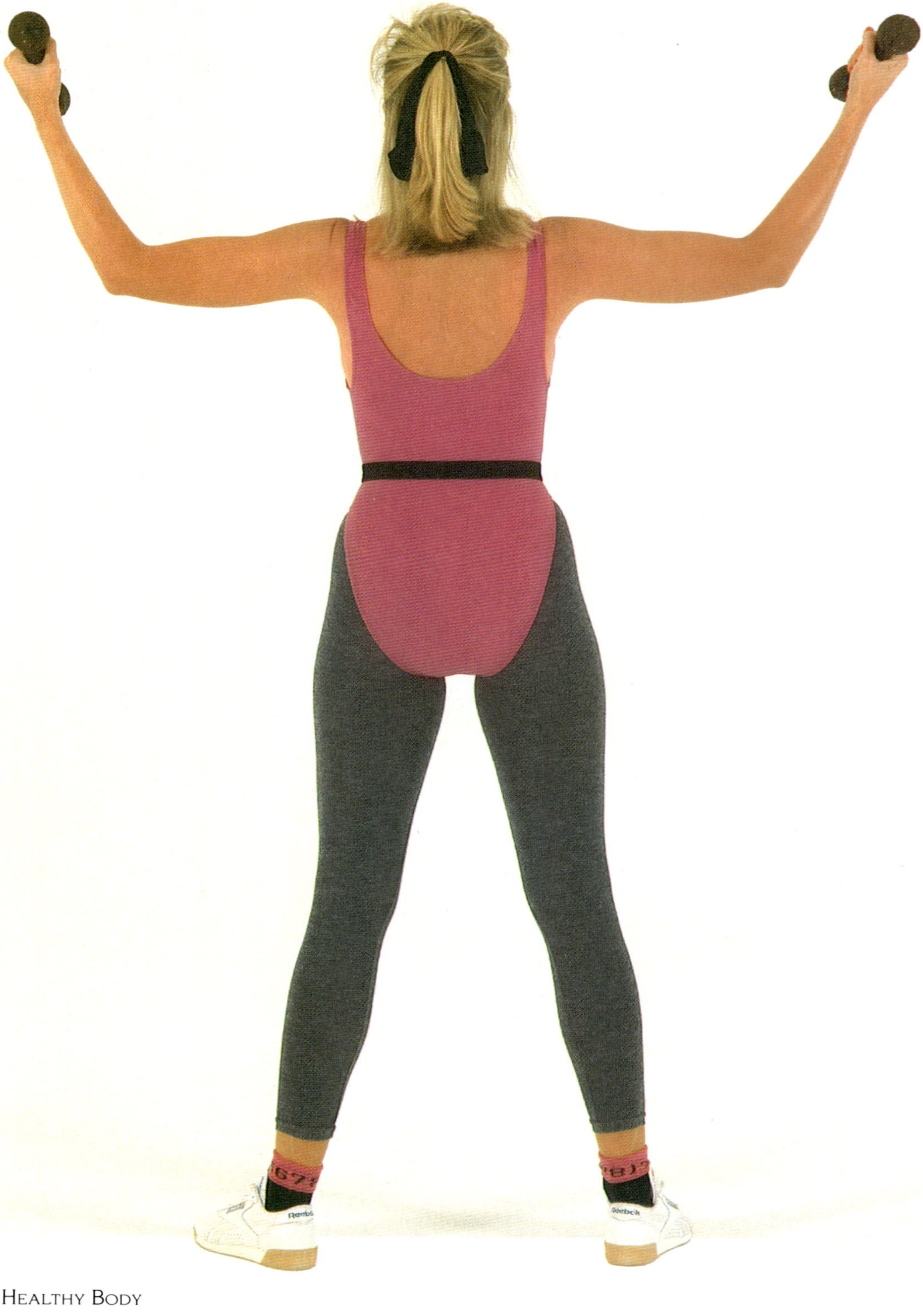

LEG TUCKS

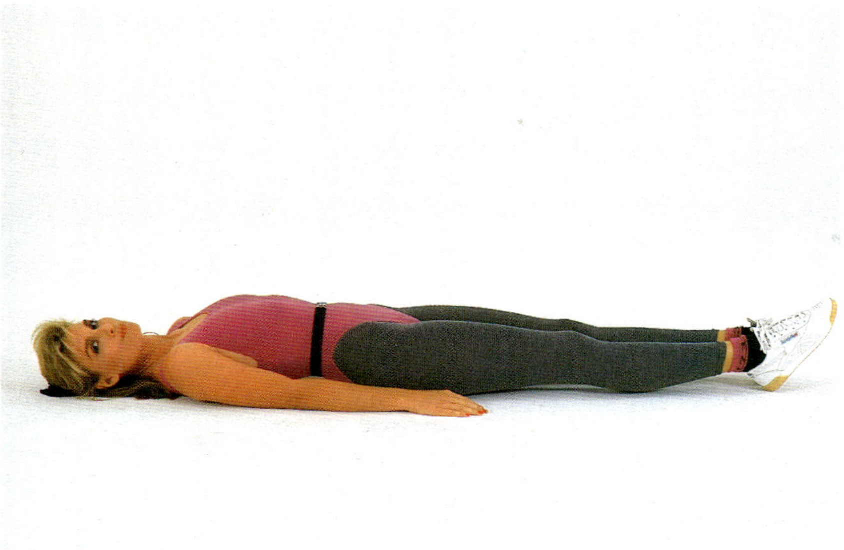
1

1. Starting position.

2. Lift your right knee up to your chest, hold with your arms for five seconds, then relax. Repeat five times. Do the same with your left knee. This exercise limbers up a stiff back.

3. Bringing both knees up to your chest, curl your back up and roll your body from side to side. Make sure to touch the ground with your knees on each side as you roll. Do 20 rolls.

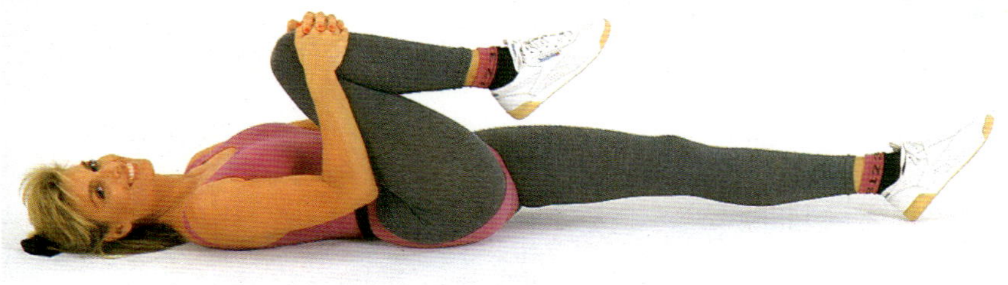
2

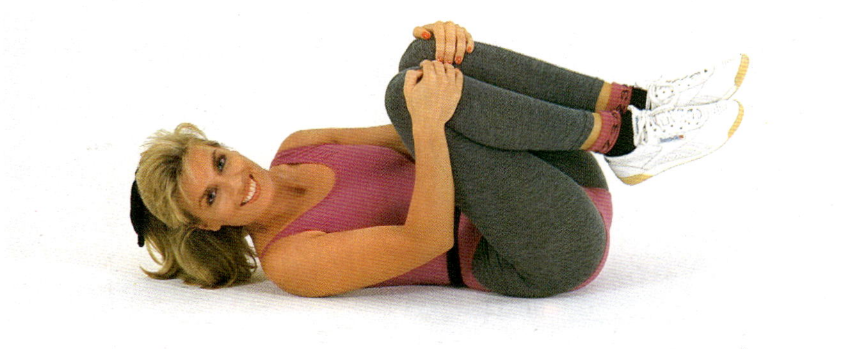
3

PELVIC TILT

1. Starting position.

2. Bend you knees up and firmly tighten your buttock muscles. Hold for five seconds, then repeat five times. Make sure to keep your lower spine flat against the floor.

3. Keeping your knees bent, slowly lift your bottom and pelvis up off the floor as high as you can. Hold for five seconds. Relax and repeat.

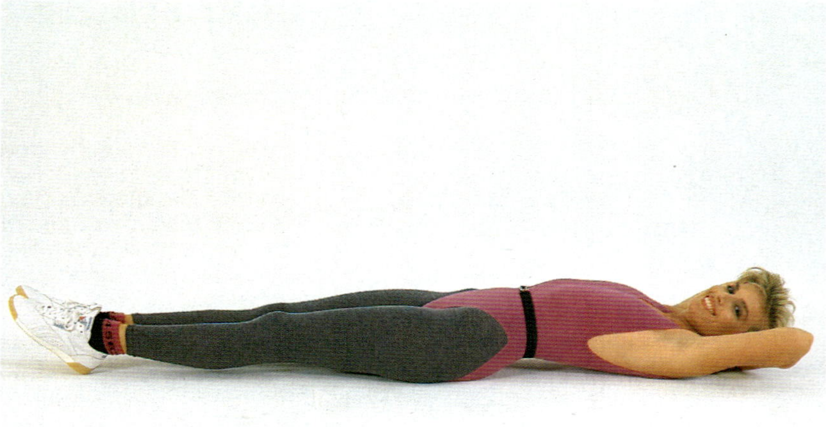

1

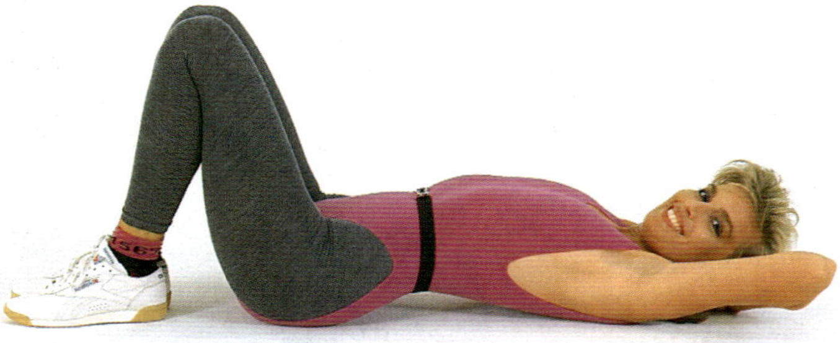

2

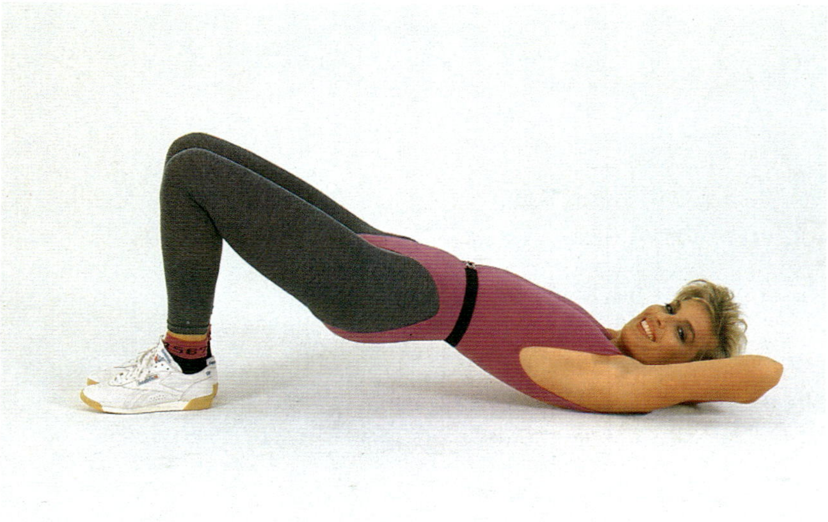

3

AERIAL SCISSORS

1. Starting position.

2. Start this exercise slowly as it is quite difficult. Always keep your lower back on the floor and maintain good balance. Slowly scissor legs up and down ten times. Eventually you will be able to bring each leg down very close to the ground without touching it. But start with just dropping each leg a few centimetres.

3. Raise both legs until they are straight again, then slowly scissor legs across each other — alternately right leg over left, left over right. Do 10 scissors. Bend knees to your chest, then your feet to the floor.

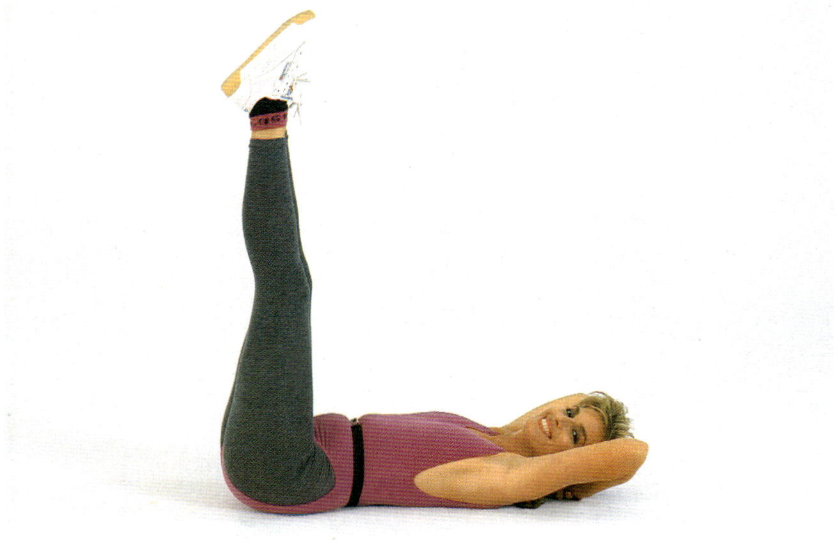

1

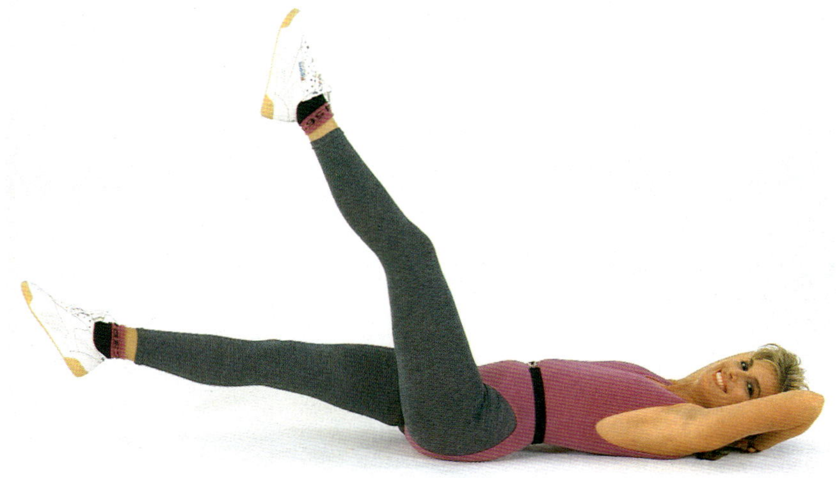

2

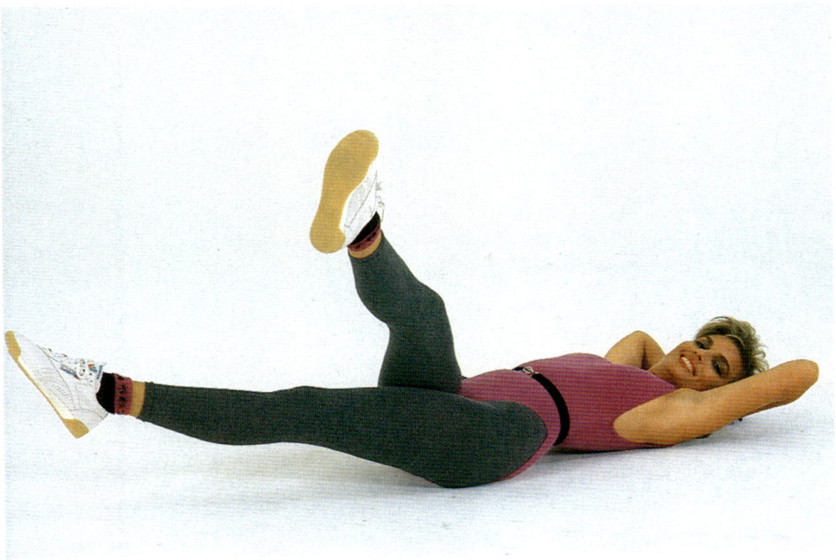

3

KNEE ROLLS

1. Starting position.

2. This exercise massages the spine and strengthens the thighs and knees. Take an ankle in each hand. Keep your right knee up and roll your left knee inwards, down to the ground. Bring your left knee up and roll in your right knee. Roll each knee five times.

3. Pull both knees up to your chest. Kick out from the knees 20 times, alternating legs.

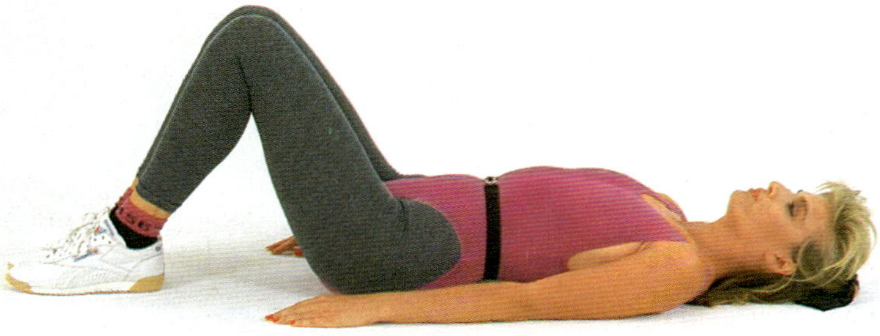

1

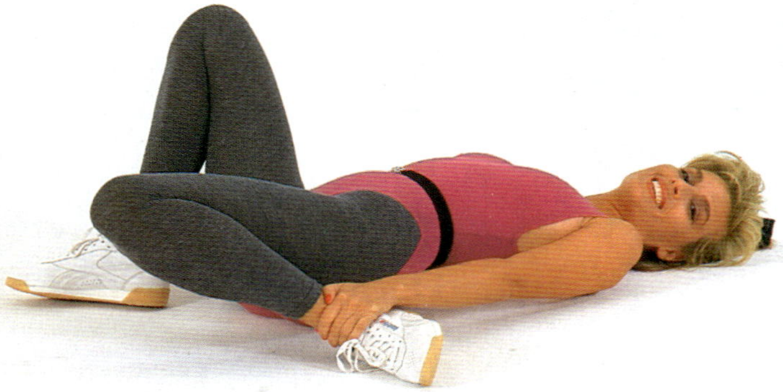

2

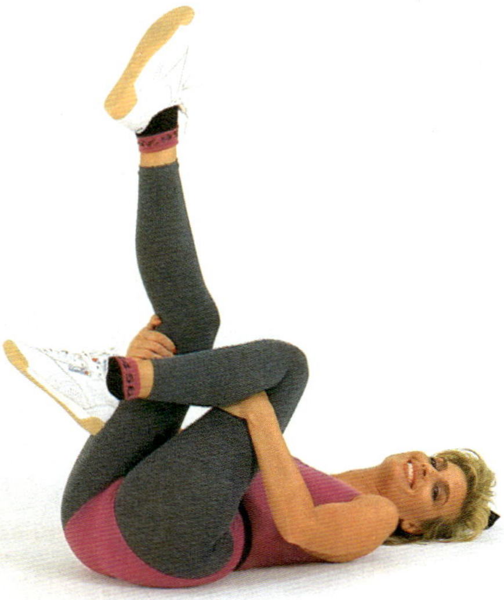

3

BANANA SCISSORS

1. Starting position.

2. Keeping your left leg straight, slowly raise it from the hip as high as you can. Don't lift your pelvis to raise your leg. Return left leg to the floor and repeat the exercise with your right leg. Do 10 lifts with each leg.

3. Repeat the exercise, lifting both legs at once 10 times.

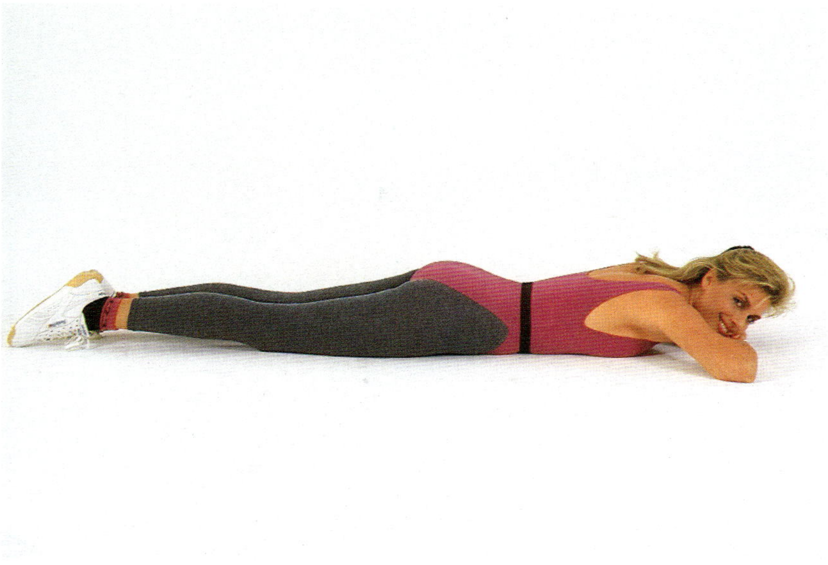

1

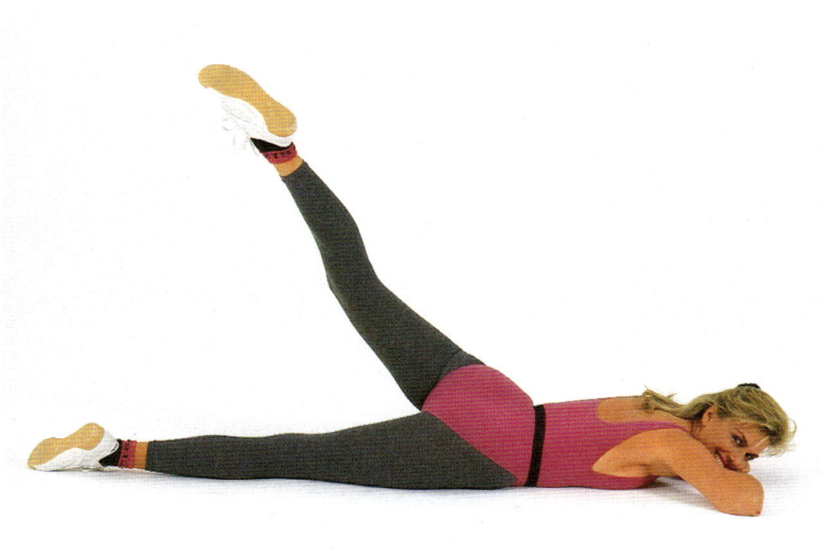

2

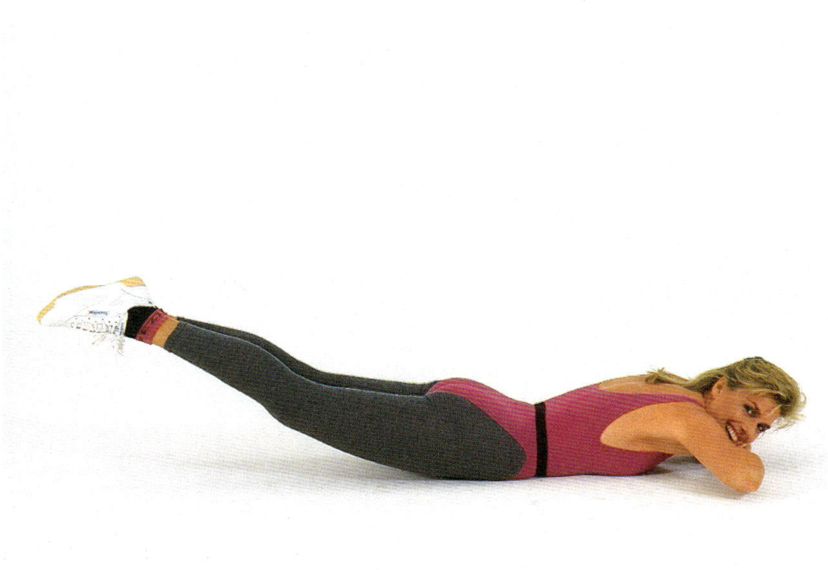

3

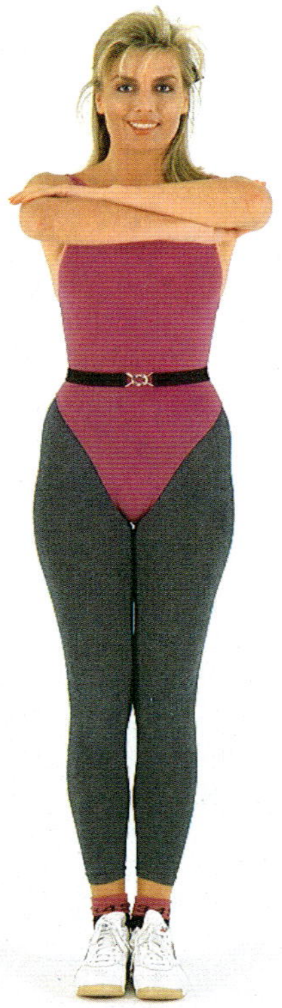

1

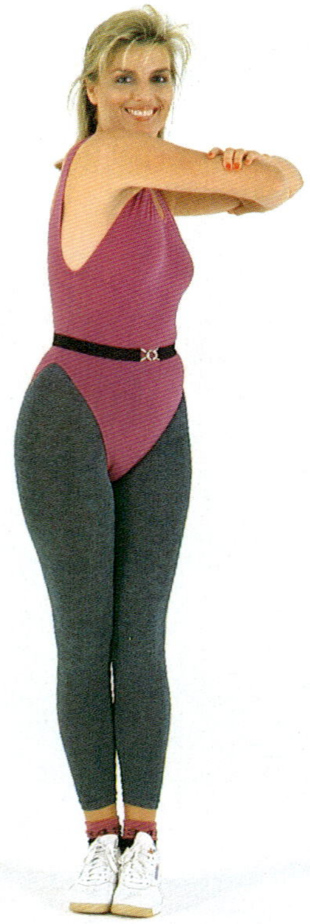

2

WRESTLER GRIP

1. Starting position.

2. Clasping arms together, swing your upper body around to the left as far as you can, then swing around to the right. Swing in each direction 15 times. Make sure you keep your arms up at chest height.

3. Return to starting position. Push your right hand against your left arm and your left hand against your right arm as hard as possible. Hold for 15 seconds, relax and repeat.

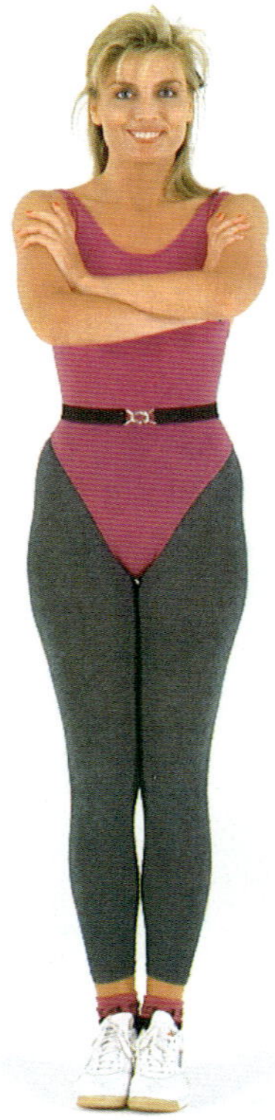

3

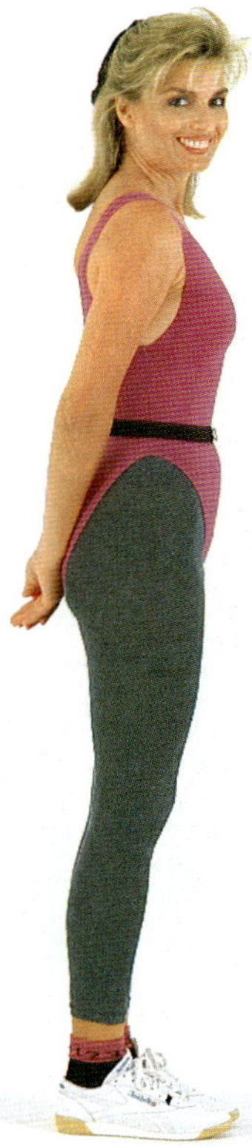

1

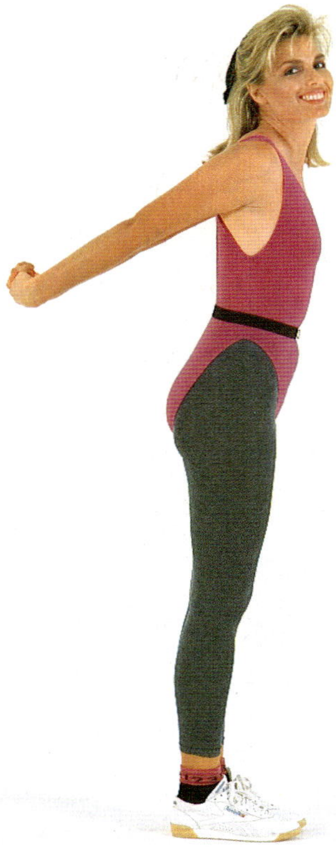

2

BACK TOUGHENER

1. Starting position.

2. While continuing to stand straight, raise your arms, with hands clasped, up behind your back as far as you can go. Hold for five seconds. Return to starting position and repeat five times.

3. This time bend forward from the waist as you bring your arms up behind your back. Hold for five seconds. Return to starting position and repeat five times.

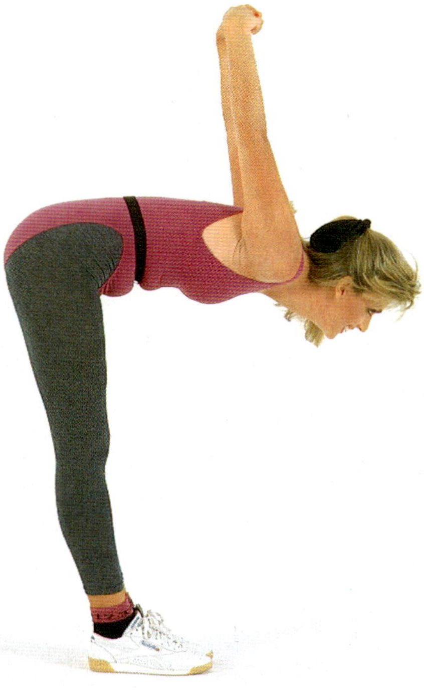

3

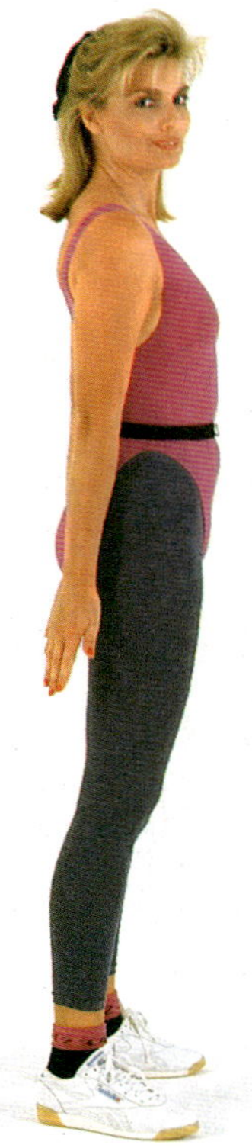

1

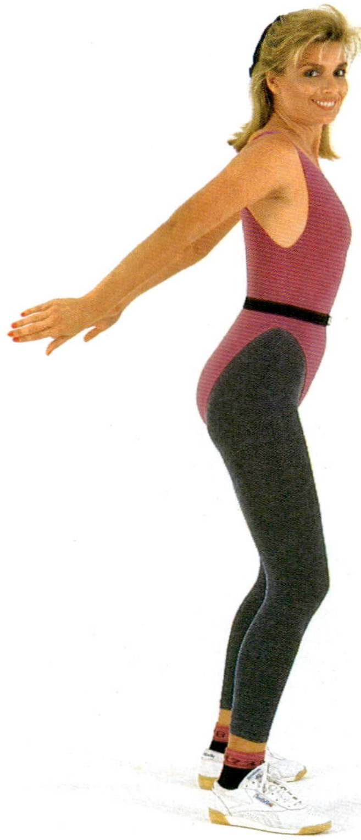

2

SQUEEZE AND SWING

1. Starting position.

2. Tighten your buttocks and the front and back of your thighs. Pull in your stomach. Hold and release. Begin with 50 rapid movements, gradually building up to 100. This exercise strengthens the back and tones up the bottom and pelvic area.

3. Return to starting position. Stretch your arms out to the sides for balance and rotate your body from the hips as if using a hula-hoop. Repeat 10 times.

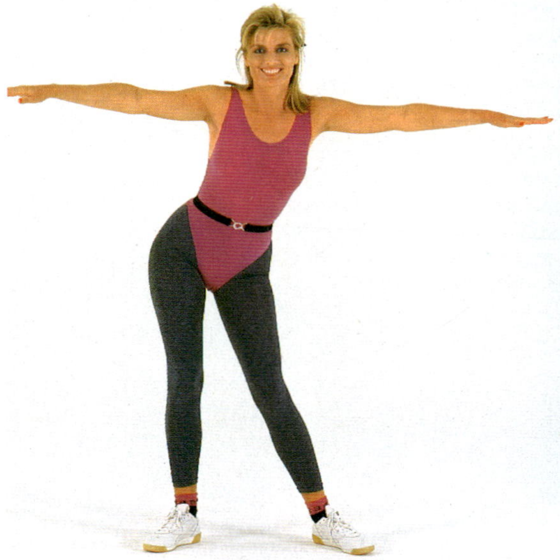

3

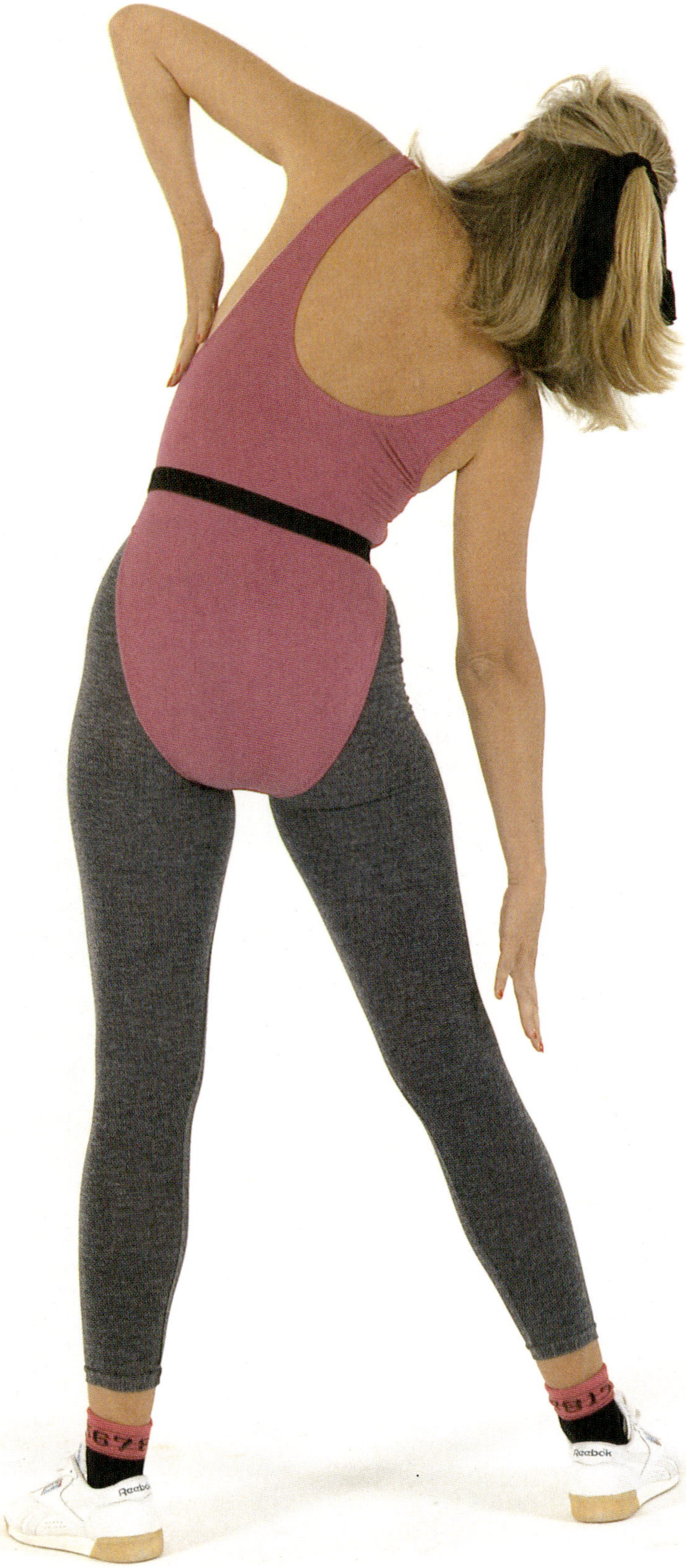
Reebok
Reebok

SPORTING WAYS

Sport is fun and enjoyable, and above all, it's a great aid to fitness. It tones you up, gives you a healthy glow, relaxes you and can become an absorbing and rewarding part of your life. The following table outlines the benefits of some popular sports. Bear in mind the message of all the exercise sections: build up slowly, exercise consistently, stop if you feel faint, exhausted or simply too strained. Sport, like all good exercise, is to be enjoyed!

Sport is great for increasing your fitness but remember it must also be fun.

SPORTING BENEFITS

SPORT	HEALTH BENEFITS	BEAUTY BENEFITS	KILOJOULES USED	COMMENT
Cycling	If you work hard at it cycling is good exercise for your cardio-respiratory system. It is also relaxing, and helps flexibility.	Improves thigh muscles and firms buttocks.	At 24 kilometres per hour you could use up about 2730 kilojoules in an hour. At 16 kilometres per hour this drops to 1640; at 8 kilometres to 1010.	Its fun, faster than walking and builds up stamina of heart and lungs provided you push hard enough, for long enough.
Golf	A great relaxer, golf helps you to unwind and get rid of tension. It's a non-strenuous, gentle exercise with a lot of walking.	Quite good for flexibility of arms and legs. Allows you to get lots of fresh air.	About 840–1010 kilojoules an hour.	Not a sport to improve endurance or muscular development. Benefits are probably more psychological than physical.
Riding	Good for overall fitness and legs, thighs and buttocks. Relaxing and good tension-easer.	Improves grace and deportment.	A gentle trot will obviously use less energy than a canter — but the horse does most of the work so you won't expend many kilojoules.	Moderate/low energy expenditure on the whole, but can be invigorating and satisfying.
Sailing	Dinghy sailing is a hard physical sport. It quickens reactions, and exercises back, legs and stomach. Cruising is much softer; it doesn't call for so much exertion.	Makes you look healthier, but if you don't want to look weather-beaten, use a strong protective sunscreen.	Up to 1680 kilojoules in a more strenuous hour.	Not recommended if you have a weak back. You need to train properly and you must be able to swim 45 metres in light clothing, to sail with a reputable club.

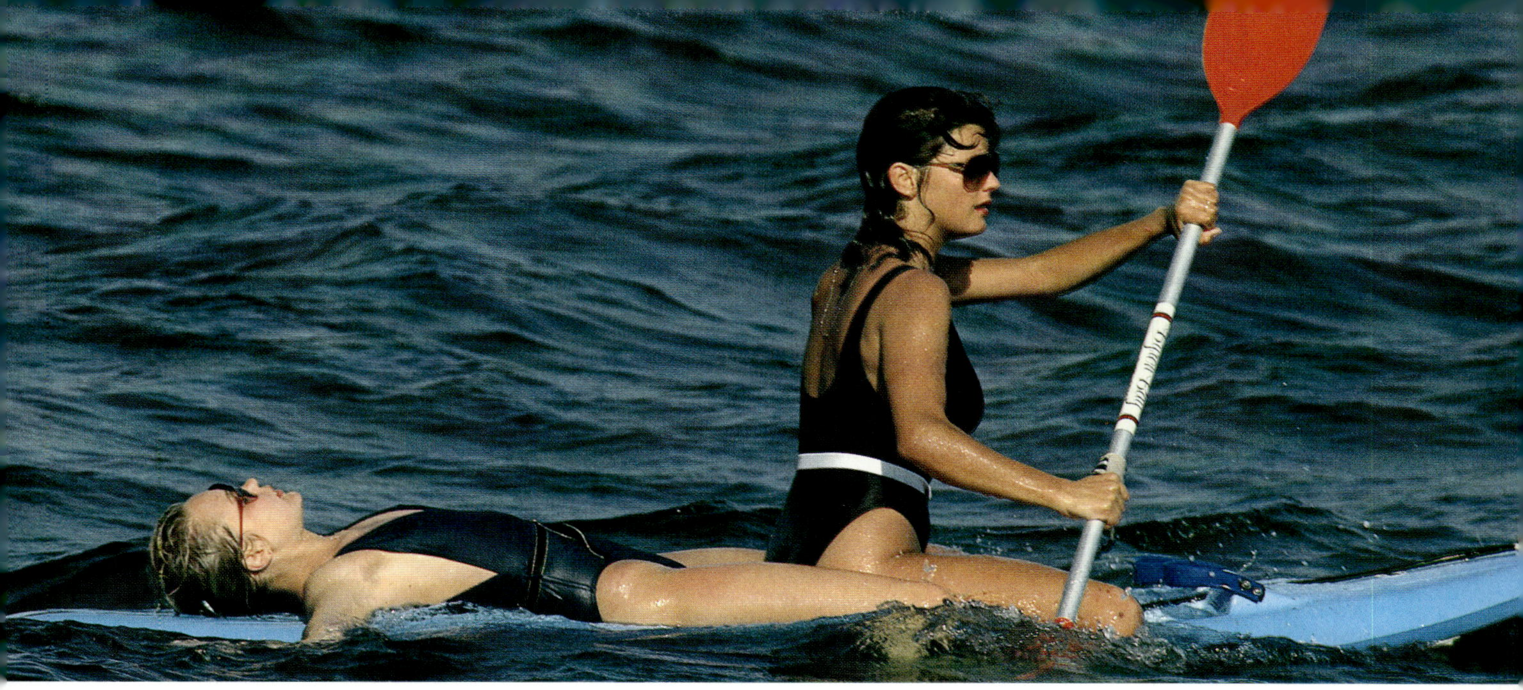

Roller-skating	A good exercise for heart and lungs.	Helps tone and trim thighs, calves, buttocks, waist and hips.	About 1512 an hour.	Great fun — especially roller-disco. Make sure your boots and skates fit.
Squash	Excellent for stamina and very good for suppleness. Helps work off frustrations. Provides good muscle work-out.	Relaxing — because it works off tensions, you feel and look more at ease. Helps suppleness.	In half an hour, the usual length of play, you could use up as many as 1260 kilojoules.	Fast and furious, squash can be exciting. It may be expensive, and you need to book courts well in advance.
Swimming	An all-over body toner, swimming develops stamina, suppleness and strength. Good exercise for older people, or those with rheumatism or arthritis, because the body is supported.	An excellent exercise for the pectoral muscles supporting the breasts. Breaststroke is good for hips and knees; backstroke and crawl for shoulders and trunk.	1170–2940 per hour depending on intensity of effort.	Try a variety of different strokes to exercise different groups of muscles. Build up slowly to two or three 20-minute sessions weekly. Don't swim within two hours of a big meal.
Tennis	Develops balance, enhances alertness, strengthens hand/eye co-ordination. Unless played competitively to high standards, tennis does not really stretch the body significantly. Good exercise if you are out of condition.	Gives you an outdoor glow. The bending and stretching is good for your waist and legs, and makes arms and shoulders more supple.	840–1680 an hour depending on how much you put into your game.	Good social sport for all ages, but not recommended if you have back trouble. To play it really well, you need to be an athlete. Even if you're not, however, it's great fun.
Water-skiing	An exhilarating sport in warm weather in a warm sea. If you don't have strong thigh muscles, you'll need to develop them.	Toning for the legs, especially fronts of thighs, and back, shoulders and stomach muscles.	Probably not more than 250 kilojoules in 10 minutes.	Not recommended if you have high blood pressure, heart problems, or if you are not at all fit.

relaxation

Although you may not always be aware of it at the time, modern stress and the tensions of twentieth-century life are probably the greatest enemy of your looks, not to mention your general well-being.

Stress of course is nothing new; for hundreds of years, human beings have lived and coped with wars, plagues, fires, famine, poverty and a host of other factors that created upheaval and unrest. But it has now been medically proven that it's not so much the major upheavals that are harmful to us, but the nagging day-to-day irritants that build up, often unnoticed, eventually causing chronic worry, anxiety, depression, anger and, most damaging of all, nervous tension, which have no opportunity for outlet and release. The final result is that this tension gets 'stored' in the body, particularly in the nervous system, leading to such familiar stress symptoms as insomnia, migraine, backache, indigestion and many other chronic ailments.

The chemical cause of stress isn't hard to understand. When we are suddenly faced with a stressful situation — say an exam, an interview for a job, a family quarrel, a bad traffic jam — the body automatically puts itself on to 'full alert' releasing large quantities of extra stress hormones such as adrenalin and noradrenalin into the bloodstream to provide extra energy, increasing the heart-beat and breath rate, raising the blood pressure and the pulse rate, speeding up the digestive system, and increasing the flow of blood to the muscles to increase their power. This is what scientists call our primitive 'fight or flight' response that for thousands of years has ensured survival and evolution by preparing us against attack. Our ancestors, however, never wasted their survival 'kit'; when the moment of danger had passed or the kill had been completed, this emergency response immediately switched itself off and the body returned to a normal and relaxed state.

The problem today, however, with modern pressures and stresses is that they very often don't resolve themselves; bad traffic is commonplace, pressures at work or at home often build up rather than blow over, with the result that our body frequently switches over to a tense state — and very often stays that way until physical and mental exhaustion causes us to break down and become ill.

No one nowadays is immune to the ill effects of stress. Even very young people can suffer from the pace and pressures put upon them by modern life. Also, the fact that people are less inclined to take exercise, eat too many of the wrong foods, have bad posture, and swallow medicines to deal with all sorts of aches and pains means that they are usually very ill-equipped to control the amount of stress in their lives.

However, although we may have largely lost the art of relaxing naturally, practising stress control is relatively easy once you've found a method that suits you, and you make it an integral routine of your daily life. It's no use practising relaxation or breathing exercises every now and again and expecting to feel cool and calm. Just like exercising to keep fit, relaxing should become a way of life and a ritual that you look forward to. What's more there's little mystique attached to relaxation. All you need is a quiet room, total privacy for 20 minutes and a good imagination! Instead of seeking relaxation from outside sources, like watching TV, drinking and smoking, it should come from within as a form of self-awareness and control. There are a number of different systems which you can use to help you become more

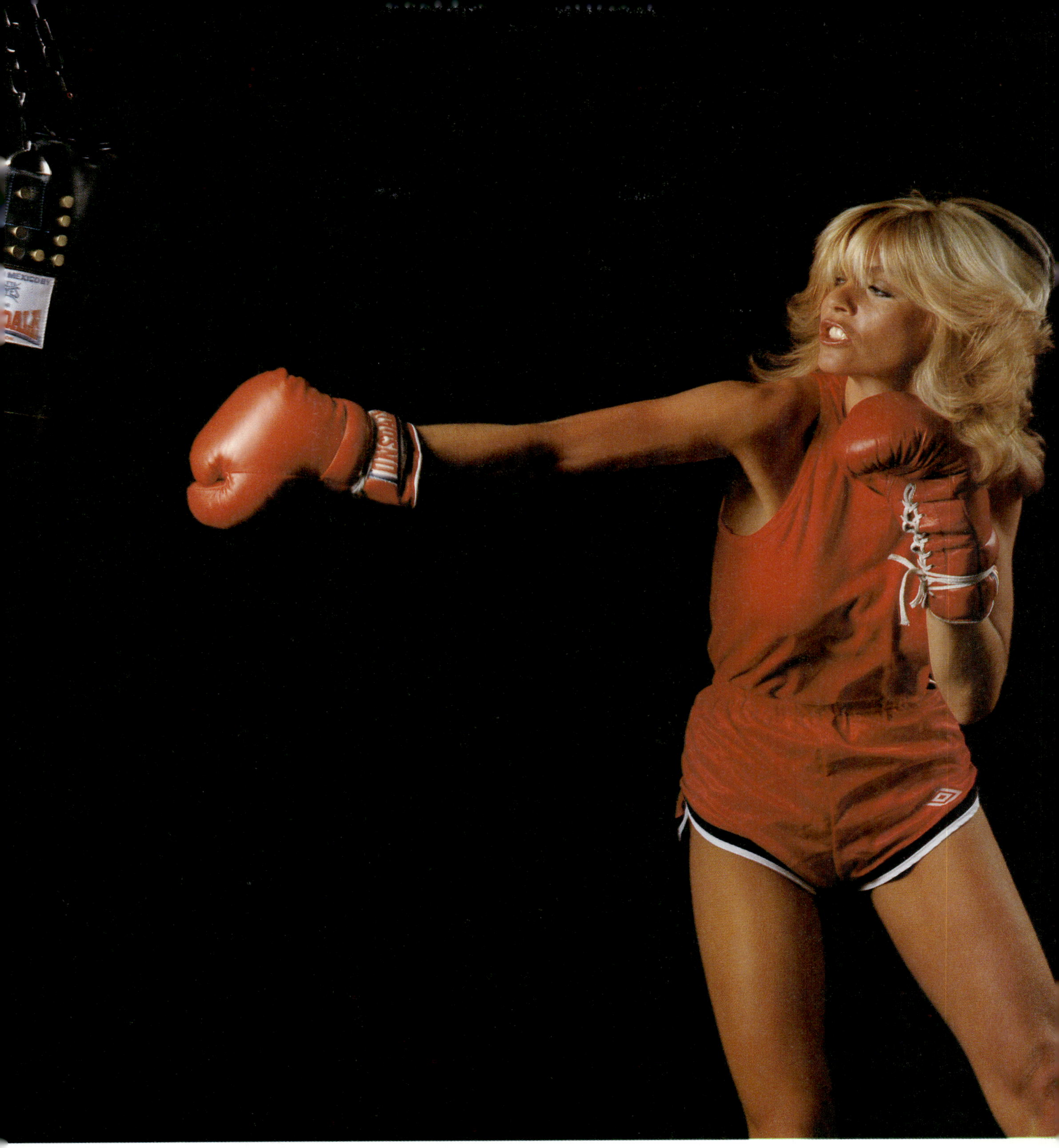

relaxed and more able to cope with stress: yoga, meditation, bio-feedback, self-hypnosis are all tried, tested and highly successful methods, but most require a definite period of study and the help of a teacher. Doing simple relaxation exercises to turn off physically and mentally at home can prove just as effective, providing you do them regularly, preferably at the same time every day.

Stress, tension and aggression — inevitable results of our lifestyle today. Relaxation can help to combat stress and safeguard looks and health.

COUNTDOWN TO PERFECT PEACE

Put aside 15–20 minutes and avoid any disturbances such as phone calls and knocks on the door. Choose a well-ventilated, quiet, slightly darkened room with enough space for you to lie flat on the floor. Put on some quiet background music — something slow and rhythmical — loosen all tight and restrictive clothing and take off any jewellery. Now prepare to switch off: this should be the one and only goal in your life at this particular moment.

1 Lie with your palms upward, knees loose, feet relaxed and slightly splayed apart.

2 Become aware of your breathing. Are you taking short shallow breaths, using only the top of your chest? This is one of the most common signs of tension. To correct your breathing, imagine as you inhale that your abdomen is a large vacuum; you're taking air into this space, blowing it out like a balloon. Then, as you exhale, feel the air travelling back through your chest and let it out through the throat, hearing yourself breathe out. At the same time lower the jaw and let the tongue rest on the lower teeth. Repeat this gently for a few minutes savouring the rhythm and sensation of your breathing.

3 Begin to think of relaxing each part of your body in turn: feet, calves, knees, thighs, stomach, back, chest, shoulders, neck, arms, hands and face. Imagine that tension is coiled up in each of these parts of the body like a spring. Try to make each coil gradually unwind, until all the tension has disappeared, saying to yourself 'tense . . . relax' as you feel the muscles relaxing and becoming limp. Try to relax the lower part of your spine, so that it lies flat against the floor.

4 Now that you've isolated and driven tension out of every part of the body (check that there isn't still some stubborn muscle harbouring stiffness and stress) it's time to move into isolating and relaxing the mind. Concentrate on one particular and beautiful restful image — a lake, stream, mountains, the ocean — and at the same time visualise one predominant colour. 'Hold' the imagine in your mind, creating an inner space that's filled entirely with your basic image and the colour that you've chosen. At this stage you are at a fairly advanced level of relaxation, when the pulse rate begins to drop and your body is at the same stage of rest as during deep sleep. Once you can reach this state fairly easily and regularly, then you'll find that you can control your body and its response to stress far more effectively. Mastering body control of this sort even means difficult goals such as dieting and giving up smoking become far easier to achieve.

Relaxation exercises are first and foremost designed to strengthen your 'stress defences', and wind down the body if it's tense and tired. They are also an ideal way of overcoming sleeplessness and headaches, two common and disturbing by-products of a stressful life which almost all of us have suffered at some time.

We all take sleep very much for granted — that is until our sleep patterns start to go awry, leading to 2 am waking and disrupted, fitful sleep that makes you feel more tired than refreshed, or simply the inability to drop off! Insomnia in itself is of course pretty harmless. No one ever became ill or died through lack of sleep since the body *does* eventually go to sleep when it is tired enough. Also, it's a common misconception that we all need the same amount of sleep. Eight hours' sleep is by no means a norm that applies to every one of us. How many hours you find you need to sleep depends entirely on your metabolism, your age, your body type, the amount of mental and physical energy you expend, and your lifestyle generally. Sleeplessness, however, is a very clear warning that:

☐ You are too tense and worried about the day's activities to be able to unwind sufficiently.

☐ You are suffering from a minor complaint like indigestion which means that a part of your body is working and not at rest.

☐ There is something worrying you subconsciously and your sleep is disturbed in an attempt to resolve the problem.

☐ Your environment is unsuited to restful sleep — an uncomfortable bed, too much or too little fresh air, too much noise or light.

Learning to relax should help tremendously in clearing your mind, unwinding the body and so preparing you for a good night's sleep. Don't embark on the exercises immediately before going to bed, 6 or 8 pm is about the latest time you should do them. Taking exercise helps to make you healthily tired and works off any stored tension — but again not just before bedtime. Having a warm bath, reading a book, listening to some soft gentle music, can help make you feel more sleepy and drop off more easily. Try not to eat a big meal late in the evening, since it's heavy going on your stomach and digestive system. Hot milky drinks, however, can often make you relaxed and sleepy, as milk contains an amino acid that helps the brain produce certain important 'sleep' chemicals. Camomile is a soothing herbal alternative, while peppermint tea helps settle the digestion before going to bed. The most damaging thing you can do to your health is of course to take sleeping pills or tranquillisers. Not only can they become addictive, but they are not a solution to the problem, as they mask the true causes of insomnia and produce an artificial form of sleep which can often leave you feeling drugged and woozy the next morning. Above all, too much worry about not sleeping can encourage those wakeful nights. Changes in the weather, pre-menstrual tension and changes in diet can all affect the way you sleep, and the less you worry about sleeplessness the sooner the problem will pass.

Headaches and migraines are a much more unpleasant offshoot of nervous tension and generally are harder to treat. A 20-minute relaxation period can positively help in easing muscular tightness and so help to shift headaches. Simple neck and head rolling exercises can loosen tight muscles at the back of the neck and the tops of the shoulders, which generally trigger headaches. Migraines, however, may be directly linked to certain foods you eat — in particular chocolate, cheese, orange juice, wine, dairy produce — so you may need to do some detective work on your normal diet. Headaches and migraine can also be a problem just before and during your period, so make sure you relax and get plenty of rest at this time. If you do suffer from persistent and troublesome headaches consult your doctor about the problem.

POSTURE — USES AND ABUSES

Sloppy, incorrect posture is also guaranteed to load your body with extra tension. For instance, most of us are guilty of sitting slumped or curled up like a sack of potatoes on a chair at some time or other during the day. Our breathing becomes shallow, the lungs are unable to expand, the neck and shoulders get tense and the chest area is constricted. Extra strain builds up if you spend a lot of time typing or writing in a distorted position and the same goes for standing over long periods. Waiting for trains and buses in the freezing cold, or queueing in shops and stations is inevitably tedious and a bit of a strain on the legs, but you'll take a lot of the slog out of standing if you correct your posture — weight evenly distributed on both feet, stomach pulled in, back straight but not rigid because all backs have a natural curve, shoulders, neck and arms relaxed. By all means shift your weight from one foot to the other, but don't push your hip joints or buttocks out of alignment as this is not only ugly, but can lead to lower backache and poor circulation.

How do you rate your walking style? Do you walk slowly, dragging your feet, shoulders slumped and back slouching forward, eyes downcast, so that they never take in the sky, trees, tops of buildings, or other people? Bad posture becomes glaringly obvious when we're in motion, because it distorts the smoothness, rhythm and alignment of the body. We often carry things in a clumsy way, allowing heavy shopping bags to dislocate shoulders and arms, or outsize handbags to tip-tilt the upper half of the body and create backstrain. The longer you are unaware of such bad habits the more restricting they become, putting a brace on the body and making it rigid when it should be free. The first part of you that suffers if you have bad posture is your back. After all back pain accounts for more sickness and absenteeism in this country than any other complaint, a problem which could be often avoided if we paid more attention to correcting our posture.

Exercise techniques based on physical realignment such as the famous 'Alexander Technique' rely entirely on restoring health by teaching you to move and stand without putting strain on the body. Poor posture also saps the body of energy; walk with your head high, back upright, with a spring in your step, legs swinging out from the hips and you are less likely to get bogged down with aching feet and general fatigue at the end of the day.

There's even a correct and incorrect way to sleep. While a soft mattress makes the body compensate for its lack of overall support by shifting and contorting into different positions, a hard mattress literally throws you into the correct position, cutting down on disturbed sleep, cramps and backache. Remember also not to strain your back when pushing heavy objects or bending down to pick up anything from the floor; try to use your stomach muscles not your back to take the strain out of extra physical exertion. When bending down to pick up a heavy suitcase or a bag of vegetables, keep your body upright, stomach in, and bend at the knees only, taking the full weight of the object you're lifting up with you as you swing back into a standing position.

MASSAGE — THE OLDEST THERAPY IN THE WORLD

The origins of massage date back thousands of years. The use of scented oils to heal, relax and calm the body dates as far back as the civilisations of ancient Greece and Egypt, and today different forms of massage have become popular in the treatment of everything from hair loss and skin problems to anxiety and tension. Nor does massage necessarily involve spending lots of time and money on professional treatments. Everybody can learn the basics of different massage techniques; after all, in China, Japan and India massage has been recognised as a home therapy for centuries, that members of a family practise on one another to stay fit and healthy, as well as to treat minor aches, pains and illnesses. Anyone, even a child, can master the principle of massage and use it amongst family and friends.

The very simplest massage method comes from China and is based on the guiding rules of acupuncture, except that you use finger pressure instead of needles. Acupressure (or *shiatsu* as it is called in Japan) works by stimulating the body's various reflex points — there are over 800 dotted all over the body — and so improving the flow of energy and circulation in specific parts of the body, as well as eliminating muscular tension. The feet have a particularly dense collection of reflex points which connect to every area in the rest of the body and therefore the soles, sides, toes and tops of the feet should always get a lot of attention in any acupressure massage. By looking at a person's expression while you're massaging their feet, you can tell a lot about what is wrong with them, as each point on the foot corresponds to an organ or area of the body. The face too is covered in different points which you can treat more specifically to banish colds, headaches, sore eyes and tiredness. The hands contain many important key reflex zones such as the *hoku* point that controls pain relief. Dentists and doctors who use acupuncture instead of conventional anaesthetics always stimulate this point to prevent a patient feeling discomfort and pressing this area often gives fast and total relief for migraines.

General massage

The object of any massage is to make you feel more relaxed. It is easy for a masseuse to locate a person's main tension spots, by laying her hands flat over areas like the shoulders, nape of the neck, small or top of the back, tension in the muscles can be felt like tight cords. Relaxed muscles are rather like putty; firm and flexible, never rock hard. You can ease tension by gently kneading these muscles and rubbing them with a firm, circular motion, pressing into the flesh without pinching or hurting. Always use a fragrant oil to help make the skin soft and supple, as well as create a luxurious atmosphere!

If you are going to give a more thorough overall massage, make sure your partner is lying face down on a firm, flat surface (the floor will do), hands relaxed on either side of the body, head to one side. Begin by putting your hands on the lower back, exerting a comfortable amount of pressure, then keep pushing as you slowly follow the muscles upwards along the sides of the spine. Open the hands up over the top of the back then pull them along the sides of the body down to the waist. Start the massage like this to encourage relaxation before you begin working at specific knotted areas, finishing afterwards with the same broad sweeping movements. Massage can relieve a lot of stiffness and soreness after an all-out bout of sports or jogging, or even dancing. Whenever the muscles have been contracting for a period of time, you should stretch and massage them to help counteract muscle spasm and the risk of cramp. Patting and pinching the calves and rubbing the thighs, knees and ankles, prevents muscle fatigue and also means you won't build up ugly bunched muscles.

Recontouring massage

Because of the toning effects on the skin and muscle tissue and the stimulus of blood and lymph circulation, massage has long been recognised as the ideal therapy for figure problems such as slack and flabby muscles, rough unconditioned skin, stubborn patches of localised fat and also stretch marks. Of course there's no need to invest a lot of money in a massage course — unless you want to indulge in some unashamed pampering. One of the benefits of localised massage is that you can do a lot of it on yourself — once you've learned a few simple guidelines. The best time to massage is immediately after you've had your bath or shower, when the skin is still moist and warm. There are special ivy- or seaweed-based creams on the market, which have been especially designed to stimulate the circulation and help break down fatty tissue, provided you massage them in regularly and correctly.

The most obvious parts of the body that respond to massage are the thighs, knees, hips, waist — all areas that you can easily get to grips with.

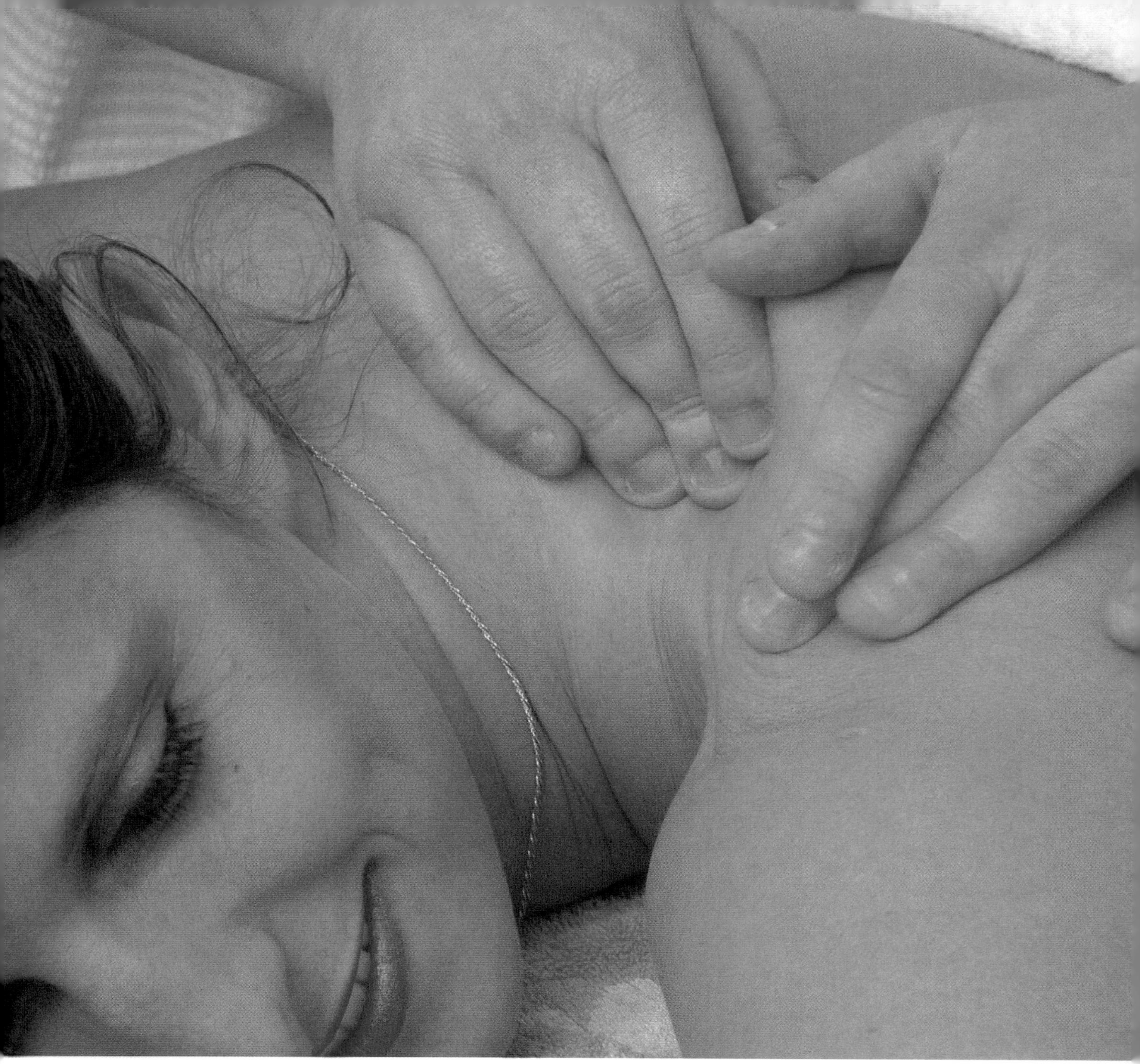

Massage is known as the oldest therapy in the world; not only for its relaxing and calming effects but also for a number of other healing properties including eliminating pain and stimulating the blood and lymph circulation.

Regular massage is the only way to tackle the problem of cellulite — those lumps and bulges at the top of the outer thigh — which may not respond to exercise or dieting. You can tell when you've got cellulite: the skin looks pitted and gives a dimpled 'orange peel' effect when you pinch it, showing lots of tiny hard nodules of fat just beneath the skin's surface. Firm circular movements with the palm of the hand encourages the circulation and the elimination of waste products in the system, while kneading, wringing, knuckling, and very gentle pinching movements help to soften and disperse the fatty lumps. Never manipulate the areas so aggressively that you bruise the skin or make the flesh red and painful. If you are trying to whittle down your thighs, or any other lumpy, bumpy areas you should give yourself at least 5–10 minutes' massage a day. Of course massage alone won't do the trick; keep a check on your diet, avoid salty and spicy food, drink plenty of water

— six to eight glasses per day — and cut down on coffee, tea and alcohol. Bathtime can also double up as an opportunity to massage. Use a rough hemp mitt or a friction glove to whip up the circulation on buttocks, thighs, hips, stomach and keep the skin silky and smooth. This will also help to open the pores and soften the skin in preparation for your main massage after your bath.

Acupressure points

Press each point for a count of 30 seconds with your middle finger or thumb.

1 To relieve headaches, press both of your temples about an inch from the edge of the eyebrows.

2 To clear stuffy nose and blocked sinuses, press the points running along the sides of the nose, starting at the nostrils and working up to the corner of the eyes. Lastly, press the 'third eye' point right betweeen the eyebrows.

3 To refresh tired eyes, press the front, centre and outer edge of each eyebrow. Then repeat on matching points underneath the bottom eyelids.

4 To relieve toothache or neuralgia, press the point right in front of your ear at the bottom edge of the cheek bone.

5 For general faintness, or to reduce a craving for food, press the centre of your upper lip about one centimetre below the nose.

6 To control migraines and tension headaches, press the *hoku* point on the top of the hand. To locate it, crook your left thumb and place your other thumb at a slight angle onto the fleshy part between the thumb and index finger and squeeze hard.

Feet

There are literally dozens of reflex points all over the soles, sides, backs of the feet and on the base of each toe. Simply covering the entire area of both feet with lots of firm pressing movements with the edge of the thumb helps to relax and invigorate you when you're tired and tense, while also providing a delicious foot treatment. If any part of the foot feels sore or particularly rigid keep pressing and making tiny semicircular movements with your thumb to get the circulation going and to disperse any built-up waste matter that has accumulated.

YOGA FOR FITNESS AND HARMONY

Many people make the mistake of thinking that yoga is only for the very fit. Unfortunately all those pictures of lithe double-jointed girls in advanced yoga positions suggest you have to be a contortionist to take it up in the first place, but nothing could be further from the truth. Yoga is the oldest form of keep fit in the world and its present day appeal is certainly due to the fact that *anyone* can take it up at any time in their lives and experience tremendous health benefits. Yoga is unique in that it not only exercises and strengthens all parts of the body, including the internal glands and organs, helping them to function more smoothly, but at the same time it encourages deep mental relaxation and improved circulation, through emphasis on special breathing techniques. Yoga literally translated means union, therefore the entire body gets stronger through practice, not just one isolated part of it. What's more each person creates their own level of fitness, so you can benefit from yoga whether you're 17 or 70, fit or unfit, used to exercise or totally inactive.

Those parts of the body which yoga strengthens dramatically are the back, stomach and lungs — simply because among the majority of use these are nearly always in pretty bad shape. If you decide to take up yoga for fitness and relaxation, you'll invariably find you can adapt a specific series of *asanas* or poses to suit your body's own needs, or alternatively you may decide to embark on a long and exploratory training which teaches you to practise the exercises as well as the philosophy of yoga more fully — including adopting a certain diet and lifestyle.

Whichever direction you decide to follow, yoga practice must be regular, at least three times a week, preferably more. It's not something you can take up now and again when you are feeling a bit sluggish. Learning physical control and stretching your body to its fullest extent means setting time aside to practise — preferably with an expert yoga teacher. Books can teach you a certain amount about the rudiments of yoga, but if you are starting from scratch it's best to learn with a teacher, otherwise you may hurt yourself, or generally misinterpret the different poses and exercises. Later, when you have mastered the basics, you can use a book to help you adopt a system to suit yourself. However, whether you practise yoga for a mere 15 minutes a day or for an hour or more, you'll find that breathing is an essential first step to 'tuning in' the body and mind to the rhythm and control of yoga.

Practised independently of any physical exercise, yoga breathing can in itself help tremendously in teaching you to breathe deeply and correctly. This helps to calm frayed nerves, clear a muzzy head making you feel bright-eyed and more energetic, increases the absorption of oxygen into the blood and therefore to the rest of the tissues and generally helps you to become more aware of your body. Try and practise yoga breathing lying down to begin with; when you have mastered the different techniques you can do them sitting, standing or even while out walking in the countryside or a park.

Deep yogic breathing

This is an ideal way to wake up the body and mind at the start of the day. It teaches you not only to use the lungs, abdomen and chest correctly but increases the amount of oxygen taken in with each breath. Place your hands on your abdomen and feel it rise as you inhale deeply through the nose. Take the breath down into the lower lung, filling the middle and upper lung, right up to the collarbones. Pause for one pulse beat, then start to exhale through the nose, emptying the lungs in the same slow smooth manner, pulling the abdomen well in towards the backbone as you breath out the last remnant of stale air. Most people feel so invigorated after they've practised their first few yogic breaths — both more alert, yet more relaxed — that they soon overcome any puny, shallow breathing habits. Finding you can increase your lung capacity is another delightful surprise which has invaluable health benefits. As you breathe in count silently up to two, hold the breath for a count of four, exhale for a count of eight. As your lungs get stronger you'll be able to build this up to counts of four, eight, 16, or even more — always remember to exhale for double the time you've held your breath. Don't do too many breaths when you first start, otherwise you might feel faint or dizzy from all that extra oxygen.

Tranquillising breath or alternate nostril breathing

This should be done in the evening before bedtime, to help you relax and sleep well. Place the right thumb against the right nostril, closing it, then inhale through the left nostril for a count of eight, now hold the breathe for a count of eight, closing off the left nostril with your middle finger, then

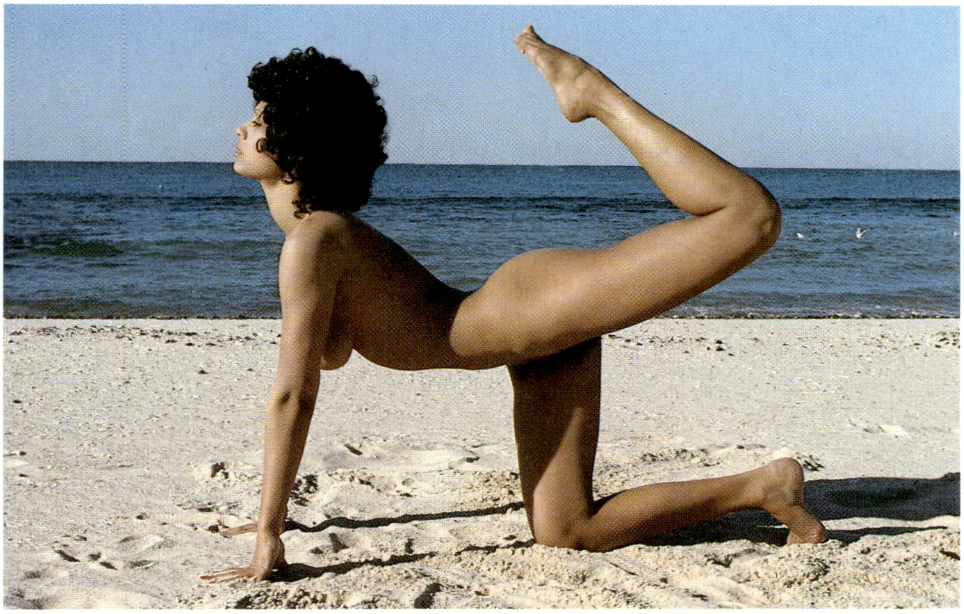

Yoga is not for the contortionist. It is something people of all ages can do to exercise and strengthen the body and encourage deep mental relaxation.

exhale through the right nostril for a count of eight. Inhale once more through the right nostril for a count of eight, hold for eight, exhale through the left nostril for eight; this completes one round. Try and keep the breathing rhythmic and continuous, repeating it for up to seven rounds. If you're tense, nervy, or headachy, this has an immediate calming effect.

MEDITATION FOR CALMNESS AND RELAXATION

If you are put off the idea of meditation by a vision of a lot of saffron-robed, shaven-headed devotees, endlessly chanting prayers in a cloud of incense, think again! You certainly don't have to join a religious sect, withdraw from the world or become a vegetarian in order to reap the benefits of simple meditation. What's more, as anyone who meditates regularly will tell you, not only does this type of 'switching off' do wonders for relaxing both mind and body, but by focusing the brain it increases mental alertness and concentration, and improves memory and overall energy. As a tool for fighting stress-related illnesses — migraine, asthma, insomnia, indigestion, high blood pressure — meditation can prove invaluable by exorcising destructive nervous tension.

Simplicity and straightforwardness are the key to meditation, which makes it a technique that's instantly appealing and freely available to just about anyone. Most forms of meditation used in the West today are variations of basic Zen techniques, as practised over many centuries by Buddhist monks in China and Tibet. If you go to a school or a centre for meditation, you may be given a *mantra* which is a short Sanskrit word or phrase chosen for its deeply relaxing effect on both your conscious and subconscious levels of thought. However, in order to meditate successfully, you can just as easily devise your own key word or rhyming phrase to help you get into a calm, reflective state of mind. Concentrating on a word or phrase is, after all, just a device to block out all other disturbing thoughts and problems which may come into your head, so just about anything will do such as 'romantic red roses', 'crisp crackly snow' or 'limpid languorous lagoon'. Have fun and

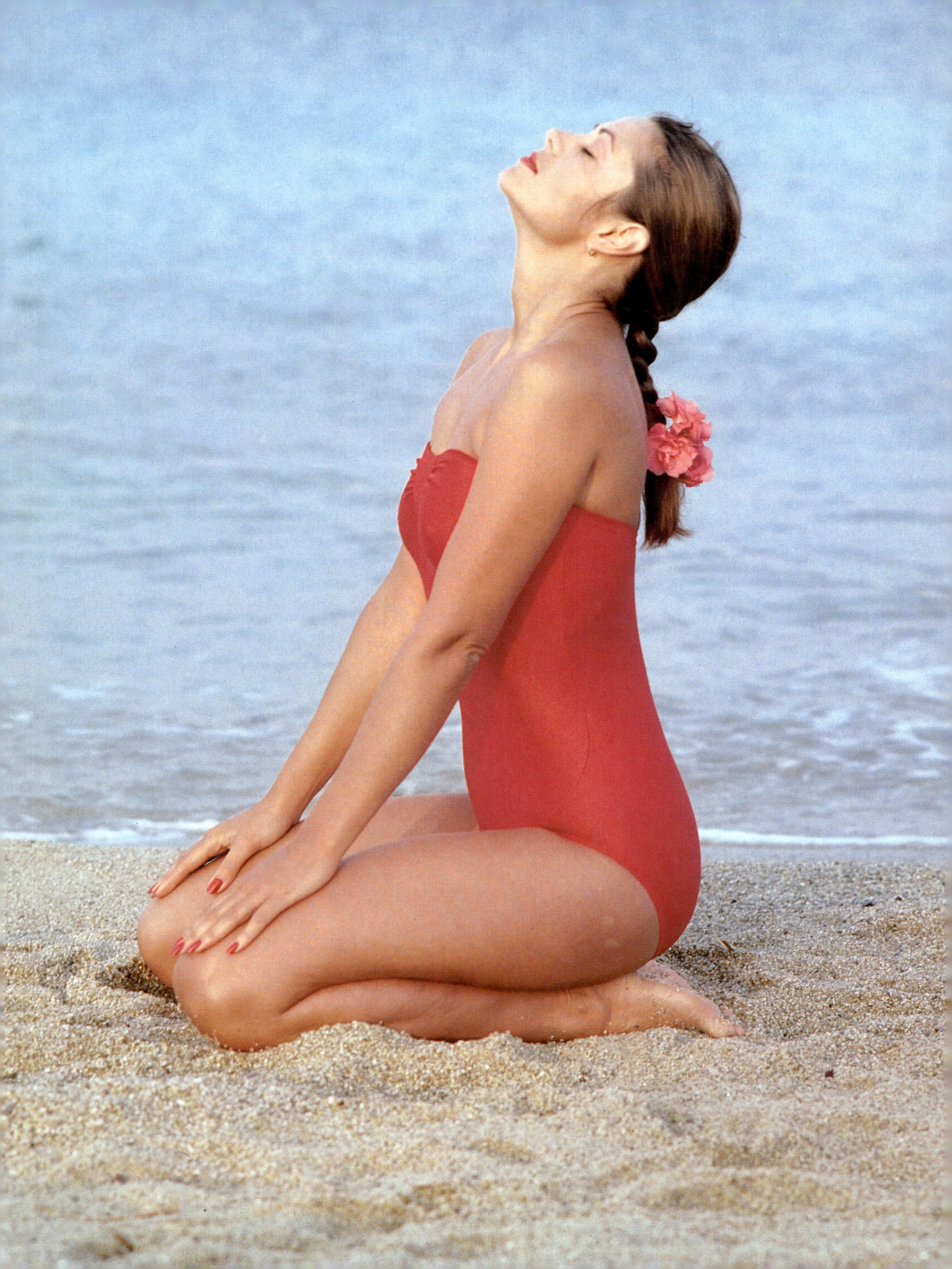

make up your own mantra to suit yourself — but when you've found one, stick to it!

A yoga teacher might suggest using the word 'one' — similar to the mantra 'om' — simply counting 1–10, or concentrating your attention on one specific object. Remember, however, hypnotic repetitiveness, not variety, is the object of your word-image, so don't get carried away with anything long-winded or fancy! When you first begin meditating, you will find that no matter how hard you concentrate on your word or mantra, your mind will start to stray to other things. Just nudge these 'intruders' gently out of your conscious mind and return your focus firmly to your key word. Eventually you will find that you can switch off and slip quite easily into a calm withdrawn state, pushing aside such worries as what to cook for supper or how much washing you've got to take down to the laundrette. Set aside the same 10–20 minute period each day for meditation. First thing in the morning, lunchtime or early evening are ideal, but not just before bedtime, because meditating recharges your store of energy and will stop you sleeping.

MEDITATION TECHNIQUES

One

Make yourself comfortable, sitting on a chair or the floor, back upright. Ensure that each part of your body is relaxed. Close your eyes and become aware of your breathing. This should be deep to begin with, it will get shallower and softer as you become more relaxed. This is not a breathing exercise however. Don't follow any particular rhythm. As you exhale each time count silently or audibly the word 'one'. Savour the sound, image and feeling of the number, it's roundness and simplicity. Continue breathing, repeating this word over and over at your own pace until your meditation period is over.

One to ten

The same rules apply as above but instead of repeating the word 'one', build up the numbers 1–10 with each consecutive breath. Visualise the numbers each time you exhale by mentally 'planting' them in the centre of your tummy. Don't anticipate or rush the next number, just let one melt gently into two, two into three and so on each time you breathe out. Take as much time as you like to breathe, count and 'see' each number.

Pretty pictures

Place one small perfectly shaped object — a flower, a lit candle, a vase — in front of you at eye level. Concentrate on this while you breathe, stare at the object, giving it your 100 per cent undivided attention. Presently it will exert a pleasant hypnotic influence over you, losing its obvious everyday form, appearing surreal, shifting its image and outline. As they become more relaxed, some people see a glow and different colours, surrounding the object, rather like a halo. Each time your mind begins to wander off onto other things, draw your concentration in closer to the object pinning it down until nothing else exists. An added benefit of this type of 'creative imagery' is that it often sharpens concentration and visual perception.

Whatever system of meditation you follow, proof of its success can only be experienced once you have finished meditating. Do you feel calm, rested, yet totally alert — all the advantages of a good night's sleep without any of the doziness? If so, your meditation is a success.

Correct posture, whether at work or play, not only reduces physical tension but also allows you to breathe properly and helps to prevent backache and other chronic aches and pains. Furthermore, it improves body contours and encourages gracefulness.

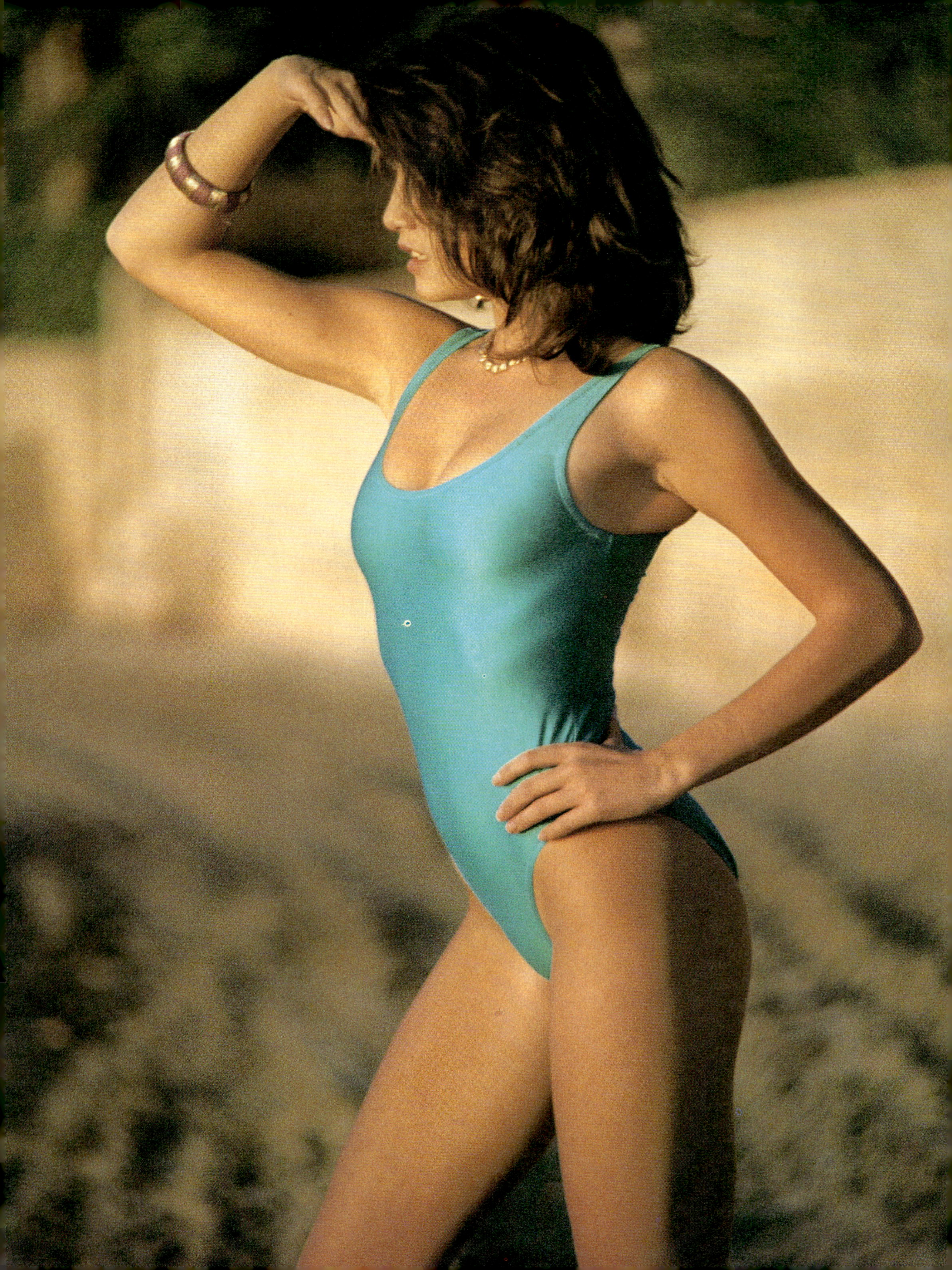

THE BEAUTIFUL BODY

The modern-day woman requires beauty routines that are simple and streamlined so she can incorporate them into her busy lifestyle. The accent of today's techniques is individuality. Each woman chooses the body-care routines best suited to her own unique needs.

Skin care is a vital prerequisite — lavishing attention on the skin will pay off in terms of a glowing complexion and will prevent unsightly blemishes on your appearance. The skin is a complex, dynamic structure which constantly renews itself while eliminating waste products, moderating temperature extremes, and protecting the system from harmful substances. It is worth looking after — particularly as it is quick to show the effects of neglect.

Then there are the extremities — the parts we overlook but others notice. Hands and nails; legs and feet; teeth — essential to our lives yet often forgotten. Regular attention will ensure they remain in tip-top condition.

Self-expression through cosmetics, perfume and hairstyle offers infinite possibilities and the chance to change your looks with your mood. Experiment, define and alter as you wish. There are no rigid rules — you do not have to be a slave to fashion. Understanding your face shape and selecting those features you wish to disguise or promote are essential — then indulge your creativity.

As women age their beauty routines must adapt to the changes in their bodies. Experimentation is still the key — a constant process of defining and redefining who you are and who you want to be. Age brings benefits — notably the asset of 'knowing oneself'. Serenity derived from self-confidence is apparent to all.

The beauty routines you choose can be as simple or as complex as you wish — so long as they become a regular feature of your life and you continue to examine their suitability for your unique needs.

We all have unique needs for caring after our bodies. Determining your own body beauty routine can be as simple or as complex as you choose.

skin — the bare facts

No other part of our body records shifting patterns of health as accurately as the skin. A smooth, radiant, trouble-free complexion is, as it was centuries ago, one of a woman's most valued and desirable possessions. Yet few of us are born with impeccable skin, and a good complexion more often than not needs to be cultivated with care and patience. Just as revealing is the fact that those women who are blessed with a naturally beautiful skin must work to care for and protect it almost as much as anyone else in order to safeguard its quality and youthful appearance.

The skin is one of the most complex organs and hard-working systems of the human body. Spread flat it would cover roughly 1.6 square metres, and, if you could find a microscope powerful enough, you would see that a 2 square centimetre piece of skin is packed with about a dozen blood vessels, 25 nerve endings, 100 sweat glands, hair follicles, sebaceous glands, muscles, pores and more than three million cells, all constantly dying and renewing themselves. Skin is about 20 per cent fluid, and accounts for around 2.7 kilograms of body weight. It is continuously expanding and contracting, eliminating waste matter and keeping an automatic check on the temperature of the body. As well as providing us with very pretty outer wrapping, skin is also the hardiest, most effective form of protective packaging ever invented.

ON THE LEVEL

Surface skin is made up of the stratum corneum or epidermis — a fine layer of flattened, overlapping dead cells that's continually being shed as new cells die and are pushed upwards from beneath the skin's surface. Dead as it is, the basic condition of the epidermis is what determines the aesthetic quality of your skin.

It takes about three weeks for young healthy skin to fully renew itself, but this slows down as early as the late twenties or early thirties, heralding the first visible signs of skin ageing. Beneath the surface skin lies the dermis, a priceless reservoir of moisture, protein, living cells, oil glands and capillaries, that keep the skin moist, well toned, unlined and glowing. The deepest layer, the hypodermis, contains chiefly fat cells and muscle, giving the skin of the face and body its contour and underlying support structure. In terms of preserving young, beautiful skin, scientists have now established that what really counts is how promptly and efficiently cells renew themselves, the balance of moisture in the epidermis, and the strength and suppleness of the collagen fibres and interweaving elastic fibres which determine the skin's elasticity and smoothness. So, although the quality of our skin depends largely on how we care for its surface over the years, its basic characteristics, overall state and rate of ageing are thought to be determined more by the health and condition of these deeper layers. What's more, it's an established medical fact that strong sunlight, smoking, drinking too much alcohol, crash dieting, exposure to central heating and air conditioning, and prolonged bouts of illness and stress can drastically rob your skin of its moisture

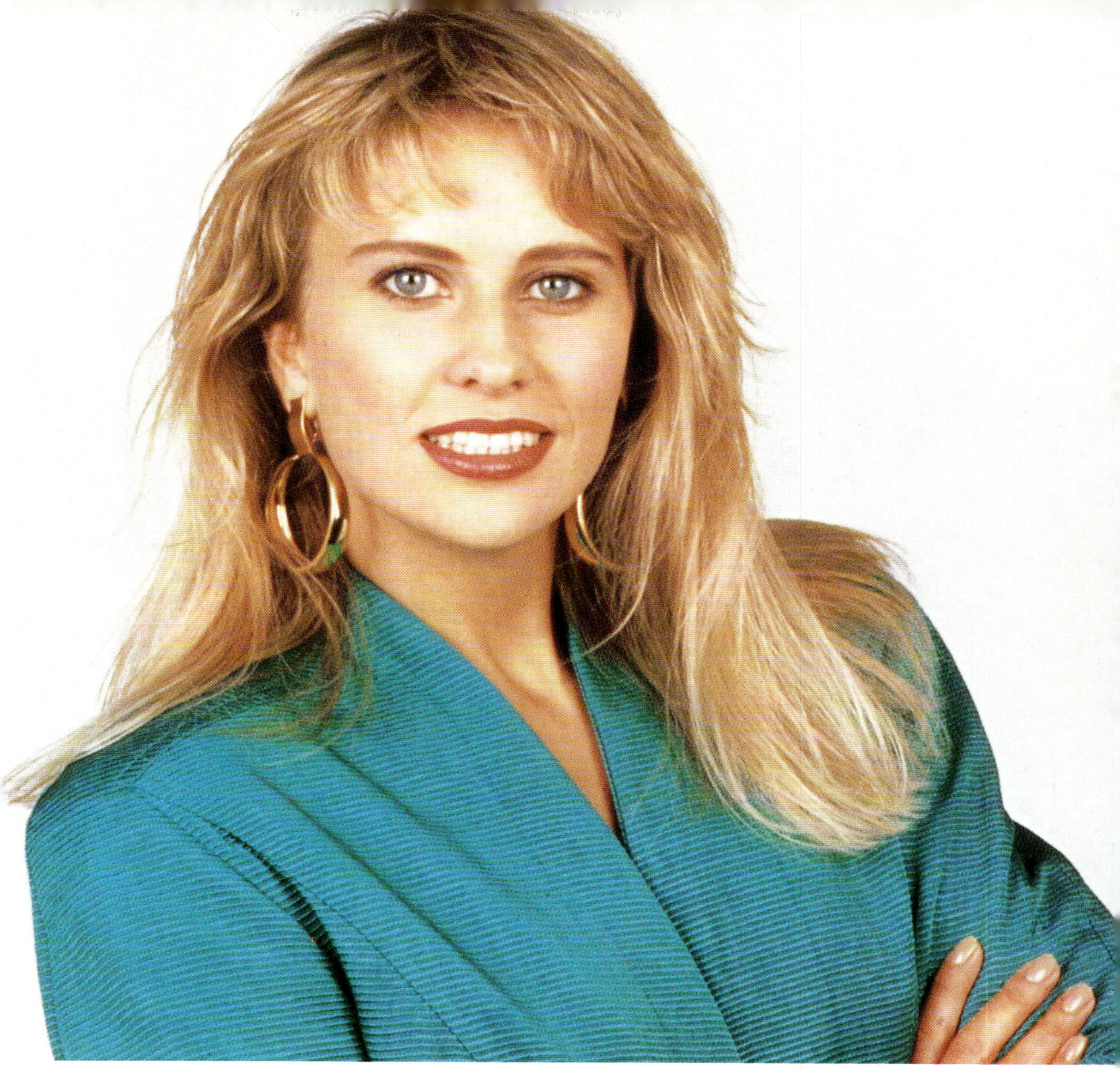

At any age, a glowing, flawless complexion is a priceless asset. It needs cultivation as well as lifelong care.

reserves and thereby cause it to begin ageing prematurely, unless you take steps to protect it.

The fate of our complexion lies more often than not in our own hands — its condition dependent to a large extent on how accurately we identify our own skin type and accordingly how careful we are in meeting its requirements in terms of proper cleansing, diet, exercise and rest.

FINDING YOUR TYPE

Just like bone structure and colouring, your basic skin type is almost entirely hereditary. It determines not only the products and routine that keep your complexion looking its best, but also provides invaluable advance warning of the sort of skin problems you may meet at some time during your life. Finding your skin type is a relatively simple procedure. You've probably heard of the tissue test and the cellotape guide which aim to identify the oily and dry areas of your face and therefore your skin type. Both are apt to be confusing and often not as reliable as plain visual scrutiny. After you have

Skin routines

SKIN TYPE	CLEANSING	TONING	MOISTURISING
oily and coloured	detergent-free soap and water and/or cleansing milk	cucumber or witch hazel skin tonic	fine, non-greasy, oil-in-water emulsion
normal	detergent-free soap and/or cleansing milk, as preferred	mild, alcohol-free tonic	will suit any type of moisturiser
dry	cleansing milk, cream or lotion, applied with cotton wool or tissue	mild skin freshener to ensure that all traces of cleanser have been removed; mineral water spray	richer, 'water-in-oil' cream or lotion
combination	detergent-free soap and water	mild skin freshener on dry areas, with stronger tonic for greasy panel	oil-free moisturiser with perhaps a richer cream for dry areas
sensitive and allergy-prone	cleansing milk or lightweight lotion applied with cotton wool	alcohol-free skin freshener or mineral water spray	lightweight, fragrance-free, oil-in-water moisturiser, preferably hypo-allergenic

thoroughly cleansed your face and applied moisturiser, wait 30–45 minutes, then take a look in the mirror. If your face is beginning to shine all over and the pores are clearly visible, you probably have an oily skin — prone to spots, blackheads and other pore problems. If only the centre forehead, nose and chin are shiny, the rest of the face matt, then yours is a combination skin — normal or dry with an oily 'T' zone. Normal skin generally looks matt with a slight peach-bloom finish that reflects the light and has no visible pores — or obvious problems. Dry skin on the other hand is often taut, fine or transparent with slightly flaky patches on the cheeks and prone to tiny lines even after you've applied moisturiser. Very sensitive and allergy-prone skin is fine to the point of translucence with a tendency to dryness, a red tone and broken red veins. This type of skin needs to be protected like precious porcelain; it may react by breaking out in rashes, spots and redness with certain, rich perfumed cosmetics. Broken veins are the real long-term problem of this skin type, so very drying conditions, extremes of hot and cold and over-vigorous, abrasive treatment must be avoided at all costs. Luckily there is an increasing number of excellent, gentle, hypo-allergenic, fragrance-free cosmetics on the market today which are specially designed to care for very delicate skins.

The darker skin tones (everything from olive to brown and black) invariably tend to be on the oily side and not prone to flakiness or extreme sensitivity. This is because on the whole dark skin is coarser and thicker than very pale skin, while the added pigmentation acts as a natural protection against the 'weathering' effects of sunlight and harsh, dry climates.

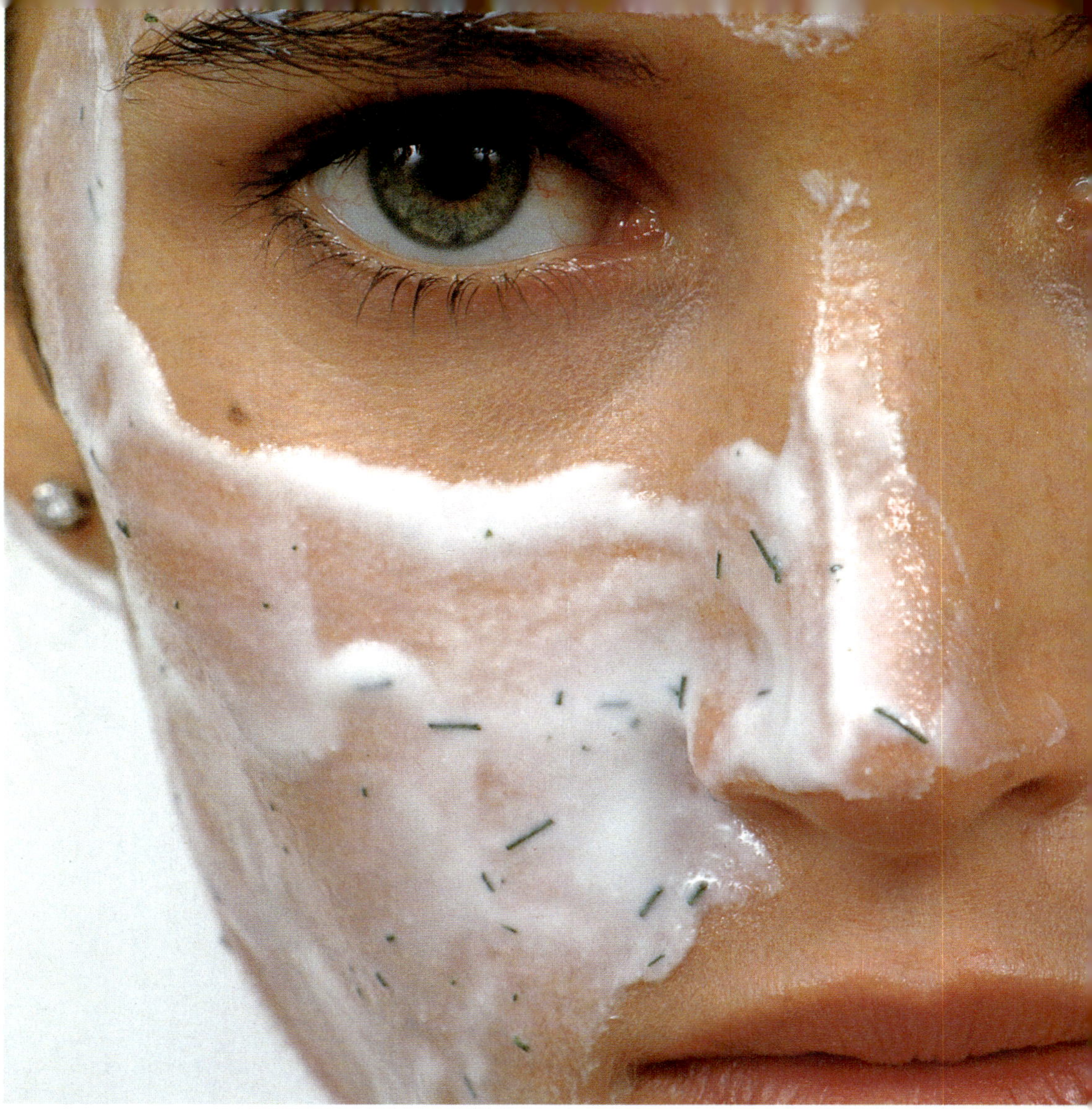

Cleansing is a necessity to remove dead cells, open pores and let your skin carry out its natural functions of cell regeneration and wastes elimination.

CLEANSING — THE TOP PRIORITY

The importance of thorough, twice-daily cleansing cannot be stressed enough — regardless of whether or not you wear make-up. Since the skin is an organ of elimination, anything obstructing this function, such as stale make-up, old face cream or just general grime, will not only result in blocked pores, which can cause spots and blackheads, but will also accumulate, leaving a drab, muddy-looking complexion. Furthermore, for any skincare product such as moisturiser to penetrate the skin's surface and get to work properly, the surface must be totally cleansed of all obstructing creams and debris.

Many people still automatically equate cleansing with soap and water, though the debate on the pros and cons of the effects of washing the face continues unresolved. Certainly you should avoid using very harsh, scummy, perfumed soap on your face, since this will only irritate and dry out the skin. However, there's little to beat a good lather and splashes of water for making the skin feel truly clean and refreshed; something leading cosmetic manufacturers have all latched onto in recent years by introducing 'soapless', or detergent-free, soaps which provide all the refreshment, lather and cleansing power of ordinary soap with none of their abrasive alkaline content, and therefore drying and damaging effects on the skin.

These new cleansing bars and complexion soaps gently dissolve dirt and excess grease removing all remnants of make-up and dirt without stripping the skin's protective 'acid mantle' — the blend of natural oils and moisture that protects and conditions the complexion. Gentler still are water-soluble cleansing creams and lotions that liquefy all traces of make-up and rinse off with warm water, leaving no oily residue. And what about the excessively dry skinned? Those women with a total aversion to the feel of water on the face can choose from a very broad range of cleansing milks, creams and lotions that whisk away make-up, dirt, and grease and are simply wiped off with tissues or cotton wool. If you use one of these cleansers make sure that you always remove all traces of lotion with a mild skin freshener or tonic.

Eye make-up, whether it is waterproof or not, is notoriously difficult to remove without leaving dark panda circles around the eyes. This is where it's worth investing in a specially formulated eye make-up remover which contains oils that dissolve mascara, eyeliner and shadow. Generally speaking, impregnated pads and clear liquid removers are ideal for removing non-waterproof eye make-up, but the heavier cosmetics respond more effectively to a thicker, oilier milk or lotion. Above all never rub, pull or stretch the delicate tissues around the eyes when cleansing — this is the quickest way to encourage lines, wrinkles, crepeyness and crow's feet.

TONICS — FRESH AND GENTLE

Skin tonics or fresheners have today replaced the harsh astringents beauticians used to recommend for 'closing the pores' after cleansing. We know now that you cannot make pores close or even tighten up for more than about 10 minutes, and while they may have a tingly, bracing effect, strong alcohol-based lotions can eventually coarsen and irritate the skin, creating surface dryness and broken veins. Gentle, alcohol-free tonics are far better for refreshing, stimulating and refining all skin types, while oily skins respond well to the natural astringent action of herbs like witch hazel or a cucumber-based tonic. Also very much in vogue these days is mineral water — the same sort you drink — in spray form. Though expensive, these sprays do actually have a very gentle and calming effect on all skins — even the very sensitive — and can be used repeatedly throughout the day. A good way to save money, however, is to decant an ordinary bottle of mineral water into a spray bottle — while lacking snob appeal the effect is exactly the same! For an added *frisson*, keep it stored in the fridge.

EXFOLIATION — GIVING NATURE A HAND

Ever thought that lizards, who shed their skin regularly, might have cornered one of the world's beauty secrets? Dead cells, trapped waste matter, clogged make-up and general debris can also too easily build up on the skin's surface into a toughened barrier of old skin which prevents treatment creams from penetrating the epidermis and creates a lifeless, lined and grey-looking skin. Exfoliation, or surface peeling, is a messy but effective extension of deep cleansing, which, if used once or twice a week, will certainly refine, brighten and soften the complexion by sloughing off this dingy curtain.

Steaming the face over a bowl of boiling water, or a facial sauna, will help to loosen impurities, open the pores and make it easier for exfoliating creams and lotions to work effectively. Suspended within these creams is a mass of microscopic granules, which will massage the epidermis, lift off dead surface skin, and refine and stimulate the layer beneath. Some exfoliators are designed to lather up and rinse off with water — use them with a soft complexion brush or a special facial 'loofah' pad to buff and polish a new glow onto the skin. Exfoliators are also particularly useful of course for softening and polishing up areas that are prone to collect patches of hard, dead skin such as elbows, heels and knees.

MASKS FOR EVERY OCCASION

Most complexions need 'revving up' at some time or another to stop them getting lethargic and sluggish, and there are few skins that don't improve from a weekly or fortnightly application of a face mask — a calculated revitaliser. Clay and other earth-based or seaweed-based 'mud packs' are ideal for oily, coarse, open-pored skins, while cleansing and tonifying peel-off masks are gentler and more suitable for refining and brightening drier skins. Masks that contain camphor, menthol and other stimulating ingredients wake up tired, stressed skin and are invaluable before a special night out. Thick gel or cream masks which don't harden are suitable for very dry

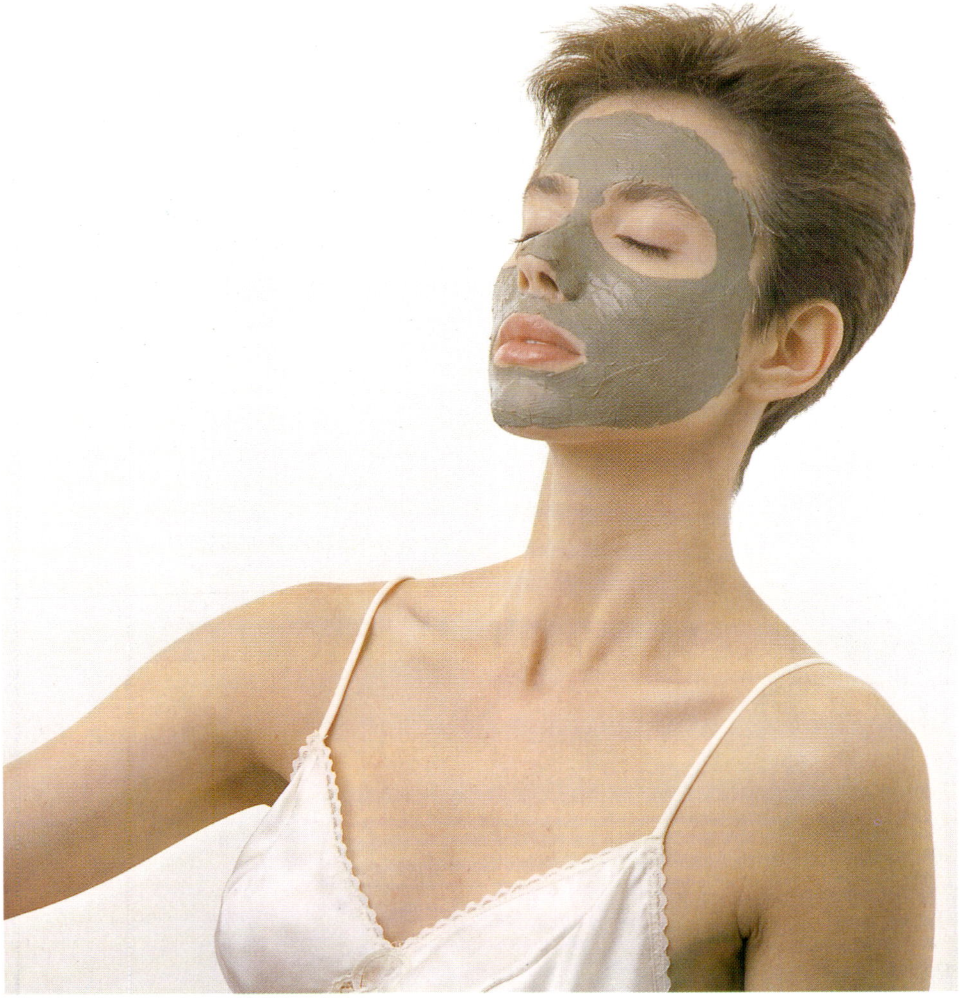

Masks are a calculated revitaliser, 'revving up' the skin to stop facial and neck tissues from being lethargic, sluggish and dull. They should, however, always be applied right down to the collarbone.

or more mature skins and can often be used right up around the eye area since they are specifically formulated to nourish even fine tissue and erase lines of tension from the face. Apply your mask all over the neck area — this is a prime giveaway area as far as signs of neglect, dryness and premature ageing go — but remember also to always extend all your cleansing, exfoliating and moisturising programmes right down to the collarbone to prevent crepey, lined, dull neck tissue.

MOISTURE — THE VITAL BALANCE

Whatever your age, your moisturiser should qualify as the basic necessity you'd choose to accompany you on a desert island. Just imagine that the upper layer of your skin acts as a moisture trap, which, as water evaporates, is constantly replenished by fresh supplies generated within the deeper skin tissues. Depending on how much you expose your skin to the drying effects of the sun, harsh extremes of weather, central heating, air conditioning and pollution, these reserves gradually become depleted over the years. Furthermore this type of assault on our skin has risen to massive proportions over the past 15 years. The result? The complexion of the 'eighties is more at risk: it gets drier and is more susceptible to tautness, lines, wrinkles, red veins, and patches of dehydration.

One moisturiser is by no means the same as another, whatever you may have heard. For instance, very fine, fluid moisturising lotions are largely composed of water — often up to 80 per cent — and act principally by protecting your skin with an invisible, greaseless film that checks the evaporation of moisture from the skin. Such moisture lotions can contain a variety of humectants — natural moisturising substances that help to attract moisture from the atmosphere into your skin. Known as oil-in-water emulsions these are ideal for protecting very young or oily skins, especially in humid weather. Richer, water-in-oil creams and lotions, however, contain a far greater percentage of oils, fats and waxes and so nourish and protect the skin more thoroughly, replacing as well as guarding moisture levels, plumping out tiny lines and wrinkles and covering the skin with a light occlusive barrier. The drier your skin — and the air around you — the harder and more efficiently your moisturiser needs to work. That doesn't mean you have to go in for heavy, clogging creams however. The manufacture and blending of emollients, water and humectants has today become a cosmetic art, and even the richest moisturisers are so refined that they're instantly absorbed leaving no tacky residue and allowing the smooth application of make-up.

NIGHT CARE — THE LIGHTER TOUCH

Not so long ago the term night cream was synonymous with thick, gooey products that ruined romance and bed linen, while doing precious little for the condition of your skin. Not any more. To be truly effective, any cream — whether worn at night or during the day — must be quickly and completely absorbed by the skin. Actually it seems there's little difference now between a deep-acting night cream and a nourishing day cream — increasingly these are designed for use 24 hours a day, making life a lot simpler. Treatment creams are generally thicker and more emollient than regular moisturisers, usually working out at about 70 per cent oil and 30 per cent water. Cold cream and lanolin are good examples of the sort of consistency to expect — but you'll find more effective lightweight products on the market. They work mainly by softening the epidermis, preventing surface dehydration — though this is much less of a risk by night than during the day — and easing away lines of tension and expression that have become etched onto the face during the day.

The aim behind the regular use of a night treatment cream is to stave off the formation of deeper wrinkles and creases. A word of caution however. There is no such thing as a rejuvenating cream or a miracle ingredient 'X' that can prevent normal expression lines from forming or which will keep your face forever set at twenty-two. Moreover, if you are indulging in late nights, drinking too much alcohol and coffee, chain smoking and getting no exercise, even the finest cream in the world will not hide the toll this takes on your skin and facial contours generally. There's no need to be lavish with night cream, that's another outmoded concept. Use it in small dots all over the face, massaging upwards and outwards without pulling the tissues.

Areas that need careful attention are the neck, forehead and the skin around the mouth and the eyes. However, since the tissues around the eyes are paper thin, lacking in sebaceous glands, exceptionally delicate and liable to dehydration, it's best to care for this essential 'danger zone' with a specially refined eye cream. These are intended to feed extra nourishment into the tissues without overloading or stretching the skin. Use only a tiny dot at a time, pat in gently with your third finger, and make sure you blot off any excess or you'll wake up with puffy, congested eyes.

Oils in general tend to be too heavy for the skin of the face — they're best left for body conditioning. In exceptional cases, oils made from the pure distilled essences of plants can be used to treat very dehydrated, tired or mature skins. These must, however, be specially prescribed for your skin type by a trained therapist, and are intended to be combined with special massage techniques. If you do like the feel of oil rather than cream on the skin, make sure you buy a pure, plant-based extract such as almond, apricot kernel, wheatgerm or avocado oil or pure vitamin E, and massage well into the skin using only a few drops at a time.

ENERGISING — THE NEWEST CONCEPT

There's a lot of talk nowadays about skin energising, using biologically active skin products. But how effective is this latest crop of treatment creams — if at all? Far from being yet another commercial gimmick aimed at luring us into spending money on our skin, they do in fact represent a very important breakthrough in cosmetic chemistry. Alternatively labelled 'energising' or 'performance' creams, these have been especially developed to penetrate the epidermis, into those layers of tissue where cell activity is rife.

With the help of the latest technology, chemists claim that they can now analyse the essential active ingredients of young healthy skin as well as isolate those substances which are believed to play the most important role in bolstering cell activity and keeping the balance of moisture topped up. These creams aim to boost the quality and renewal rate of skin cells, which is absolutely vital to the maintenance of smooth, soft, young-looking skin. Special tests also indicate just how far into the epidermis these active substances can penetrate — which gives short shrift to those dermatologists who

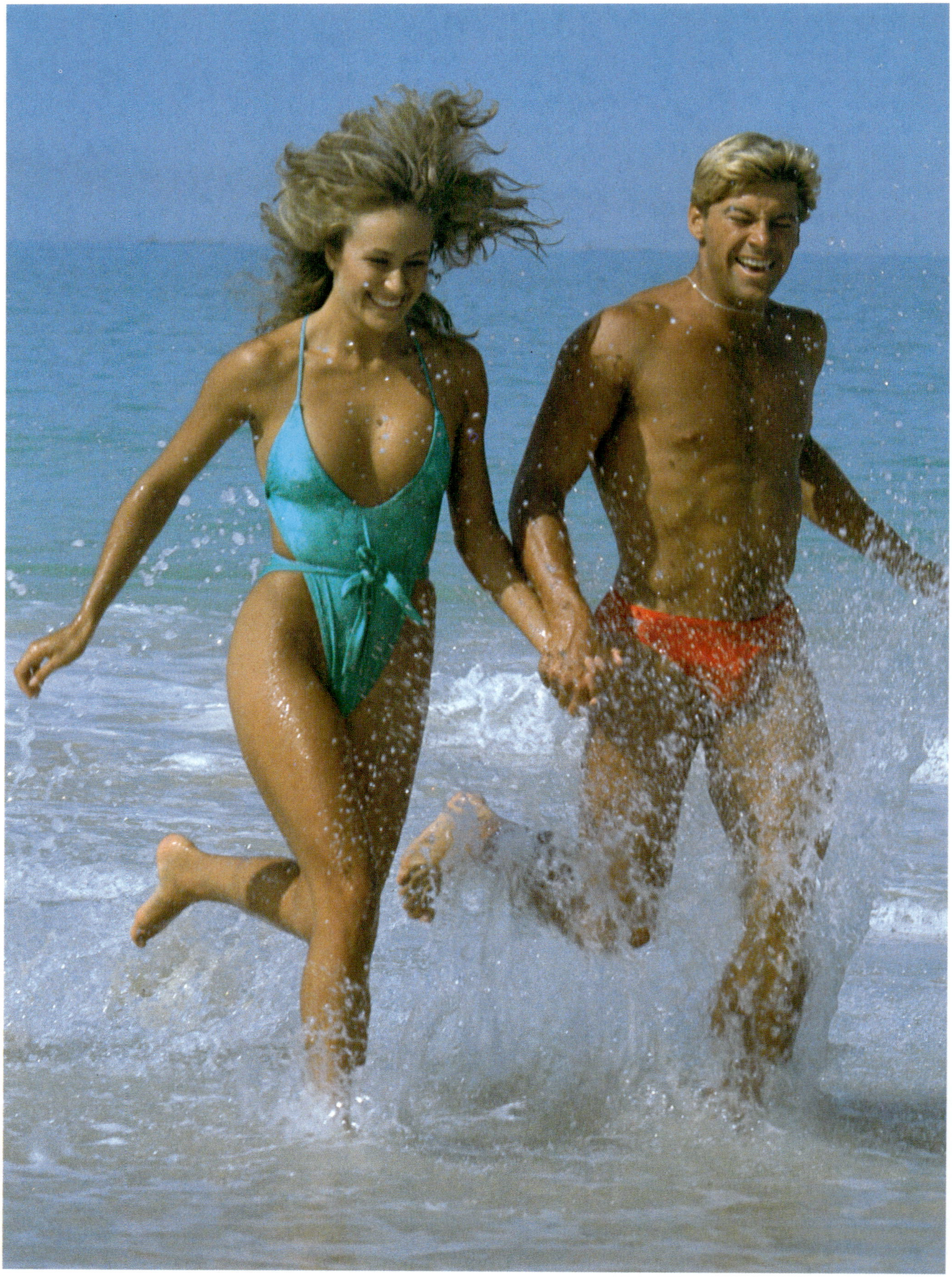

say that cosmetics cannot be absorbed by the skin. Yet far from relying on any newfound miracle ingredient, these products generally contain a complex variety of different substances to reduce the loss of moisture, slow down the destructive effects of pollution, protect the skin's collagen and elastic network fibres, and reduce the ill-effects of sunlight on the skin. Generally intended to be worn night and day beneath your usual moisturiser and nourishing cream, energisers often come in tiny phials, the contents used two or three drops at a time. Though it's too early to judge whether they can significantly slow down the march of time, they certainly have a beneficial, immediate effect on most skins, improving texture and tone, reducing existing lines and delaying the formation of new ones.

THE SUN — FRIEND OR FOE?

Bronzed summer skin still rates undeniably high in the glamour stakes. It's a status symbol and instant cosmetic rolled into one devastatingly healthy, sexy look. It's something we save up for, travel the world for, and cultivate with endless patience. Instant appeal certainly — but in the long run, what's the true value of a tan?

We have all heard an increasing amount about the damaging effects of strong sunlight on the skin. Dermatologists keep warning us in no uncertain terms that ultraviolet light is the skin's arch-enemy — and unfortunately, at least for those of us who like to look tanned, they're absolutely right. Tan now, pay later is the message, for sun damage begins slowly and deep down within the base layers of the epidermis to surface only years later in the guise of blotchy, weathered, thinning, wrinkled and prematurely dehydrated skin. Repeated overexposure to strong sunlight is the most common cause of destruction of the skin's collagen and elastic fibres, speeding the formation of lines and wrinkles, and leading to a loss of elasticity.

But worse, indiscriminate, long-termed exposure to the sun can lead to skin cancer — no matter what skin types, although those people with fair skin or who burn easily are at a far greater risk. Australia has the greatest incidence of skin cancer in the world, including the highest level of the most dangerous skin cancer, malignant melanoma. This cancer can be deadly but if handled correctly and diagnosed early is completely curable. Research has shown that in the last ten years, the incidence of melanoma has doubled.

There are three types of skin cancer, all of which are partly or wholly caused by sun damage. By far the most common skin cancer is the B.C.C., followed by the S.C.C. which is less common but grows more rapidly. And thirdly, there is the least common but most dangerous type — melanoma.

Chronic exposure to the sun not only greatly increases chances of developing skin cancer, it also means premature ageing of the skin. These ageing effects can creep up on you if you don't take sufficient care of your skin in the sun at all times and allow it to burn. Ultraviolet light is made up of three principal types of rays: longwave UVA rays which produce a tan and rarely burn, shortwave UVB rays which both burn *and* tan you, and UVC rays which are blocked out by the earth's ozone layer. It's the UVB and UVA rays which are chiefly to blame for causing degenerative changes within the skin. How your skin reacts now, as well as in the long term, to repeated exposure to sunlight depends almost entirely on your skin type and how you protect it.

The reason why some people rapidly acquire a gorgeous golden tan while others turn red and peel depends entirely on a substance called melanin. Melanin is the skin pigment produced by skin cells which secrete and distribute extra quantities of pigment in the form of a tan when stimulated by UVA rays and some of the UVB rays. In some of us, melanin production

Bronzed skins are beautiful — but are they? The effects of too much sun on skin can be far from aesthetic.

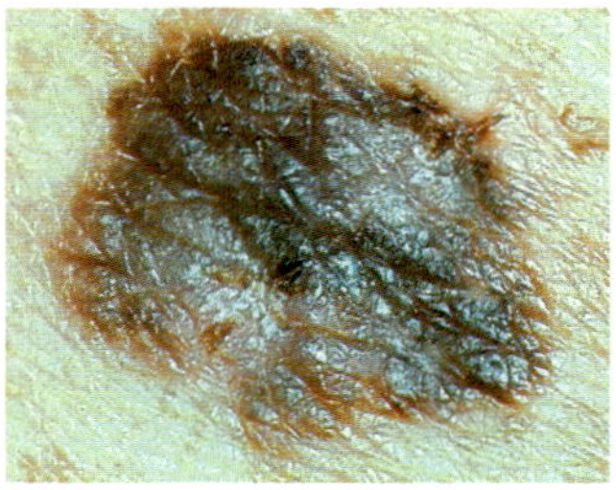

Melanoma arising from Hutchinson's freckle.

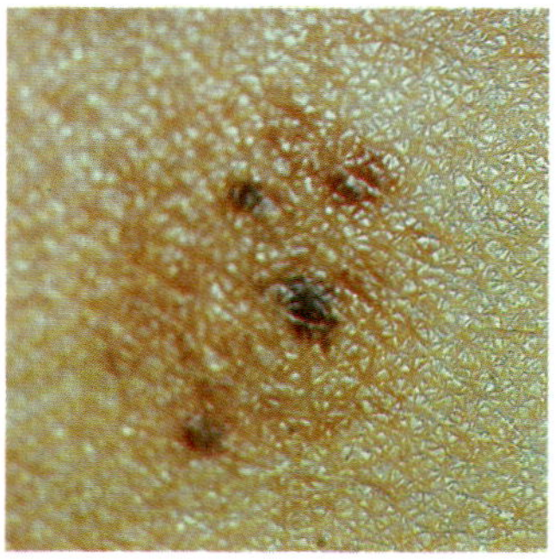

A malignant melanoma.

increases with gradual exposure to the sun, acting as nature's own inbuilt defence against sunburn. People with black skins obviously have the greatest amount of melanin, while those of us with dark hair and sallow, olive skin usually tend to produce sufficient melanin to develop a dark or medium tan. Those at greatest risk from burning are people with very fair or red hair, pale delicate skin or freckled skin whose low quota of melanin-producing cells turns their skin into prime fuel for the sun's rays.

You must avoid burning, whatever your skin type. The skin's sensitivity changes with age and general health, so don't be caught off guard. Just because you have never suffered from sunburn doesn't guarantee permanent natural immunity. Bear in mind also that taking strong medicines like antibiotics, some tranquillisers and the pill can sometimes cause a skin reaction if you go into strong sunlight.

Here are a few simple guidelines to follow to reduce sun damage on your skin, and consequently lower your chances of developing skin cancer and looking old and wrinkled beyond your years.

☐ The easiest time to burn in the sun is between 10 am and 4 pm when ultraviolet light intensity is greatest. So try to keep out of direct sunlight during this period. If you can't resist trying to boost that tan, remember it takes only 10 minutes during the heat of day in summer to develop a good tan.

☐ You are more liable to burn quickly if the sun's intensity is doubled through reflection off water, snow, concrete and even sand. When you are swimming, UV rays penetrate 20 cm below the surface and are intensified by the water droplets. Wear a water resistant sun screen.

☐ Whenever possible wear a hat and protective clothing. Thin, white clothes, particularly nylon, allow a lot of the UV rays to reach the skin. Dark coloured cotton or natural fibre blend clothes give maximum protection.

☐ Wear a broad spectrum, maximum protection sunscreen when in direct sunlight.

☐ Children's skin is more susceptible to sun damage than adult's so ensure children are always properly protected when out in the sun to avoid their developing skin problems later in life.

☐ Also, don't forget the 'delay factor'; sunburn can take anything from three to seven hours to appear, so don't be fooled if at first your skin seems to remain pallid in the sun — by evening it could well be kindled to a choice shade of lobster!

Skin damage is accumulative so each time you get burnt adds to any previous damage. Protection now means good skin later in life. For more information on properly protecting yourself from sun damage, contact either a doctor or else the Melanoma Foundation or the Skin Cancer Council in your state.

SUNSCREENS

Nowadays everybody has the opportunity to tan safely and slowly without burning. Modern sunscreens really *do* cut out the most damaging wavelengths of strong sunlight while conditioning and moisturising the skin, and more companies are perfecting very powerful screens and blocking agents that offer almost 100 per cent protection from the sun.

Sunscreen products are a rather sophisticated development in Australia. In the United States and Europe, sunscreens are graded on a cosmetic basis, ie, a protection factor sunscreen of PF 2 or 3 is suitable for dark skins while a higher PF numbered product offers more protection for fairer skinned people. However with Australia having the world's highest incidence of skin

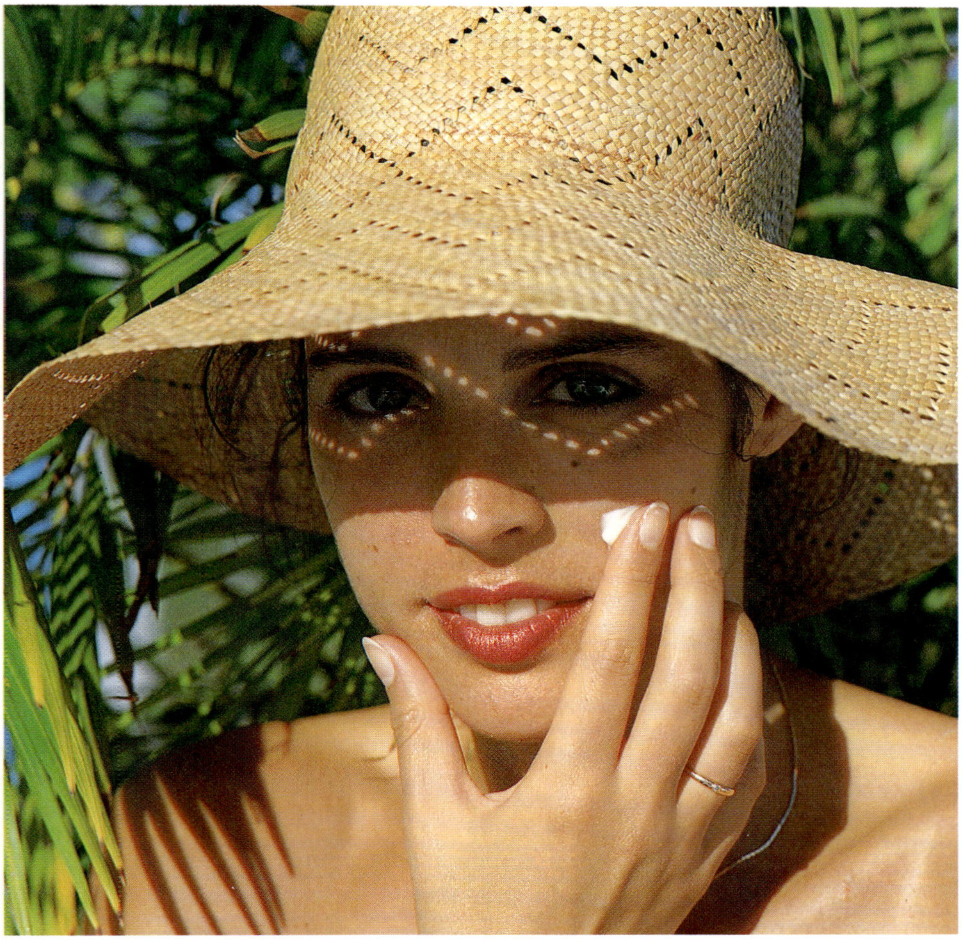

G. Marche/Australian Picture Library

A sunscreen cream with an SPF 15 and broad spectrum rating teamed with a hat is ideal protection against the damaging effects of the sunlight.

cancer, going by this artificial grading alone is irrelevant.

In sunscreen products, the SPF (sun protection factors) measures the sunburn protective properties filtering out the burning UVB rays. The SPF range varies in protection levels from a minimum of two to the maximum SPF of 15+. This SPF measures protection against sunburn but is not a measurement of protection against skin cancer and other skin problems.

Many people in Australia have the type of skin where they can get away without using a sunscreen or else one with a low SPF rating of 2 or 3. But such skin which easily tans without burning is like all other skin types in that it is not protected from the long-term damage caused by UVB and especially UVA solar rays. Long-term damage from these rays includes not only skin cancer and premature ageing of the skin but also photosensitivity due to commonly used drugs.

Most dermatologists agree there is only one type of sunscreen to use for protection against both UVA and UVB rays. These sunscreens carry a SPF rating of 15+ and a broad spectrum label. It is now acknowledged by the Standards Association of Australia that only sunscreens which filter out both UVA and UVB rays can offer total sun protection.

Some sunscreen products contain special tan accelerators which sensitise the skin to the sun and therefore encourage it to go brown slightly faster than it normally would. These accelerating agents or psoralens — such as bergamot oil — should be used with extreme caution. Some doctors have expressed the fear that they may cause skin cancer, but as they have only been in use for two or three years their long-term effects are not yet known. However, more certainly, instead of turning you an even brown, they can lead to blotchy tans which will take some time to fade. The use of these products while tanning on a sunbed is also potentially hazardous, because it can rapidly cause the formation of dark blotches which are extremely difficult to remove.

Fading creams which can be used to treat blotchy and spotty skin are available. However, before using such creams, it is wise to seek medical consultation from a skin specialist on the correct treatment for the complaint. You may be trying to fade not a simple sun spot but instead, a more serious skin problem.

Lastly, no matter how hardy and resilient your skin seems to be right now, or how much you love a suntan, do try and think ahead a few years. Repeated overexposure to the sun will inevitably increase your chances of looking prematurely aged. You have only to compare the complexion of a woman of 50 who has never been in the sun to someone of the same age — or even five to 10 years younger — who is a sun-worshipper to see that tanning rarely allows skin to age truly gracefully. Note those tell-tale areas of pigmentation, red veins, wrinkles, crow's feet, that might otherwise have been avoided, then ask yourself if that's a price worth paying for just a few weeks of bronzed glamour every year.

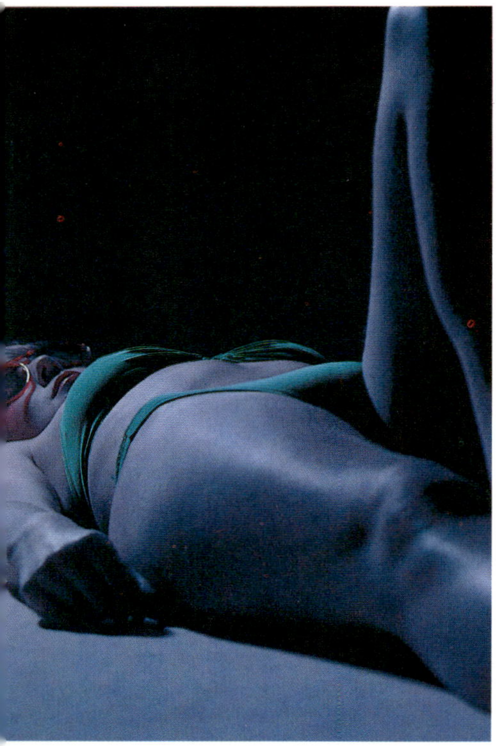

It may give you the chance to 'cheat' and have a glorious tan when setting foot on the beach the first day in summer, but the medical profession warns strongly against using sunbeds for cosmetic purposes.

FAKING IT

You may have noticed of course that there is an increasing number of people around these days with beautiful suntans who've not set foot in sunny climes. Sunbeds, which tan you fast, simply and painlessly and wreak no visible havoc with the skin, offer a valid — if expensive — alternative to roasting oneself under the real thing. They work by bombarding the body with a very high concentration of pure UVA light so that you end up tanned and not burnt. The medical profession is very much against using sunbeds to tan claiming it is a false concept and a very dangerous one. Research has shown that UVA rays do promote cancer growth. It is advised that sunbeds are used under supervision for treatment of skin problems but not for cosmetic purposes.

However, if using a sunbed to tan follow a few simple rules. Showering beforehand to remove all traces of perfume, oils, creams or cologne which could create an allergic reaction to the UVA light; using goggles to protect the eyes; and checking that you're not taking any medication that could make the skin extra sensitive.

Always go to a reputable suntan parlour or salon where the therapists are properly trained. Hygiene is an aspect of sunbed treatments that is too frequently overlooked in many salons, so check that the beds are washed down between clients. You mustn't take UVA sun treatment if you are pregnant and you should leave 48 hours between each session. A course of tanning treatments can greatly help people with fair skins gain a headstart on acquiring a tan before going on holiday and help to maintain a healthy bronzed look long after they've returned.

SKIN PROBLEMS — GETTING A PERSPECTIVE

Nearly everyone is hypercritical of their own looks — to the point of excess. Ask someone with even an apparently flawless complexion how they'd rate their skin and they'll inevitably point out some blemish or flaw you'd need a microscope to find! Of course there are certain very common, often minor conditions that many of us must learn to live with, especially those that are inherited and largely irreversible, but in almost the majority of cases these really do appear much worse and more glaringly obvious to you than to anyone else. Try not to exaggerate their importance. There is after all no such phenomenon as a 100 per cent perfect complexion.

Sallow skin

This often accompanies brunette hair, brown or dark eyes, and an olive or greasy complexion that tans easily. Unfortunately when you are not tanned it can look dingy and lacklustre. One big bonus, however, is that sallow skin is much less liable to suffer dehydration and develop early wrinkles than other skin types. Poor circulation is often a problem here so take lots of exercise, preferably out of doors. Treat your skin to regular steaming, stimulating masks and exfoliation and use a facial washing brush to keep spots and blackheads at bay.

Lines and wrinkles

Those that appear prematurely are often the spin-off from too much sunbathing, harsh weather, dry atmospheres, smoking or losing a lot of weight very suddenly. A certain number of expression lines are only to be expected from the mid-twenties on — due as much to our personalities and the faces we pull when we smile, talk, laugh and frown as to lack of skin care. Using a good protective moisturiser and night cream daily, however, will go some way towards delaying the formation of premature lines and deep wrinkles as we grow older.

Red veins

These tend to appear more noticeable on very delicate, dry skin that reacts adversely to extremes of hot and cold. So treat the skin gently and avoid drinking very hot liquids, eating very hot or spicy food and go easy on saunas, steaming and sunbathing. Severe broken veins can be treated by sclerotherapy, a specialised injection using a chemical fluid whereby the traces of blood are dried out so that they fade away and the broken capillary wall is sealed off. Milder or superficial capillaries can be treated by electrolysis which cauterises each capillary. There's little you can do to cool down a ruddy or flushed complexion except to use soothing decongesting creams and gels and a make-up shade that tones down high colour.

Open pores

These tend to be a by-product of greasy skin. There's little you can do to shrink them, just cleanse, exfoliate and refine with a mask or mud astringent to combat blackheads and spots. Use an oil-free foundation make-up base to minimise the appearance of large pores and to prevent them clogging and therefore appearing worse.

Blackheads

These are not, as often supposed, trapped dirt, but the direct result of oxygen coming into contact with trapped sebum. This is why they are often a problem for people with oily skin and coarse enlarged pores, especially around the nose and chin. Scrupulous cleansing, exfoliation, face masks and the regular use of a facial washing brush will refine open pores and prevent oil from settling, while also softening and easing out any existing blackheads. Never attempt to remove blackheads yourself at home by prodding or squeezing them, as this could lead to permanent scarring. Consult a trained beautician if you want them removed correctly.

Moles

You have nothing to worry about, providing moles don't change shape, grow dramatically or bleed. Don't try to remove hairs if they are growing out of a mole. Avoid salon treatments and consult a dermatologist if you want a mole checked or removed.

Spots and pimples

There can be virtually nobody who does not at sometime or other in their lives suffer from the occasional 'breakout' of spots either during a period, as a result of changes in the weather, using different skincare products or just plain stress and tension. The odd spot — as opposed to acne — is nothing to worry about provided you deal with it promptly to avoid cross-infection. This means meticulously cleaning the spot area, preferably with a medicated wash-off lotion to whisk away grime and bacteria, and using a medicated cream, lotion, or gel to disinfect and dry out the offending area as quickly as possible. There are some excellent deep-acting antiseptic agents on the market which make short shrift of pimples. They are generally very drying to the skin, however, so be careful not to use them too often if you have a very sensitive or dry skin. A course of brewer's yeast, rich in the B complex vitamins, can also work wonders in helping to clear a spotty skin.

Milia

Also called whiteheads, these spots of trapped oil just beneath the skin's surface show up as tiny hard bumps about the size of a pinhead — usually around the eye socket, cheekbones and generally on bony areas where there are fewer pores to allow sebum to escape. They can often result from warm weather or a change in diet and disappear later on. You can usually banish them in a few weeks with a mild antiseptic lotion.

Freckles

They accompany fair skins, auburn, fair or red hair and become more pronounced in the summer, multiplying especially if you go into the sun. Bleaching creams have little effect on them, so avoid the sun if you want an even complexion and choose a foundation with extra coverage to hide them completely.

Brown patches

Chloasma can appear while you are pregnant or after sunbathing if you are on the pill. The higher levels of female hormones in the body at this time sometimes make certain parts of the face extra sensitive to sunlight so that they come up in dark brown, muddy-looking blotches especially around the eyes, on the upper lip, across the forehead and on the cheeks. Unfortunately there's little you can do to stop them recurring, except avoid the sun or come off the pill during the summer. Try using a hydroquinone-based bleaching cream for 8–10 weeks — this can often eliminate the patches quite effectively. Alternatively, a dermatologist might be able to prescribe a much stronger bleaching agent for you. A small percentage of women, however, find that their skin becomes red and ultrasensitive to these creams, especially during very cold weather. Once you've successfully bleached away the dark areas, make sure you wear a strong sunblock over them when you go into the sun to stop the blotches intensifying once again.

Allergic skin

Often confused with very fragile, delicate skin that gets easily irritated, true allergy-prone skin is a much rarer condition and is often linked to a family history of hay fever, asthma and migraine. Tracking down the offending

A good skin routine and care taken when in the sun, will have a freckled complexion healthy and glowing. Each complexion has its own features and flaws and it is up to the individual to accentuate or tone these down.

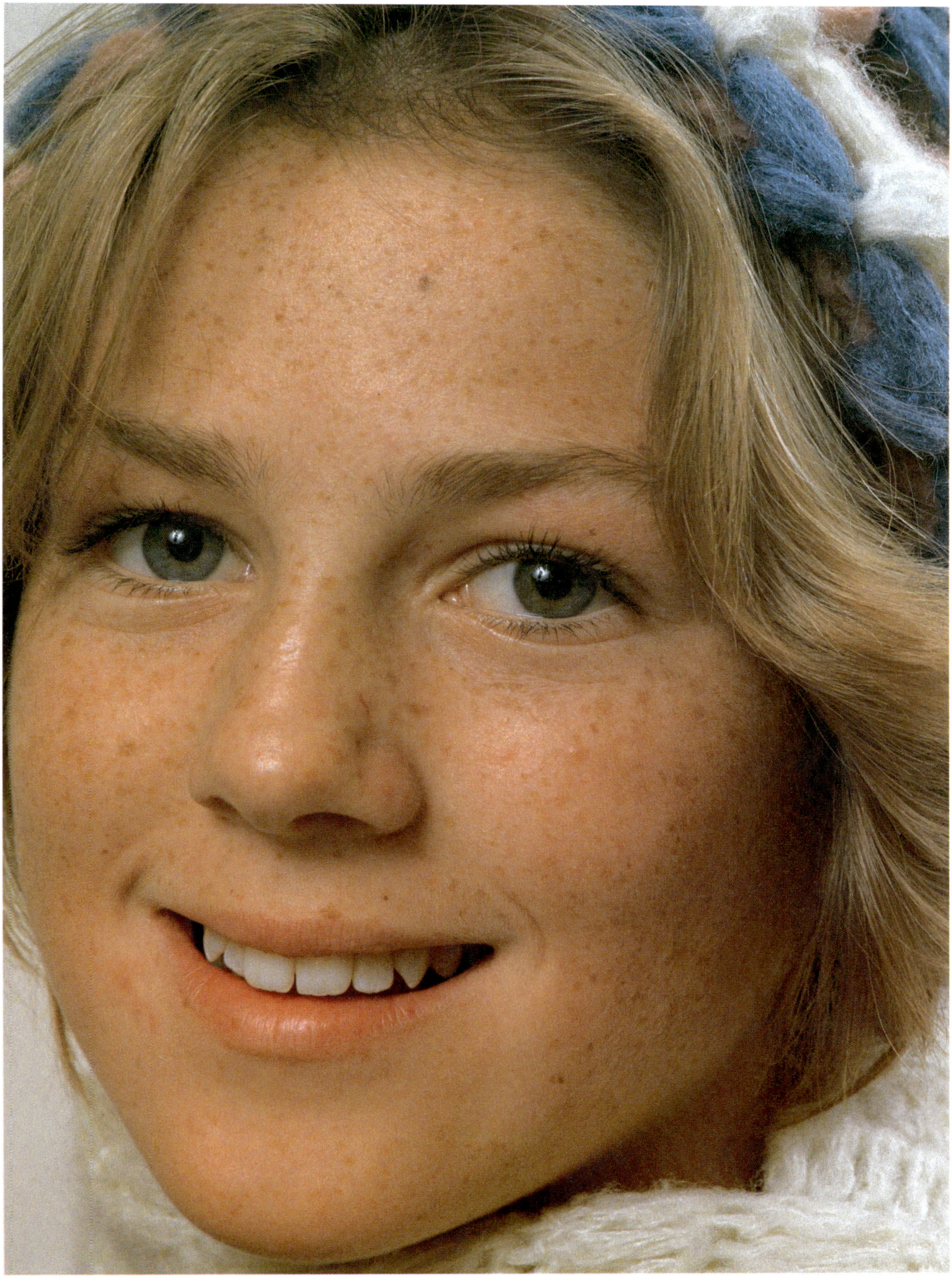

substance to which you are allergic is of course the hardest part of solving the problem — but well worth the trouble in the long run. Your doctor or skin specialist can help you greatly with this and will probably ask you to make lists of foods, cosmetics, household and other common products that you use. Obviously if you tend to develop an allergic reaction to some cosmetics you must always try out new products with a patch test in the crook of your arm and wait 24 hours to see if they suit you.

Rosacea

This is often confused with allergic skin since this is a skin that becomes sensitive and reacts violently to changes of atmosphere, sunlight, hot food and drink, becoming ruddy and developing a mass of tiny red spots. It tends to affect people whose temperament makes them excessively prone to nervous tension and stress and occasionally those who have suffered from acute acne. Doctors often prescribe a course of antibiotics to calm down the condition and it is a good idea to use skin-care products that have a cooling effect as well as a camouflaging make-up to mask the redness.

SUPERFLUOUS HAIR

Fashion does, to some extent, dictate how freely we should allow our hair to grow — the changing style of eyebrows over the decades is a good example of this; in the 'twenties, 'thirties, 'sixties and early 'seventies we tweezed our brows into pencil-thin curves, while the 'eighties has seen a return to the strong, even bushy emphasis of the 'forties and 'fifties.

Generally speaking though, most of us recoil from the idea of overt hairiness. As a result, there's an enormous range of methods and products designed to rid us of unwanted facial and body hair. Here are their pros and cons:

Plucking

Tweezing hair out is effective but time-consuming and therefore impractical on a large scale. It is a practice to be restricted to eyebrows or the odd stray hair.

Shaving

Quick, economical and popular it does have some drawbacks. Swift regrowth is the main inconvenience and means you'll have to shave legs and armpits on a daily basis if you're really fanatical about maintaining a silky smooth skin texture. Using a wet razor can cause skin scrapes and cuts and it is

A little plucking or brushing gives you smooth, shapely eyebrows.

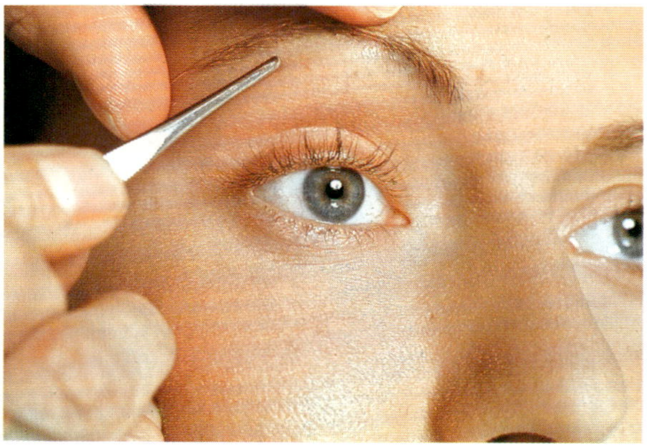

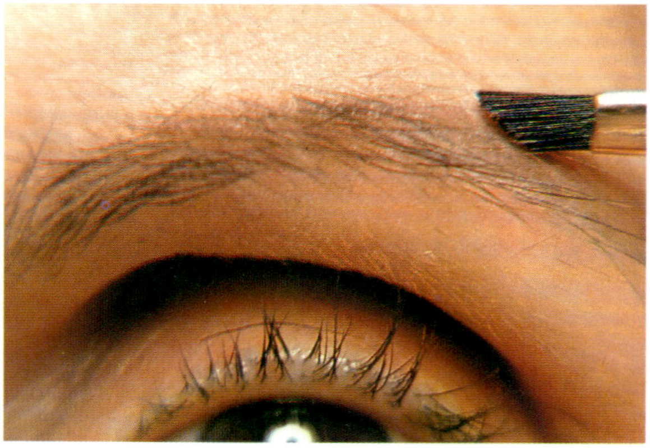

Make-up: Glenn Roberts (Elizabeth Arden)

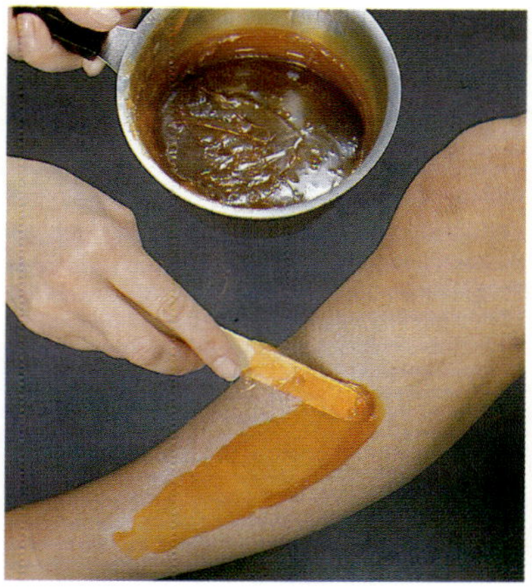

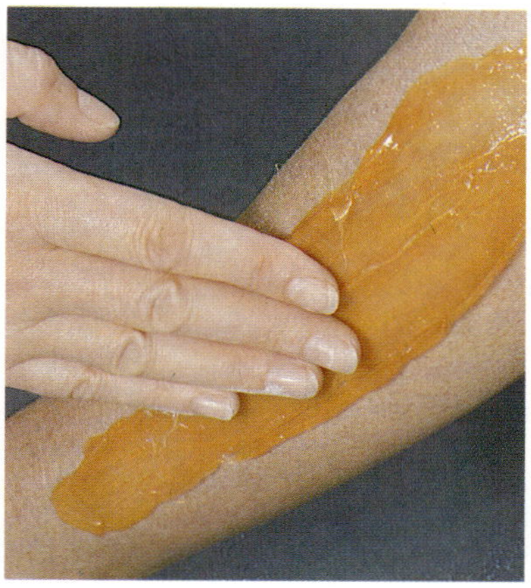

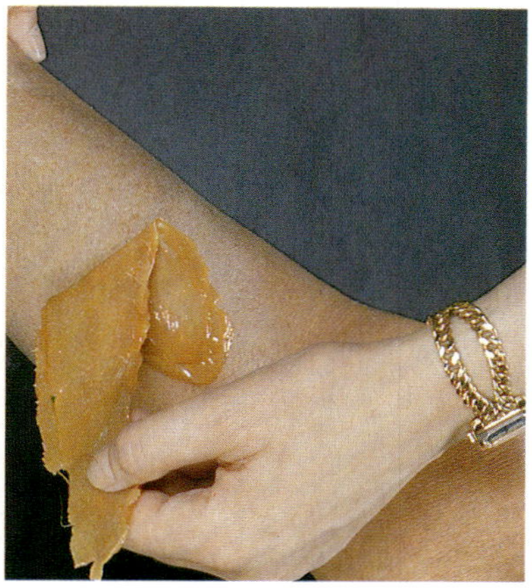

Waxing procedure step by step.

unwise to apply the majority of deodorants or anti-perspirants to the shaved area immediately afterwards, as it will sting.

Abrasive mitts

These are another version of shaving, since they also cut the hair off at skin level. They work effectively, but regrowth is again the problem and mitts may also cause skin abrasion and irritation.

Depilatories

Though these products, normally creams or lotions, are very widely used, they can cause allergic skin reactions, as they are chemically based. It is imperative to carry out a skin 'patch' test before using a depilatory product but the results normally last a little longer than shaving.

Waxing

This technique works like wide-scale plucking — hot or cold wax is spread over the area needing to be stripped of hair and is pulled off before it sets too hard, pulling out all the hair shafts that are embedded in the wax. The process can be painful, but the discomfort is very short-lived and the effects comparatively long lasting — it may be as long as six weeks before a repeat session is needed. Though beauty salons are well versed in all waxing techniques and will not hesitate to tackle even the most intimate areas, it is possible to buy home waxing kits that do the job as efficiently, given a little practice. It may be worthwhile visiting a salon to see how they do the job before attempting a waxing session at home. In the long term, waxing weakens hair follicles so regrowth gradually slackens off.

Bleaching

This can be the answer to, say, dark hair growing on the upper lip but be warned — bleaching has a tendency to coarsen hair growth so a mere downy growth could gradually turn into a full-scale moustache which still shows up in sunlight, regardless of the bleach.

Electrolysis

This is the only permanent method of hair removal, where a fine needle is inserted into the follicle and a burst of electricity destroys the source of growth. However, it is not as straightforward as this as it may take many repeat sessions to destroy all the hairs and prevent regrowth. Success also depends largely on the skill of the operator — it is certainly worth a bit of detective work to get a dependable beautician with a steady hand and plenty of experience. Risk visiting an unskilled operator and you may end up suffering acute pain and permanent scars.

body parts

Looking after hands, feet, legs and teeth really is a never-ending battle. Being healthy and following good eating habits go hand in hand with beautiful nails, problem-free legs and strong teeth and gums.

From practically the day we are born, our hands are exposed to sunlight, harsh treatment and weather, with little or no protection. They are immersed in water many times a day and often not thoroughly dried. Chapping, chafing and dryness result, particularly in cold weather.

The combination of work, exposure to the elements and the ageing process means that many hands are not a pretty sight and often belie an otherwise youthful appearance.

It is a great pity when you consider how proud many women are of all the rings, engagement, dress etc, on their fingers that they fail to look after the hands that bear them. Many of the world's most beautiful stones are displayed on hands which resemble wizened claws.

Then there are feet which in most cases definitely show signs of being the worse for wear. Considering that the poor old feet have to carry people around for what most hope will be quite some time, everyone tends to take them very much for granted. Feet and legs should receive just as much care and attention as hands.

When it comes to teeth, although, 'here decay and gone tomorrow' is no longer the norm, the dentist can't do it all. It is amazing how many people will put so much time and effort into their diets and exercise routines and then promptly forget all about their teeth. As outlined in this section, a thorough daily cleaning routine and attention to what you eat is essential to everyone's dental health.

FOCUS ON HANDS

Instantly eye catching, totally expressive, our hands are frequently overlooked and even abused. Considering the onslaught of water, detergents, weathering and grime we subject our hands to, they should merit the most devoted, well-thought-out of all beauty routines: too often, however, they tend instead to be one of the earliest and cruellest giveaways of age, accumulating marks of time that after a certain age are extremely difficult to erase. Yet all of this could be avoided provided we all followed a few simple home rules.

Gloves are undoubtedly one of the finest beauty aids. The more sensitive and dry the skin on the backs of your hands the more important it is to remember to wear rubber gloves whenever you immerse them in detergent. Cotton-lined rubber gloves are a good idea if your skin is very sensitive, as they are more comfortable and less likely to cause irritation. These will cut out about 70 per cent of the main causes of dehydration. The reason why our hands dry out so quickly and easily is that there are no sebaceous glands to keep them supple.

Wear cotton gloves when gardening and doing housework and leather or woolly ones in cold weather. Each time you wash your hands, massage plenty of rich hand cream into the tissues and never wash your hands in very hot water. Barrier creams contain a particularly high concentration of protective ingredients like silicone which provide more intensive and long-lasting protection against water and detergents. Warm olive oil is ideal for coaxing the moisture back into dry hands; soak them thoroughly for half an hour every week to treat splitting nails, and to condition the skin and cuticles. To bleach out stubborn stains and yellowish discolouration rub them with half a lemon. There's unfortunately very little you can do to get rid of the brown 'liver spots' which sometimes appear in middle age. No one knows what actually causes them, though they are possibly due to a malfunction linked to frequent and prolonged sunbathing.

NAILS — THE BIG CHALLENGE

Beautifully long, strong nails need patient cultivation and a certain amount of know-how. The reason why so many women suffer from weak, splitting, peeling or brittle nails is quite simply because they are unaware of how easy it is to inflict damage on and around the nail itself. The visible portion of the nail, just like the skin's surface and our hair, is made up of tightly compressed dead cells that have grown out of the living nail bed — the matrix — which is rich in blood capillaries and nerve endings that nourish the nail tissue. The condition of your nails therefore is a pretty accurate reflection of your general health including the medicines you take, your diet and stress levels. Prolonged illness or emotional shocks, for instance, can show up in ridged, thin, weak nails; a problem that only becomes noticeable sometime after the event because nails take anything from four to nine months to grow out fully. Your nails will also tend to reflect dietary deficiencies in protein, vitamins A and B complex, iron, magnesium, zinc and calcium.

As long as your health and eating habits are well balanced there is certainly plenty you can do to build up strong healthy nails from outside. Use cuticle cream regularly to nourish and soften the cuticles as the tissue is fundamental to protecting the smoothness and strength of new nail growth. Never jab, prod, push or cut the cuticles with a sharp object and steer clear of dissolvent creams as these only coarsen the skin and make it look messier. It is important to keep the cuticle pliable and free of the actual nail plate, otherwise it impedes growth and causes marks or indentations. Excessive acidity, which generally stems from diet, is one of the most common causes of vertical or horizontal ridges, splitting and breaking nails. Furthermore, if acid collects on the surface to the nail along with the body's natural oils, the nail cannot absorb any nutrients you apply. A good technique for keeping cuticles in tip-top condition is to gently lift the skin with a hoof stick using circular movements, and then to remove the underlying acid layer to promote healthy growth. This must be done by a specialist — although follow-up care at home is relatively simple. Avoid soaking hands and nails in warm soapy water, this dries out cuticles and nails. Try to relearn the art of buffing to bring a natural sheen and strength to the nail plate. An emery board is far kinder to your nails than a file, but make sure you file in one direction only using the soft side; don't file the sides as this weakens the structure.

Provided your nails are basically healthy, keeping them long, shiny and impeccably manicured is a matter of abiding by a few simple rules:

☐ Avoid chipped, peeling nail varnish by applying it correctly in the first place. On a clean nail, apply one layer of basecoat and two layers of colour, allowing each layer to dry thoroughly.

☐ Remember that pale and frosted lacquer will show up bumps and ridges more than plain varnish.

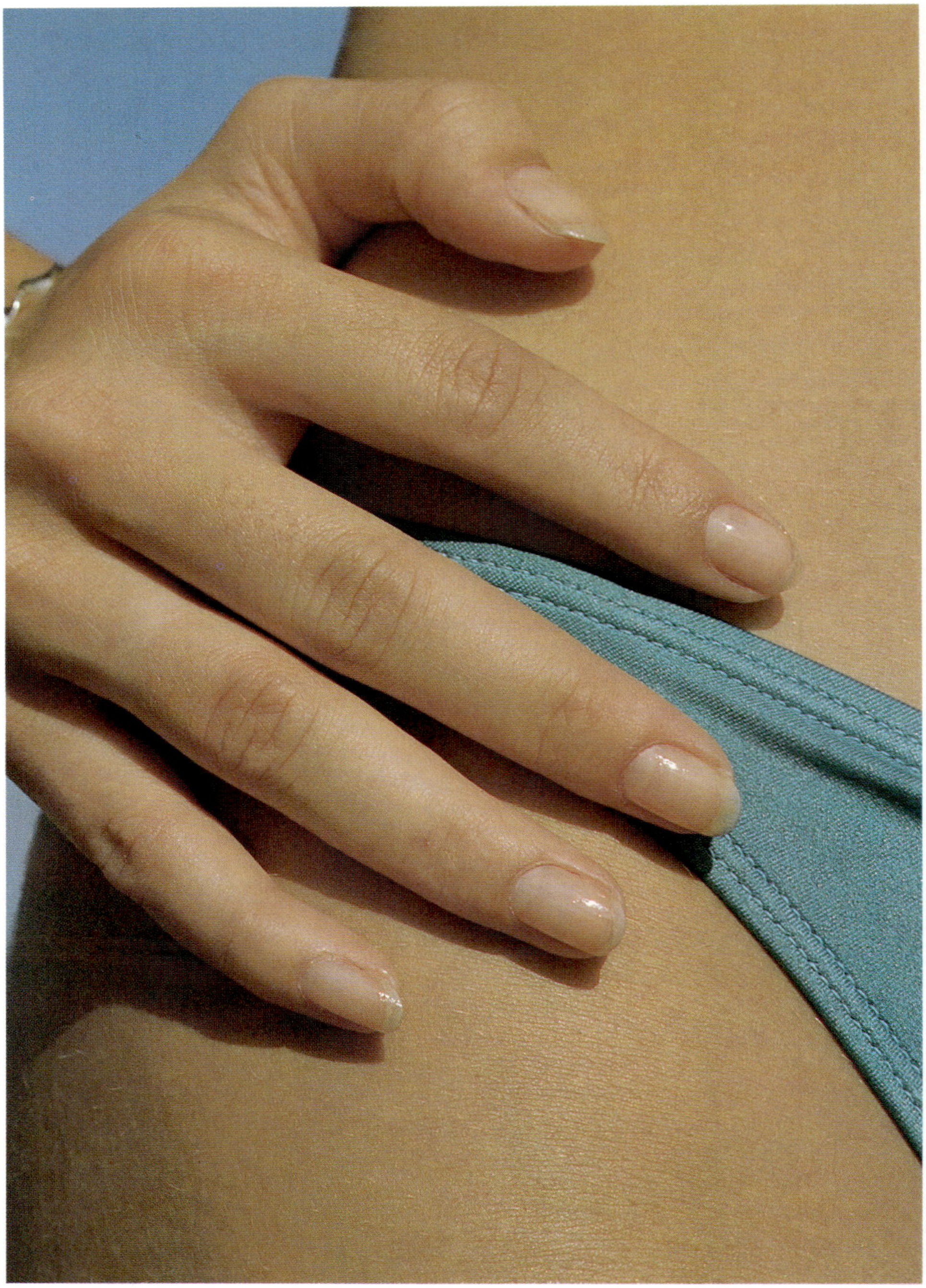

Hands — the big giveaway of age.

☐ Use clippers, not scissors to cut the nails. Scissors put a strain on the nail, eventually weakening it.
☐ Keep a phial of instant nail glue on you at all times to patch up any new crack or split in the nail.
☐ Steer clear of artificial nail-building techniques or false nails generally. These involve the use of very powerful chemicals which not only weaken and wear down the remnants of your own nails but can also cause fungus infections and a risk of allergies.
☐ To slim down the appearance of broad, flat nails, apply a strong shade of nail lacquer down the centre of the nail leaving a narrow unpainted strip on either side.
☐ Always use nail varnish remover that contains oil. Cheaper, oil-free brands dry out the nail and cuticle.

☐ To strengthen nails, opt for regular use of a really top quality cuticle oil or cream rather than a nail hardener which only treats the tips of the nails.
☐ Ridges are often caused through damaging the nail bed or cuticle, so take care not to treat them roughly. Ridges can be filled in with special preparations (though these have a drying effect), treated at a salon, or smoothed away with buffing.
☐ Scrubbing the nails with a hard brush can cause them to separate from the nail bed and so weaken them. Clean instead with a cuticle stick or a special nail sponge.

LEGS — TOPS IN THE GLAMOUR STAKES

For instant sex appeal and glamour there's little to beat a long slinky pair of legs. If you want to know how yours rate, stand in front of a full-length mirror, wearing medium-heeled shoes, feet together. Do your legs touch at the tops of the thighs, knees and ankles, leaving three gently curved gaps between each point of contact? If so, your legs are well on the way to model-girl proportions. Legs should be lean and lithe, not sticklike and skinny — and certainly not covered in bulges and bumps.

Exercise those legs

By keeping muscles firm, massage and regular exercise rather than dieting are the greatest leg shapers. The form of exercise is up to you, but if it is too boring it won't last long.

Some people prefer to exercise with outdoor sports. Swimming is particularly good for leg muscles. Indoor types may prefer aerobic dance classes or a set routine of leg exercises to be performed at home. Studio workouts with weights can be very helpful for legs and it should be stressed that women undertaking weight training, if properly taught, will never develop large, unfeminine muscles.

Cycling is particularly good as a leg exercise whether it is done outdoors or on a stationary exercise bike.

Walking instead of driving whenever possible is obviously a good move and running is currently very popular. When running or jogging, it is very important that you wear the right footwear and do warm up exercises before your run. Joint and muscle problems are common complaints seen in over-enthusiastic joggers.

So, if you have problem legs, there has never been a better time than now to take the first steps towards improving them. Never before have so many exercise options been available.

Varicose veins

This circulatory complaint is often hereditary and can occur even at an early age. Warning signs are cramp, irritation, burning, swelling of the leg beneath the knee and throbbing, clearly defined veins. Avoid standing around for long periods, don't wear tight socks or stockings, try not to cross your legs while you sit, and never jog or exercise on hard surfaces like concrete. Put your feet up whenever you can and wear fashionable lightweight support tights. Also try to switch heel heights during the day and massage your legs with a cooling gel or cream to get the circulation going. Being pregnant, overweight or prone to constipation can make varicose veins worse. If yours are particularly severe you can have injections to treat them or an operation to remove them completely.

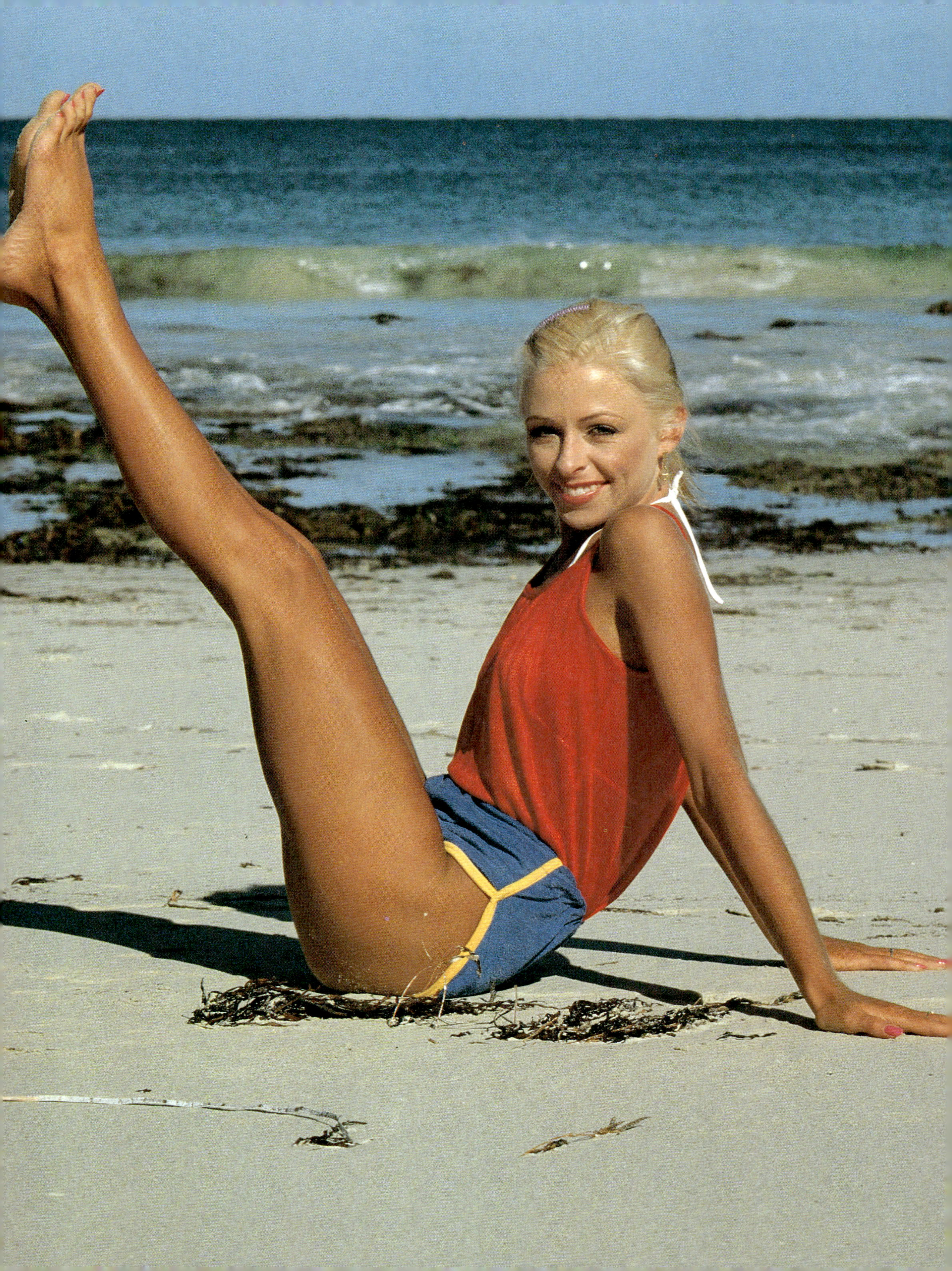

Broken capillaries

Broken capillaries resemble tiny, spidery bluish-red lines on the skin. A range of different treatments is now available to relieve the problem. With medical treatments a doctor injects a sclerosing agent then bandages legs firmly to keep the capillary walls flattened. Beauticians, using a machine like the one for electrolysis, give the affected area small charges with an electric current which destroys each little capillary.

The argon laser is the latest weapon in the battle with broken capillaries. The red colour of the capillaries (often seen first as a fine network on the inside knee) attracts the green light of the laser and the capillaries are cauterised.

Water retention and swelling

A sign of poor circulation, it may be a special problem just before menstruation when the body tends to retain fluid. Wear support tights to protect against the risk of varicose veins, don't stand in one spot for long periods and put your feet up when you can. Make sure you drink enough water to eliminate waste products from the system. Eating less salt can help to combat water retention, but if the root cause is hormonal imbalance your doctor may have to treat this.

Cellulite

Hard, slightly pitted flesh and lumps and bulges on the upper thighs and buttocks, which won't go away even when you lose weight, are generally caused through fluid retention and an accumulation of toxic waste in the tissue. Regular massage with a rough bath mitt or hemp glove and a special ivy- or seaweed-based cream can work wonders in decongesting and breaking down these fatty deposits. Also try to eliminate most of the salt and spices in your diet and drink at least six to eight glasses of water or herb tea a day. The best exercises to shape up and firm the thighs are swimming, fast walking, dancing and gym exercises.

SPOTLIGHT ON FEET

Most of us are born with perfect feet — yet 90 per cent of people develop foot problems of one kind or another before they reach the age of twenty. The majority of these occur when the correct balance of the foot is misplaced. Through wearing ill-fitting shoes and walking incorrectly the muscles and arches become weakened and the ligaments overstretched, creating excessive pressure on parts of the foot. This friction can lead to the formation of calluses, corns, and more serious conditions such as enlarged toe joints and bunions. Ignore these early warning signs at your peril! Supremely eloquent, your feet speak volumes on your general well-being. For, as we all know, foot problems are not confined locally but tend to lead to back problems, aching legs, headaches and general ill-temper! Yet damage to the feet is by and large self-inflicted, through such passing whims of fashion as platform soles, very high heels or stilettos, which thrust the weight forward onto the ball of the foot, and tight, narrow or pointed toes that crunch up the toes into a vice-like grip. This is one case where it's certainly not worth considering the short-term advantages of fashion trends over long-term health and comfort. When you buy shoes therefore, bear in mind a few cardinal rules:

☐ A well-fitting shoe should be 1.5 centimetres longer than your foot, allowing plenty of room to wriggle your toes around.

☐ Shoes must fit perfectly round the heels.

Swimming, gym work, cycling, walking and running combined with massage are great leg shapers.

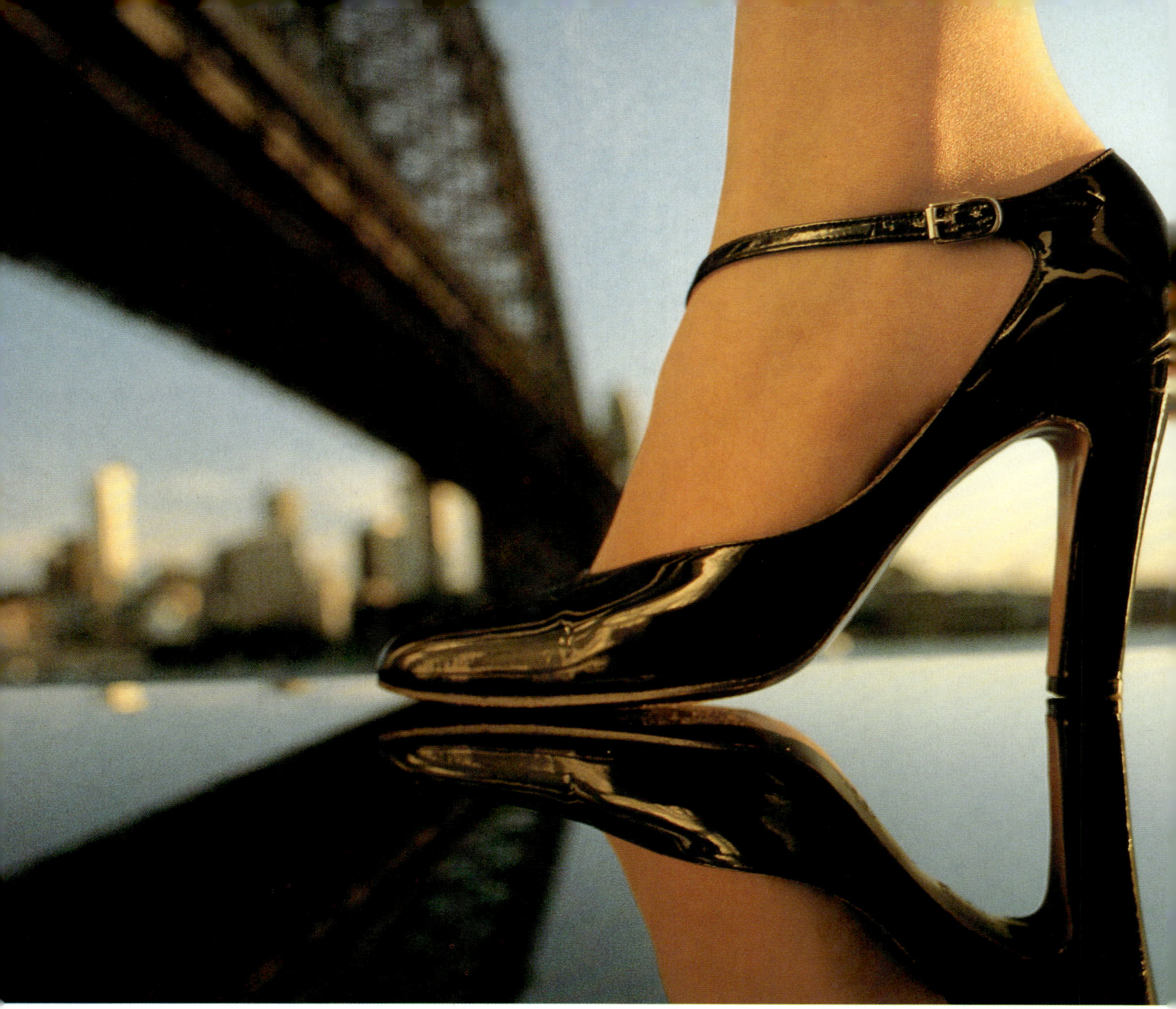

Your feet speak volumes on your general well-being.

☐ They must give firm support to the arches.
☐ They mustn't pinch, rub or squeeze any part of the foot. Don't expect new shoes to 'give' with wear. They probably won't.
☐ Avoid synthetic fibres which 'draw' the feet making them sweat and swell in all weather. Choose soft leather or fabric.
☐ Socks, tights and stockings must also fit well, allowing room for movement. If they are tight and restricting they can be just as damaging as ill-fitting shoes.

Foot care

Simple foot care can be attended to on a weekly basis. Feet should be soaked for ten minutes or more and then toenails cut and pumice applied to roughened skin. Regular elimination of rough skin with a pumice stone helps prevent the formation of calluses.

It is easier to cut toenails after a bath when they are soft since the nail is porous and absorbs moisture. Toenails should never be filed after soaking in water as they can become very jagged. After soaking the feet, you can also peel off some of the dead cuticle, thus freeing the nail. Dead cuticles can be dry and hard and tend to catch on stockings. Cream should be liberally rubbed into feet to ward off dry skin. (Like feet, elbows also need regular softening with a loofah, body brush or buffing pad in order to skim off accumulated dead skin and prevent chafing from woolly sweaters. Keep them silky soft by massaging body lotion or hand cream into the skin after your bath.)

Footnotes

Corns If the dreaded corns appear, you must go to a chiropodist for treatment before they become a more agonising, deep-rooted problem. There are other reasons for corns but basically they are caused by continuous pressure on the toes. This creates hard layers of skin and forms the painful corn. Felt pads, plasters and 'buffer' sponges can minimise the pressure of shoes and protect tender spots. Walking barefoot and wearing sandals wherever possible helps to encourage mobility of the joints and relieve muscle tension and cramps. But for many, the best way of eliminating corns is by not torturing feet and cramming them into ill-fitting and pointed-toe shoes.

Bunions Your chiropodist can give you special exercises to attempt to straighten out the big toe if you think you may be developing a bunion. Bunions may be inherited but here again footwear is the more likely culprit. The bunion occurs at the joint at the top of the first metatarsal (the big toe). Bunion sufferers should note that high-heeled shoes, by placing the foot in an unnatural position, force the metatarsal to take most of the body's weight. Once very large, inflamed and painful bunions have developed you may need to have an operation to remove them in order to make walking less of an agony.

Calluses Although calluses can develop on other parts of the body they are often found on the feet. They tend to be formed when skin builds up to protect soft areas. Although they are composed of thick layers of skin, often similar in appearance to corns, they can be treated more easily. Callused feet should be soaked in water for as long as possible, abraded with pumice or something similar, and rubbed over with cream. If the calluses do not respond, consult a chiropodist, but first, check your footwear. It is pointless treating the callus if you are still wearing the cause.

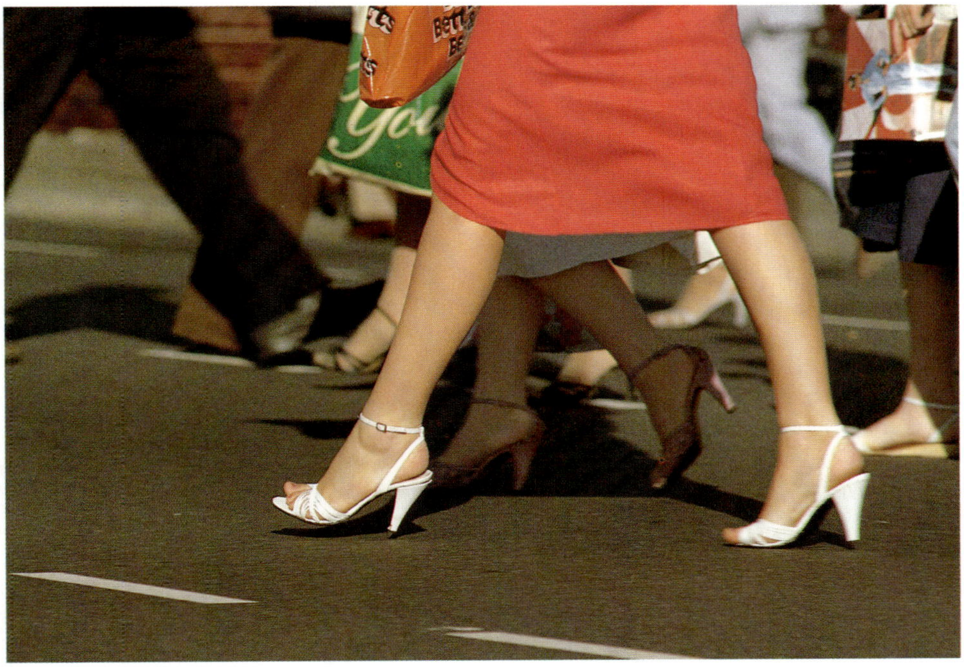

The rigours of a normal working day are enough for our feet to develop some very painful and long-term problems. Take care when buying shoes and ask yourself if the pain and discomfort is really worth it when considering a pair of ill-fitting but highly fashionable shoes.

Fungal infections Verrucae (a form of wart) and athlete's foot are both fungus infections that need immediate attention. Dark toenail polish can be the cause of trouble here. As the toenail is porous it can absorb the dye from the nail enamel and since few people renew their toenail polish as often as fingernail polish, the colour can go through the nail and cause it to lift away from the nail bed. It is important for feet to be exposed to the air and going barefoot or in open, leather sandals as often as possible is wise.

Fungal infections thrive in enclosed, moist conditions such as those created by synthetic socks and enclosed synthetic shoes. These highly contagious infections flourish in warm, moist, unhygienic surroundings — particularly in crowded areas like swimming pools and public changing rooms — and can be passed on by clothing, socks and towels. Verrucae must be professionally removed to prevent them growing or multiplying.

If you notice the skin between the toes splitting, peeling or developing a rash (athlete's foot), bathe frequently and use an anti-fungal powder or spray on your feet and inside socks and shoes. There are special athlete's foot tinctures which will clear up the infection in a few weeks.

Ingrowing toenails Usually caused by cutting the nail too low at the corners and wearing ill-fitting shoes, they must also be treated by a chiropodist before they dig deeper into the nail bed.

Swollen, perspiring, throbbing feet and ankles are something all of us suffer from at one time or another, especially during hot summer months. Regular bathing, powdering and a cooling foot-refresher spray help to take a lot of the daily punishment out of walking on city pavements. If your feet really feel they've walked their final step, steep them in hot Epsom salts or splash them alternately with cold and warm water about 20 times to reduce puffiness.

TEETH AND GUMS

It's a paradox that while women — and men — will spend time, money and a lot of effort on personal freshness, general grooming and every aspect of their outer appearance, oral health and hygiene by comparison qualifies as the poor relation! Yet strong, healthy, sparkling teeth and firm, well-shaped gums are surely an integral part of everyone's appearance, projecting charm and verve every time we smile or laugh.

Avoiding trouble

The reason why tooth decay is a national malady in so many western countries is that we eat an abundance of sugar and sweet food, especially between meals and do not brush our teeth regularly or effectively enough to undo the subsequent damage. Caring for teeth and gums begins in very early childhood and is in fact a relatively painless, uncomplicated routine:

☐ Avoid eating sweets, chocolates, biscuits and chewing gum between meals. Sugar rapidly combines with the bacteria found in saliva to form acids which systematically weaken and erode your teeth. If you do eat something sweet, brush your teeth as soon as possible afterwards.

☐ Brush both teeth *and* gums correctly. Hold the brush at an angle against the point where the teeth meet the gums and wiggle it against the surface with tiny circular movements. Concentrate on tiny areas at a time, resist large sweeping movements and brushstrokes and make sure you cover the outside, inside, sides and biting surfaces of the teeth.

☐ Learn to trace every last vestige of plaque. Plaque is the villain of teeth and gums. It is made up of a fine sticky film consisting of bacteria and saliva

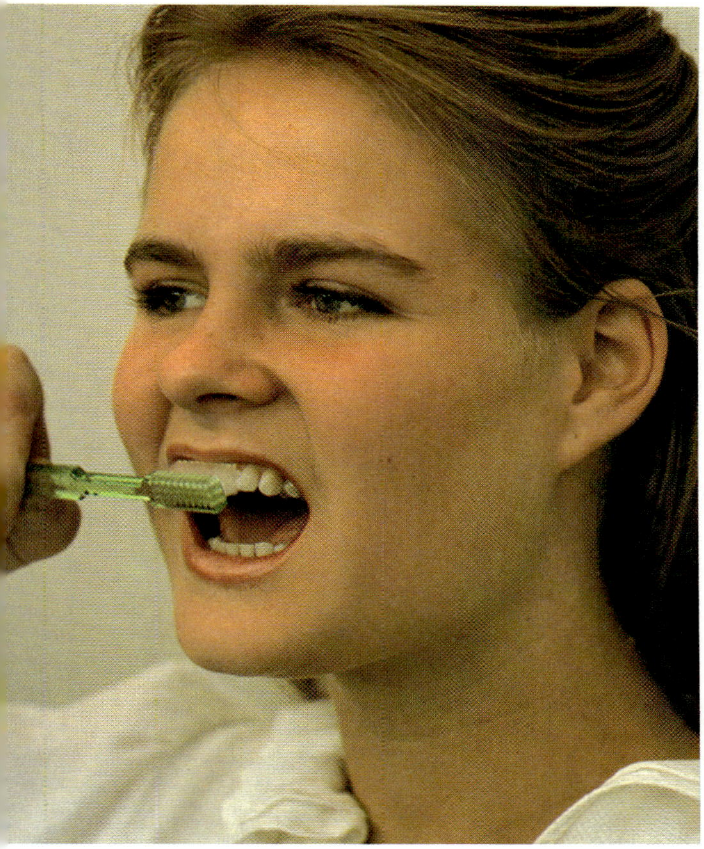

Dental Health Foundation

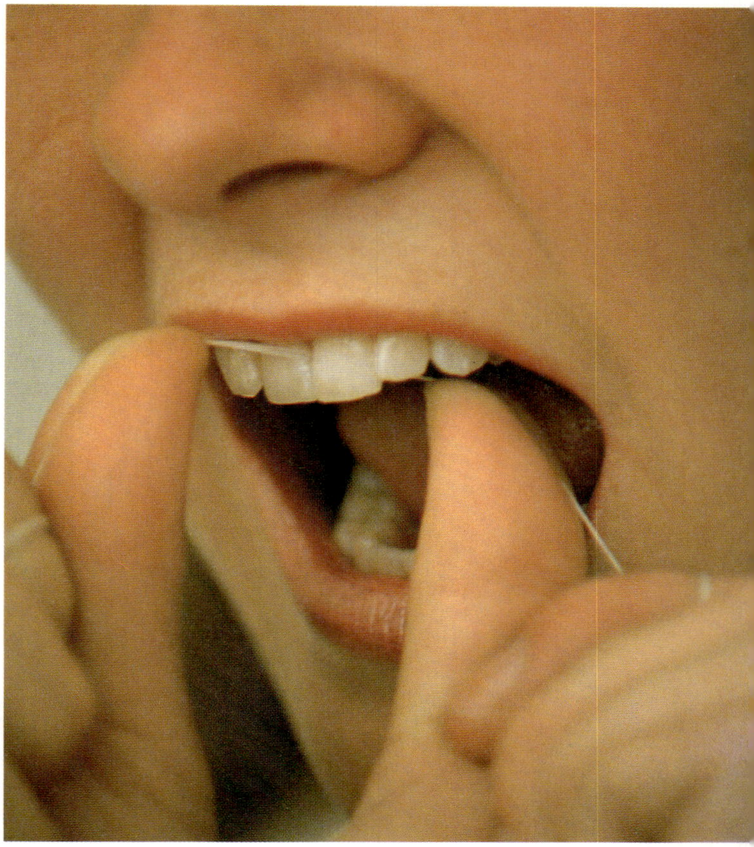

Dental Health Foundation

which adheres to nooks and crannies like gum margins, biting surfaces, and between the teeth. Plaque combines with particles of food — sugar in particular — to form acids, and unless it's promptly removed this lethal combination eats away at the surface of the tooth and causes decay. Since it's difficult to be sure you've banished every vestige of plaque, use a disclosing tablet (available from chemists) which dyes plaque red or blue so you can trace and brush it off completely. Use these tablets twice or three times a week.

☐ Add dental floss and gum massages to your dental 'kit'. They remove plaque and tiny bits of food from between the teeth and help to strengthen gums.

☐ Use a medium or soft toothbrush and change it every three months. Always buy toothpaste with added fluoride as this helps to strengthen the resistance of your teeth against the acids that cause decay.

☐ Take time to brush teeth properly. Ideally you should clean them after every meal — but few of us have sufficient time or opportunity. Never skimp brushing before bedtime, for most of the damage caused by food particles and acid build-up occurs while you are asleep. One five-minute assault a day, plus one or two slightly shorter brushing sessions should protect against tooth decay and weak gums.

☐ Gums are every bit as precious as teeth themselves. Watch out for bleeding while you brush as well as swelling or pocketing of the gum tissue which causes a tiny gap to form between the tooth and edge of the gum. These are signs that the gums are not sealing firmly against the tooth and therefore allowing plaque to filter through between the gums and teeth roots. If this hidden damage continues for too long, eventually the bone which holds the root will be eaten away, loosening the teeth. This is the main reason why so many people over the age of 35 have their teeth extracted. Correct brushing and flossing will help to prevent your gums from weakening.

When cleaning teeth, brush downwards from the gum. Use dental floss (above) to clean between the teeth.

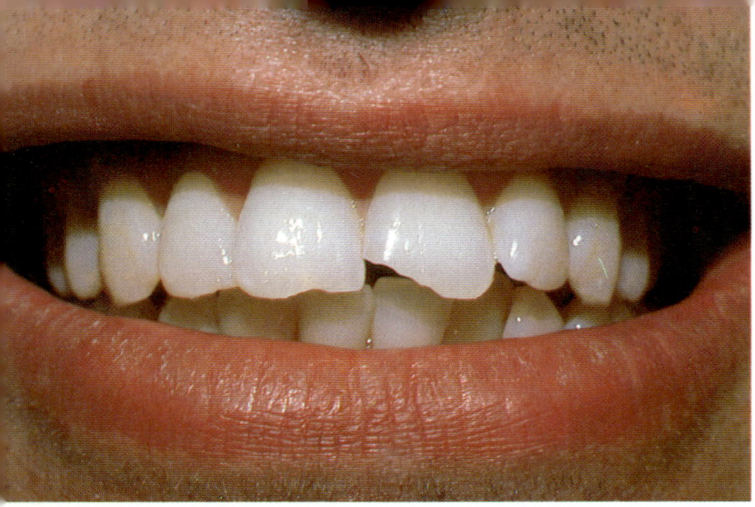

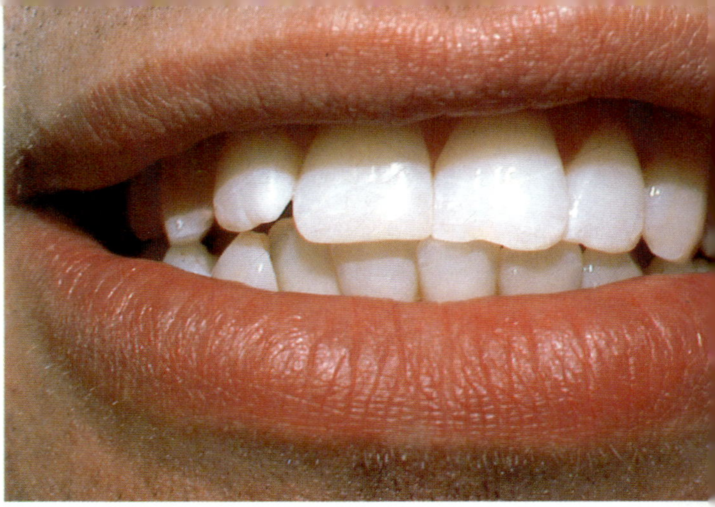

Chipped teeth can be made as good as new.

MAKING THE MOST OF YOUR SMILE

Dentistry has progressed in leaps and bounds over the past few years, no area more so than in the realms of cosmetic techniques. With injections, intravenous sedation and relative analgesia (a light gas administered to help you relax) on hand to take the pain and discomfort out of dental care, more and more of us are becoming adventurous in the type of work we're willing to consider to improve our smiles.

Light-cured veneers

This is a thin plastic cover which is moulded into place to conceal staining on a tooth or minimise the gap between one tooth and the next. It is simpler and less expensive than crowning and also takes less time.

Dentine bonding

Instead of deep fillings, which can mean drilling healthy teeth, this technique simply involves filling the gaps at the tops of teeth with a bonding material.

White fillings

These were once advisable only in front teeth as the material used wasn't strong enough to stand up to the pounding chewing surfaces received, but now tougher, white amalgam is available to banish that silver smile.

Bridges

Plates or dentures were once the only alternative to gappy smiles if you lost a few teeth. Now some really modern bridges come to the rescue. The Rochette bridge comprises false teeth bonded to real ones by tiny wings which are invisible as you talk or smile. The Maryland bridge works in the same way but is held in place with a fine metal strand instead of wings.

Tooth straightening

Nowadays adults as well as children are prepared to wear braces and bands to have their teeth straightened. The advantages of this are not only cosmetic — re-aligned teeth can cure migraine problems and have all sorts of beneficial side effects for oral health.

Crowns

Chipped, cracked or discoloured teeth can be very effectively treated these days with crowning; the original tooth is simply filed down to a point and covered with a cap, usually made out of porcelain bonded to gold.

beauty tips

A few decades ago nice girls didn't wear make-up and plain girls just stayed plain. Now, however, the use of make-up is universally accepted and refinements in modern cosmetics have allowed women to master that most elusively challenging of effects — the natural look. As the ultimate art of illusion, successful make-up consists of enhancing features without obvious artifice and de-emphasising flaws and defects — making eyes larger and

Subtle understatement: the natural look with sophisticated allure. The shades and formulas of today's cosmetics allow ample scope for subtlety and experiment.

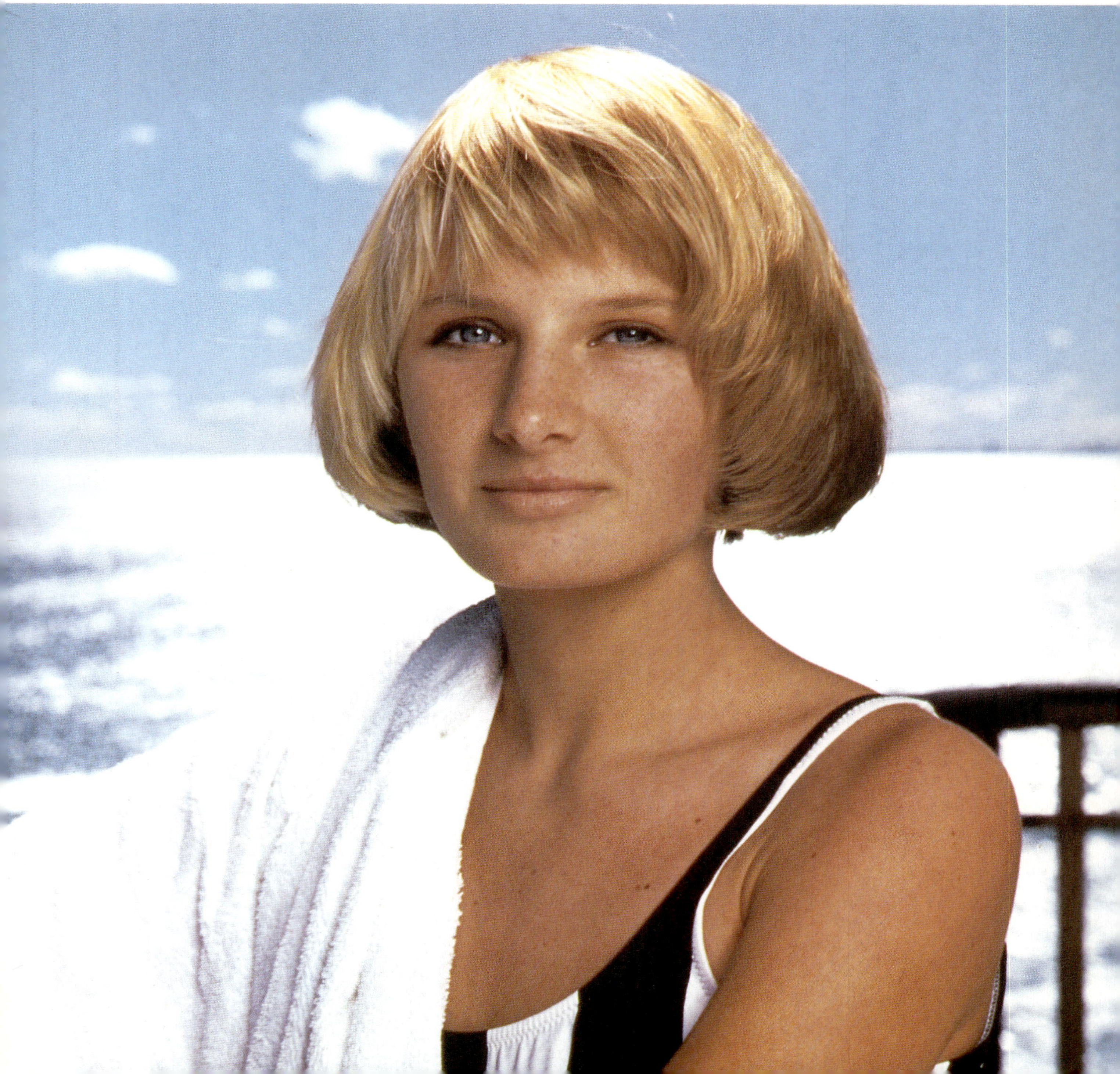

more radiant, the mouth fuller and softer — without ever seeming over-made-up. Mastering the natural look, explains renowned visagiste Olivier Euchaudemaison, artistic director of one of France's leading cosmetic companies, means studying your skin tone, face shape and individual features in minute detail in order to determine which skin products will best embellish your looks without overwhelming or distorting them. Successful make-up, he believes, is perfecting the art of the possible.

FOUNDATION — YOUR SECOND SKIN

You must never try to change your skin tone completely. The main aim of effective foundation is to enhance it and camouflage its less attractive characteristics. Remember, when choosing foundation it's best to test a little on the inside of your wrist where the skin comes as close as possible to that of your complexion. Ideally, however, you should rub a little into your jawline and look at it in daylight to find a shade which matches your skin. Although skin tones vary tremendously, they can be broken up into certain principal groups:

Ivory — very pale, translucent skin that generally accompanies black, dark brown, or auburn hair. Choose a matching foundation.

Cream — a light, slightly peachy beige that is the typical 'English Rose' complexion which needs a foundation that's either a fraction lighter or darker.

Fair — a delicate blush-like tone that tends to go with blonde hair. Try and match it exactly.

Pink — a rosy complexion which can become ruddy, often accompanying red hair and freckles. A beige will tone it down subtly.

Olive — usually teams with brown eyes and brown or blonde hair. It can look sallow in the winter. Pick an olive foundation or a warm biscuity beige for a healthier look.

Brown — this may vary from a suntanned complexion, to light coffee or very dark brown. Darker tones often don't need foundation, otherwise try and match it exactly, avoiding tan or bronze shades with a pink or brick-orange pigment.

Feel and texture

The type of foundation you choose depends to a large extent on your skin type, the 'feel' of foundation on your skin, as well as the effect you want to achieve. The choice is enormous today. There are ultra lightweight tinted moisturisers which add a mere trace of colour to the face and are perfect for young, unblemished skins and a very unmade-up look. Fine fluid foundations that give a lightweight but even coverage to the complexion are probably most suitable, while thicker cream foundations give a more opaque coverage hiding tiny flaws and problems such as broken veins and scars. Heavy pan-stick foundations and all-in-one cream powders have long passed out of fashion but they are still available and you may find them useful for camouflaging deeper scars, birthmarks and other blemishes.

An invaluable standby in your make-up kit is concealer stick or cream — a matt buff-coloured product which will erase and soften dark circles underneath the eyes. Use sparingly and blend in well after applying foundation.

Apply liquid foundation with a latex make-up sponge for a smooth, even finish. Cream foundation or pan-stick needs blending in with the fingertips. Having achieved a perfect and even colour tone don't ruin it by topping up

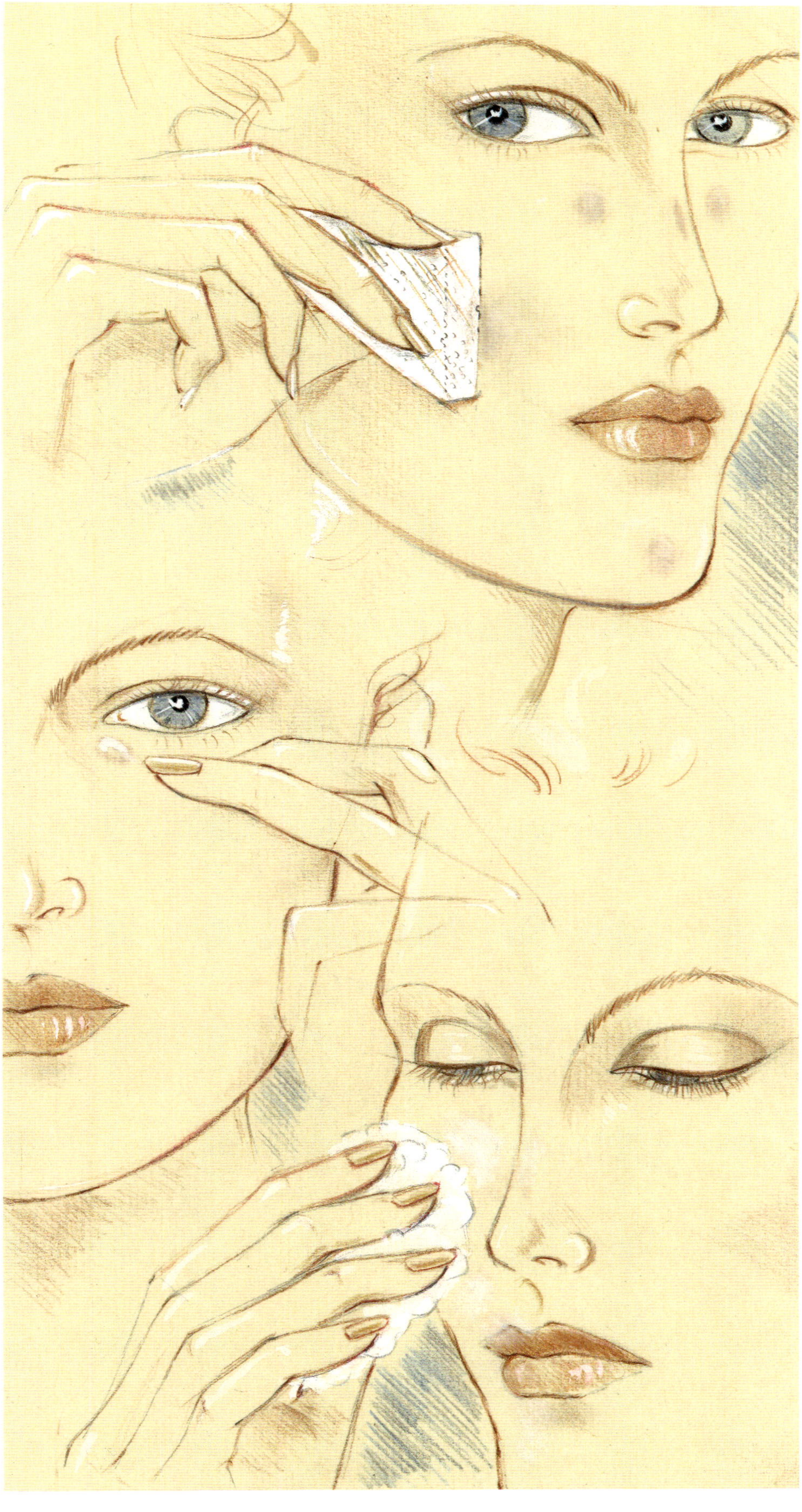

Smooth on tinted liquid foundation with a damp latex make-up sponge.

Minimise dark circles beneath the eyes with tiny dots of concealing cream, blended well into the skin where the shadow falls.

Press loose powder firmly onto the skin, skimming off any surplus.

To apply blusher correctly, press the thumb and forefinger against the bony structure of the cheek which lies at an angle between the middle of the ear and the base of the nose. Apply colour along this line and also dust beneath it.

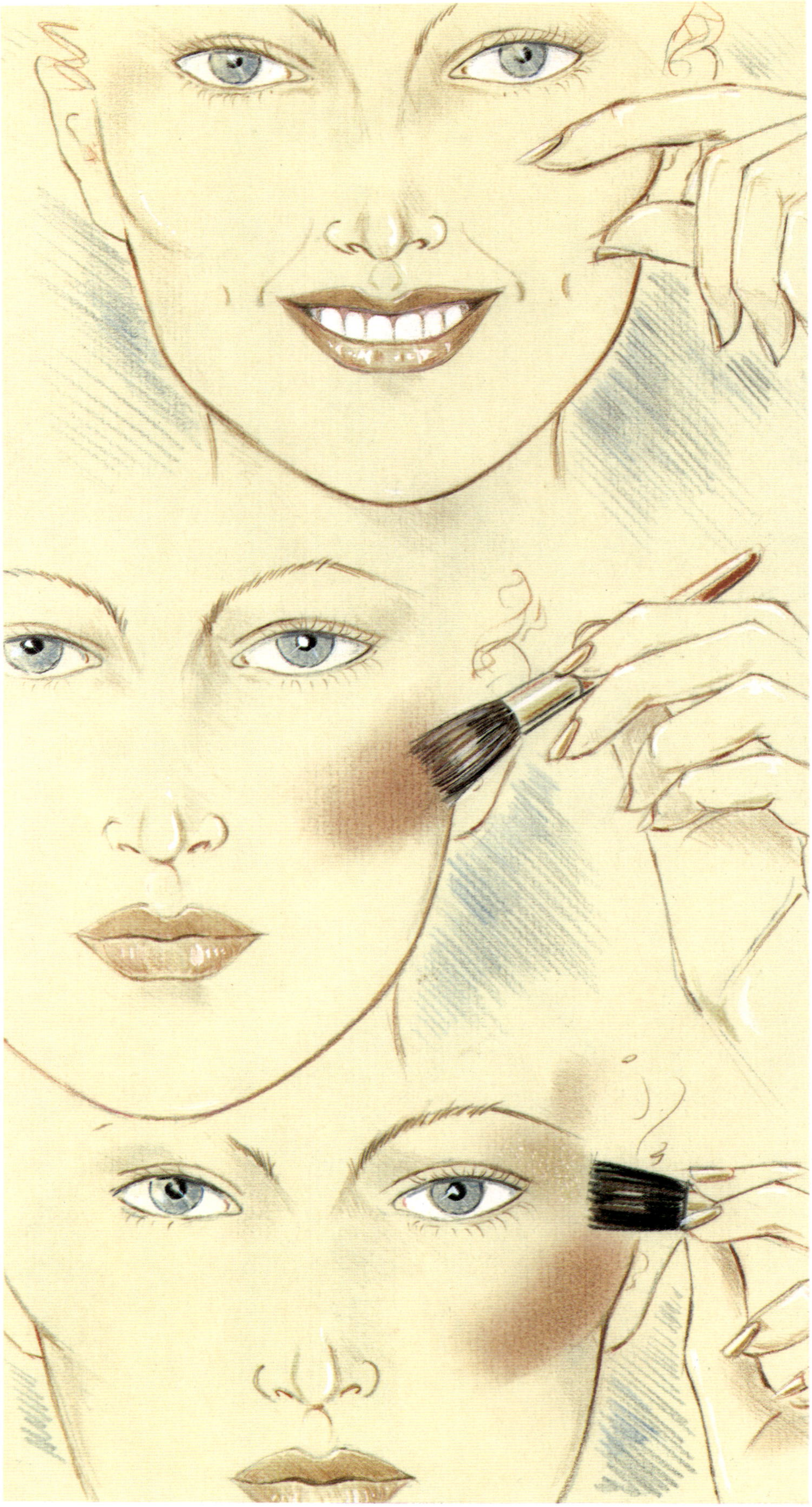

To accentuate the bone structure further, lightly trace a paler, frosted blusher or highlighter along the upper crest of the cheek near the eyes and around the temples, up to the hairline.

with tinted face powder. This is gradually becoming a relic of the past since the suspension and distribution of pigment in creams and liquids has been so refined and perfected as to appear totally natural. Colourless, translucent powder should be pressed into the skin with cotton wool or a flat powder puff to 'set' the tone you've achieved, creating a matt yet radiant effect without any trace of colour 'build-up'. Use loose powder when you first apply your make-up and pressed powder for repair jobs and renewing make-up during the day.

CONTOURING — LIGHT AND SHADE

The use of blusher can be as simple or as complex as you wish. For a healthy, natural outdoor look simply flick a trace of powder blusher, gel or cream rouge onto the fullest part of your cheek. Pinky brown, damson or tawny peach are the most flattering shades, but take care they don't clash with the clothes you're wearing. Cream or gel rouge goes on *over* your foundation but *underneath* your powder, powder blusher glides on *over* your powder. Hollowing or sculpting a round face or very full cheeks can be achieved with a sludgy-brown, matt powder.

EYES — YOUR MOST STUNNING FEATURE

Before making up your eyes, study them carefully in the mirror — their shape and size, whether prominent, deepset or droopy, and the overall impact they create facially. Large, dark, well-shaped eyes with dark lashes are a natural attribute that need relatively little contouring or definition to bring them into focus; small, deepset eyes, however, need extra embellishment.

As far as eyeshadows go, browns and greys are the perennial classic shades that every woman can wear successfully, but be more selective when choosing brighter colours. Blue, turquoise or purple look stunning on blue, grey or greeny grey eyes; marine colours — olive green or moss — intensify hazel eyes; warm cinnamons, beiges, pink or mauve-tinged shades add warmth and sparkle to brown eyes. Powder shadow is hard to beat for easy application and staying power. Cream shadow goes on like silk but tends to crease and shine after a few hours. To avoid 'sweaty' lids powder well before and after.

The mascara you use depends largely on the sensitivity of your eyes, the length and thickness of your lashes and the effect you want to create. Waterproof mascara prevents smudging and running and is great if you lead a hectic, busy, outdoor or sporty life, while it also makes lashes longer and thicker. Special 'building' mascaras with added ingredients to coat and lengthen the lashes can irritate the eyes and prove hard to remove, though the effect they give is pure Hollywood glamour! There are special conditioning mascaras to stop the lashes turning brittle and to encourage growth, and if you have particularly sensitive eyes — and skin — or wear contact lenses, look out for hypo-allergenic eye make-up. Always apply two coats of mascara, allowing each application to dry thoroughly.

DAYTIME EYES

Refresh sore, gritty or red eyes with eyedrops.

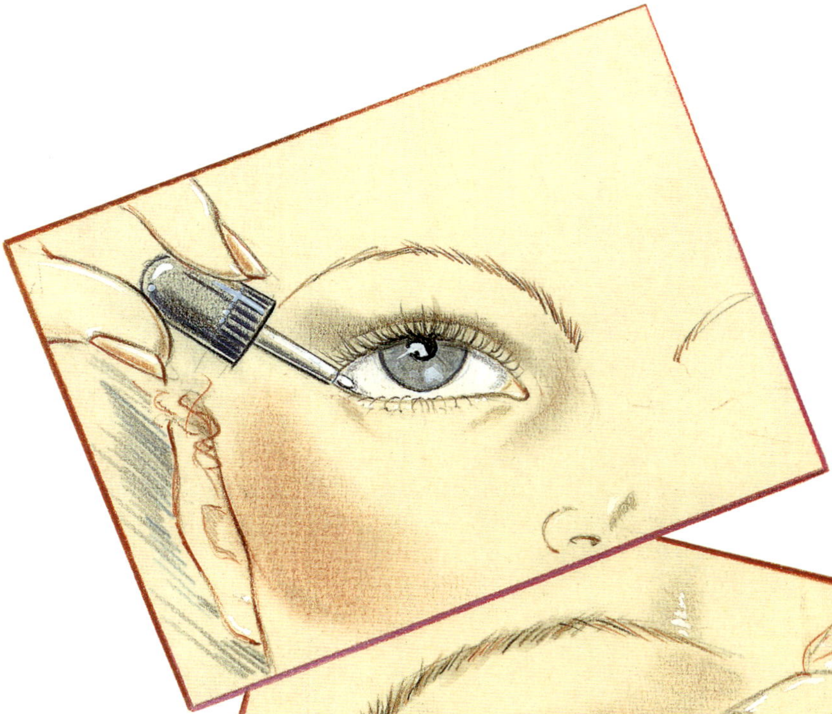

Apply a muted browny-beige, soft grey or sage green powder shadow over the entire eyelid with a sponge applicator, dove-tailing the colour out and up towards the browbone.

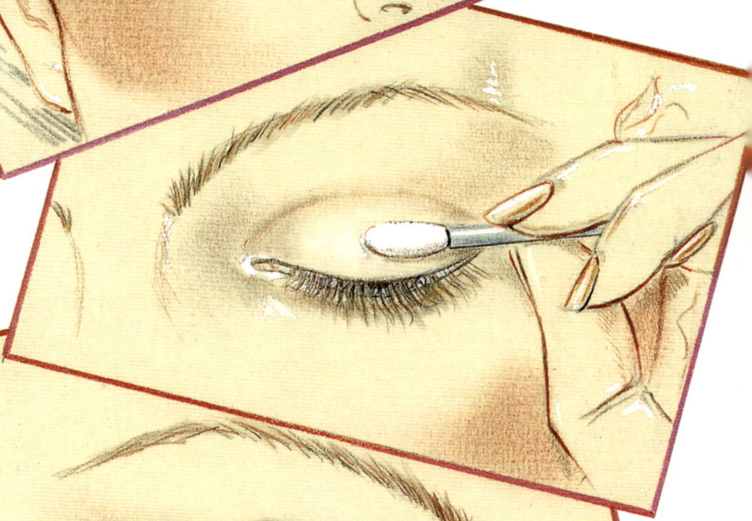

Trace a very fine crayon line along the base of the top and bottom lashes to emphasise the shape of the lids and focus the colour and sparkle of the eyes.

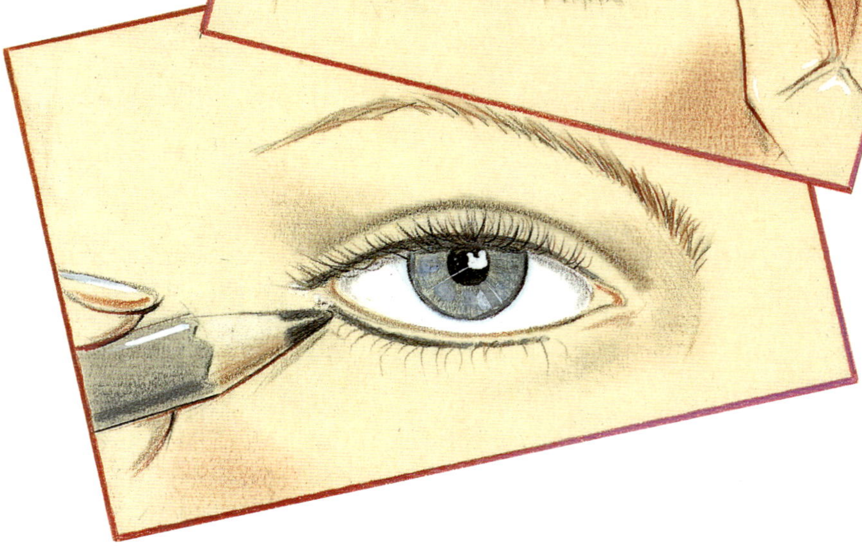

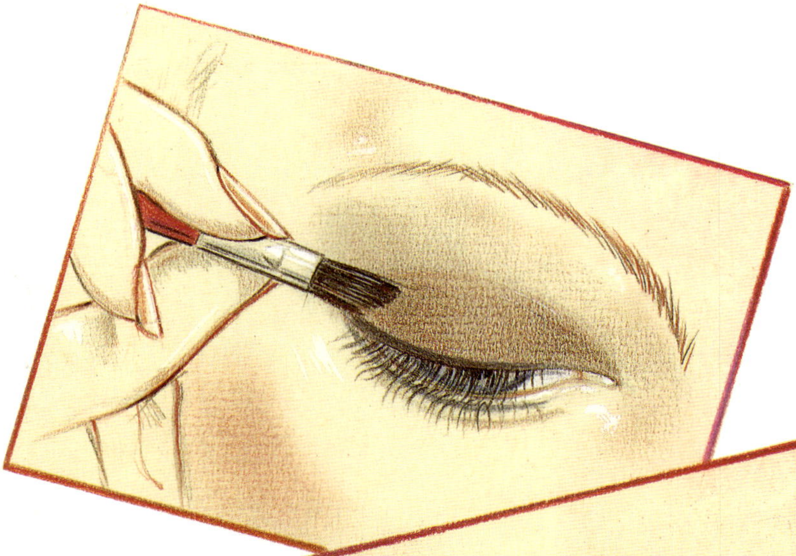

For extra definition, apply a dark, frosted shadow over the eyelid, smoothing a darker shade into the natural creaseline, to add depth to the eye colour.

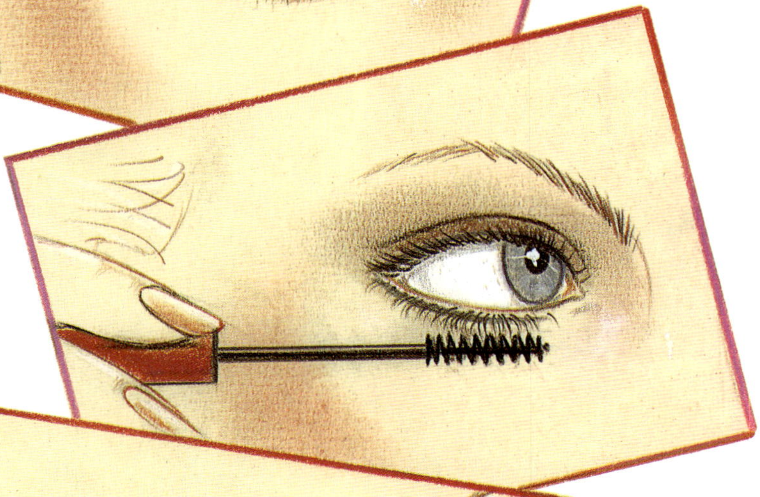

Two coats of waterproof mascara on the top and bottom lashes 'open' the eye and give a soft starry effect. To build up thickness and length without smudging, allow each application to dry thoroughly.

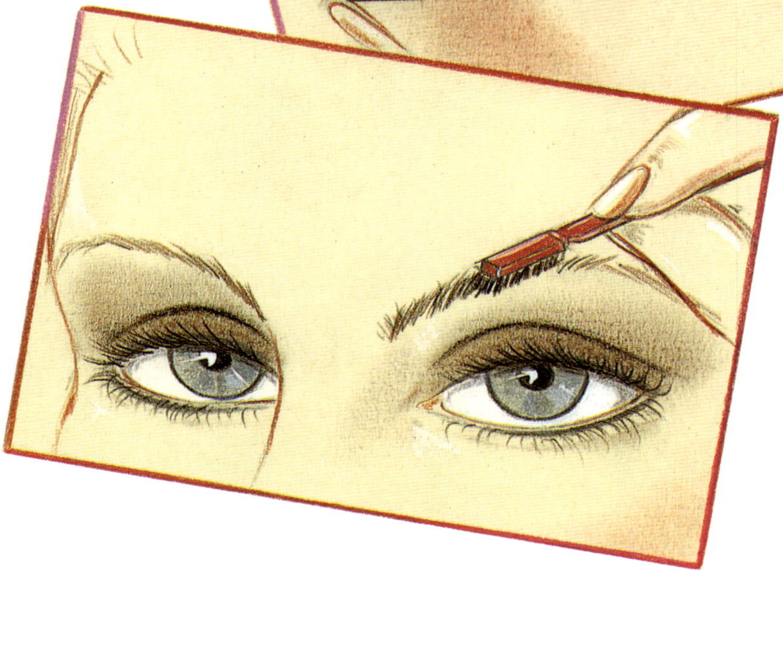

Tidy eyebrows by brushing them upwards into a gentle arch with a baby's toothbrush or a dampened mascara brush. Add a touch of vaseline to control thicker eyebrows and add shine.

EVENING GLAMOUR

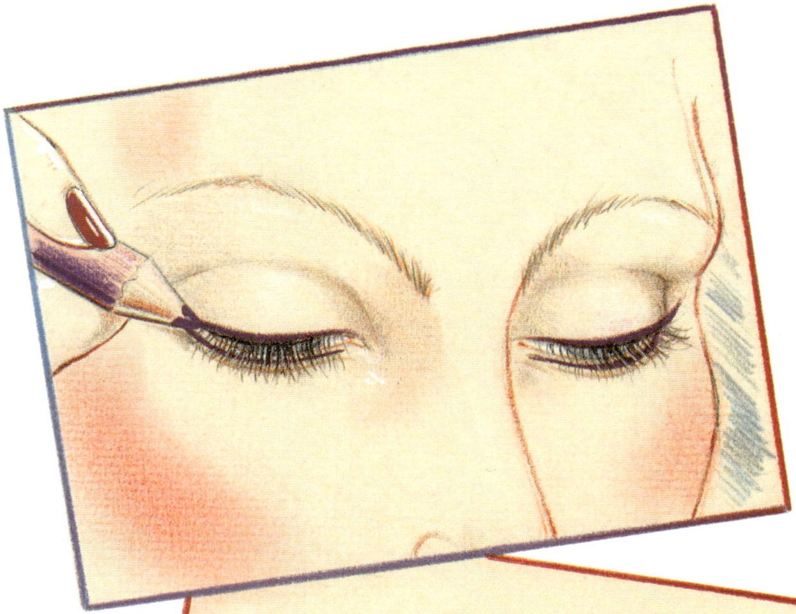

Define the eyelid by tracing a very fine pencil line or a thread of liquid or cake liner along the upper lashes extending this slightly at the outside corner.

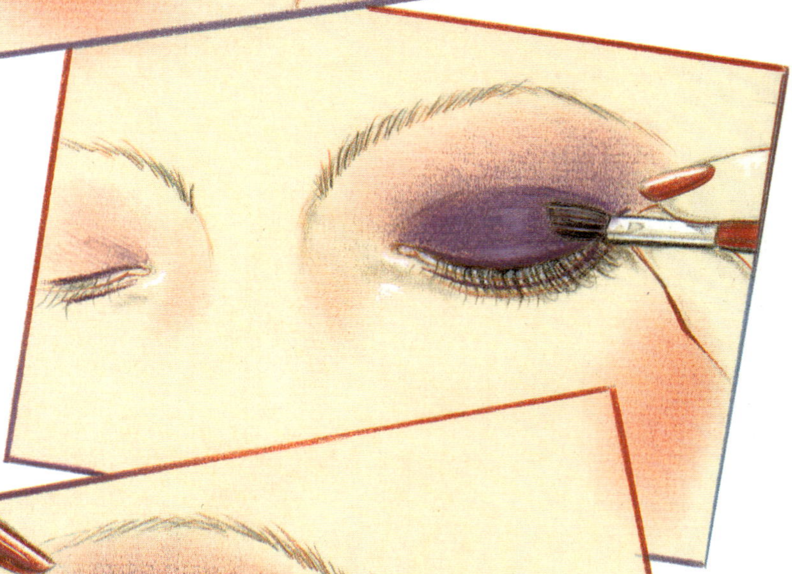

Blend a mid-tone vibrant shadow over the entire lid, using a damp brush for extra depth of tone.

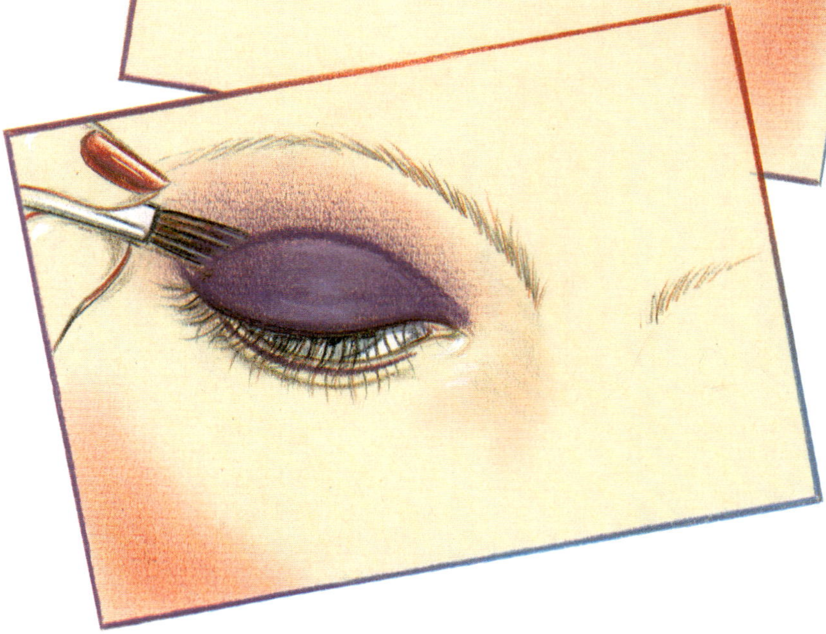

Accentuate deep hollows with a darker, smokier shadow in the creaseline, gently blending and fading out the colour towards the browbone.

Very pale frosted shadow or highlighter on the crest of the browbone projects bone structure, adding sheen and sparkle to both skin and eyes.

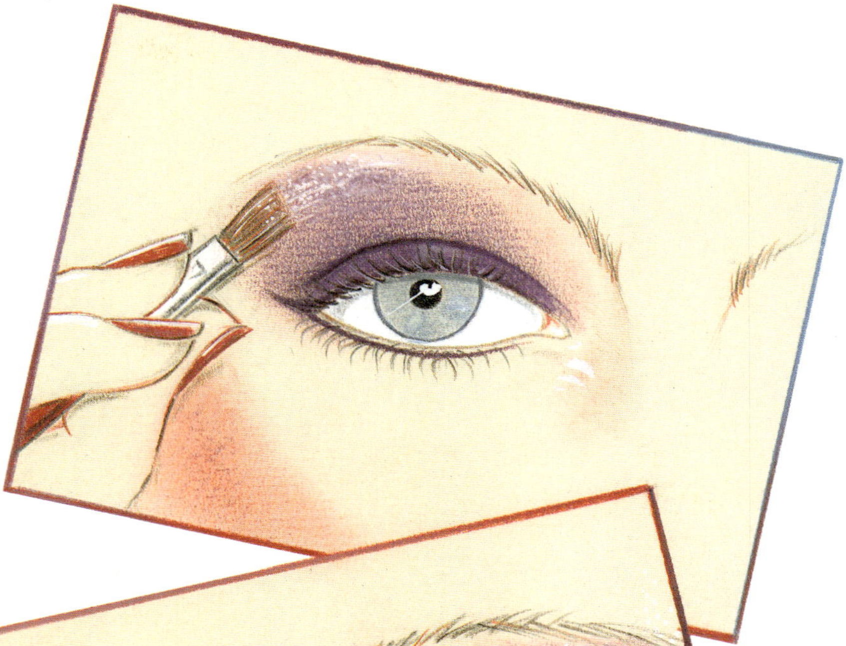

Single, false eyelashes build a thick, romantic fringe around the entire eye without hardness or giveaway baselines. Grip each lash with tweezers, dip base into a drop of surgical glue, press firmly against your own top or bottom eyelashes. An excellent trick for 'filling in' gaps in sparse lashes.

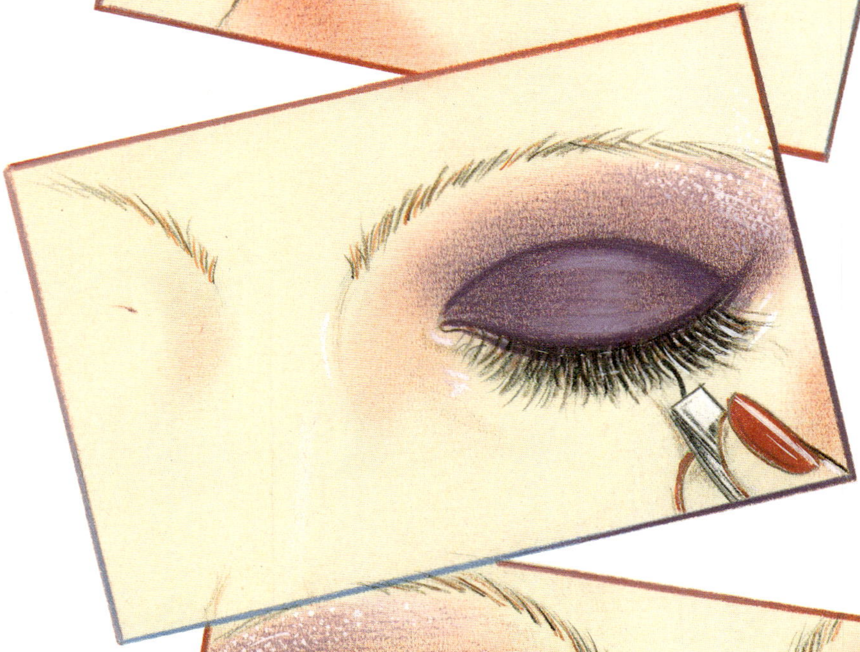

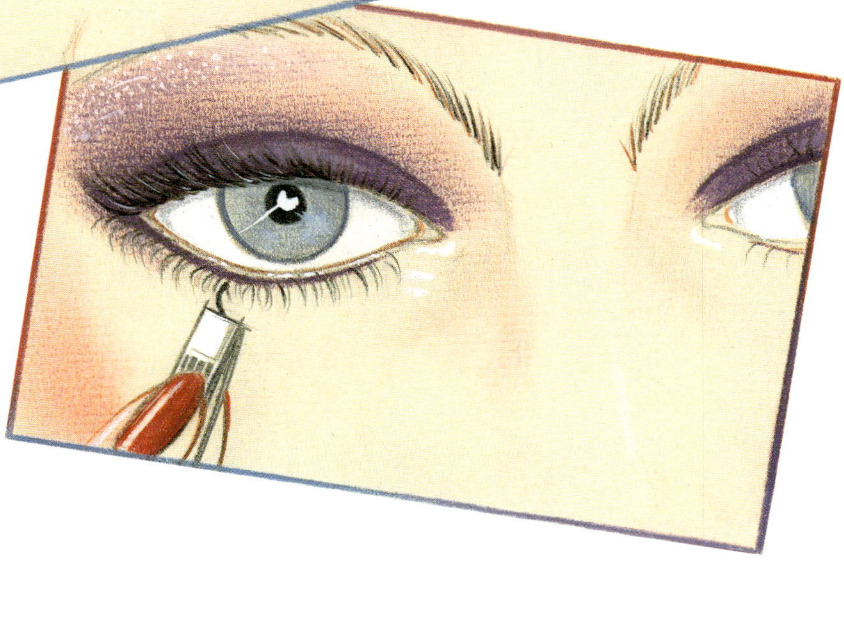

LIPS — SOFT AND LUSCIOUS

You can improve significantly on thin, flat or small lips, building up the shape and roundness of your mouth with lip crayon, using a pale brown or a colour that's one shade darker than your lipstick. Alternatively outline the lips with a firm, pointed lip brush. Full lips can get away with just about any shade of lipstick no matter how bright or bold. A smaller mouth, however, looks softer with the subtle pinks, beiges, peaches and browns as well as frosted shades. Wearing a slightly paler shade on the inside of the lips makes a small mouth appear fuller. If you prefer a natural look use a transparent colourless lip gloss, a lip tint that gives a bare hint of colour or lip salve to stop your lips from drying out.

To prevent the new softer texture lipsticks and pencils from 'creeping' into the fine lines around the mouth, extend your foundation and powder right down to the lips and then trace a good outline with a crayon or lip brush over the powder.

For a perfectly shaped, neat lip line first trace the outer contours with either a browny-beige lip crayon or a lip brush dipped in your usual lipstick. Do not exaggerate the lip line or go too far outside your natural shape. Next fill in main colour with a flattish lip brush. Finally, blot well with tissue to 'set' the colour and shape.

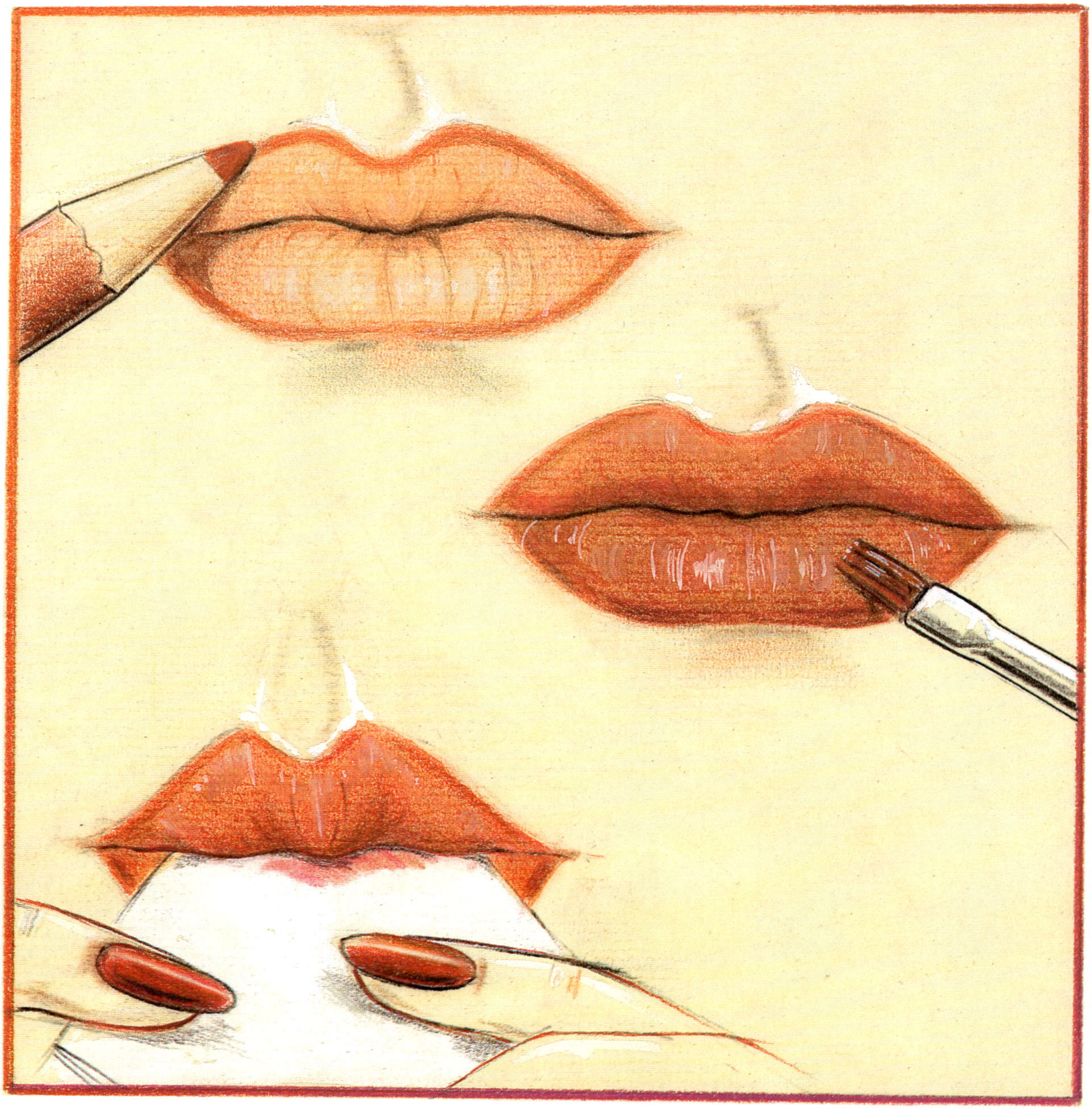

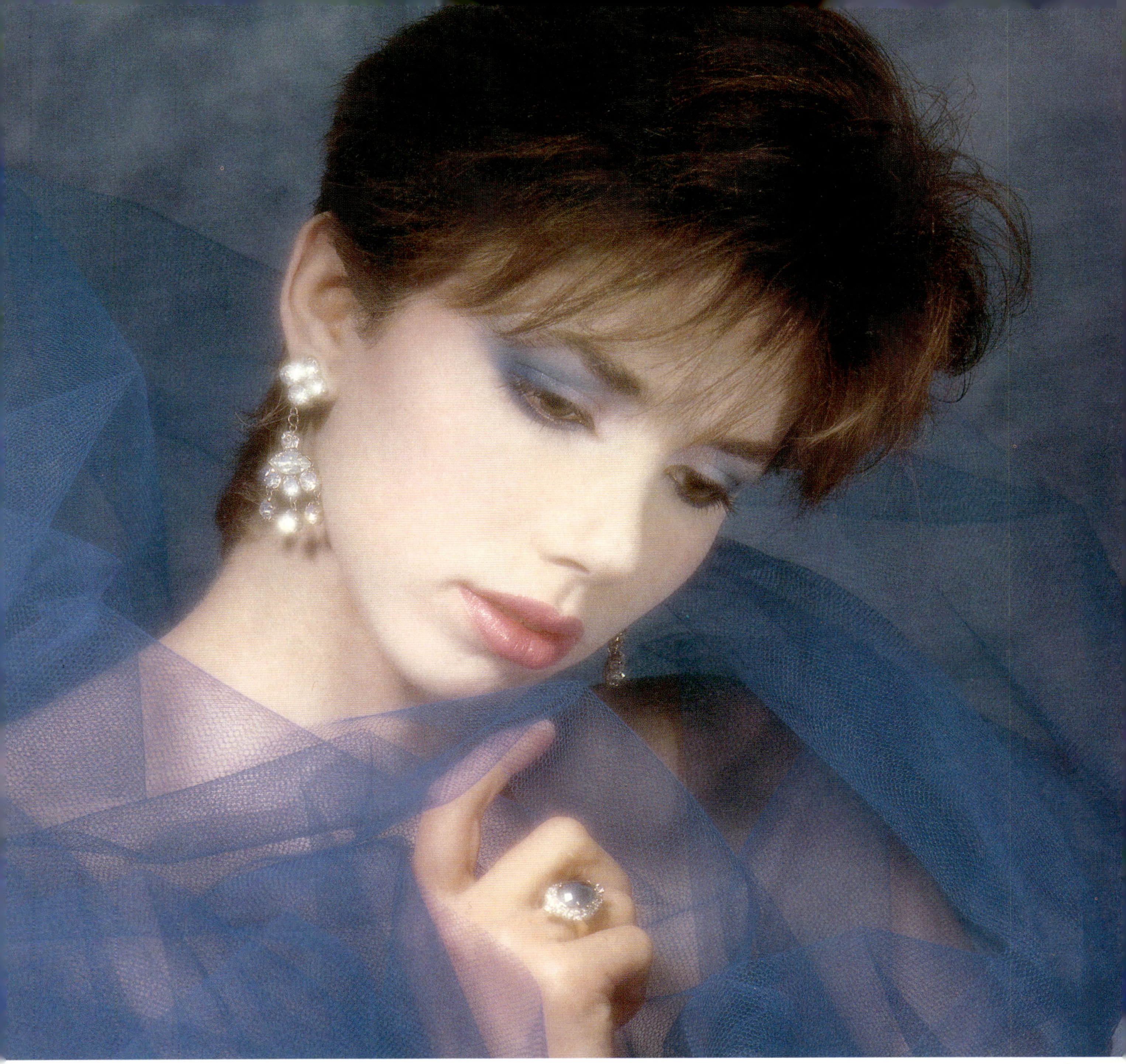

PARTY LOOKS

It's party time and the shades you would normally shun for day wear are ideal for the nightlife.

The essential rule to remember for evening make-up is that strong lights sap your complexion of its colour — so with all your cosmetics choose a slightly warmer shade than you normally wear during the day. Blusher comes into its own in the evening — experiment with stronger pinks and peaches and build up the colour more intensely. Little pots of multicoloured iridescent powder which you can buy will create a rich and diverse juxtaposition of colours on the eyes. Lips can get away with deeper or brighter, more electric lipstick tones in the evenings; shades that might look hard or garish in daylight come into their own after dark, when the soft colours you normally wear appear washed out.

TOOLS OF THE TRADE

From a variety of different brushes to sharpened pencils, these tools are all necessary for that natural, long-lasting and truly professional look.

Once you've found the products that suit you, expert application becomes the key to successful make-up. It's impossible to achieve a natural-looking, long-lasting and truly professional finish without using the correct 'tools'. It's worth investing a little extra money in these since good quality brushes will last far longer than the cheaper variety while allowing you to carry out all the tiny subtleties needed to master a particular look.

Brushes

These are the most important item in any make-up kit. You'll need a full, soft, slightly flattish brush to apply blusher and a second one for your highlighter in order to avoid colour or glitter 'spillover', as well as a very fine, pointed lip liner and a flat wedge-shaped brush made of slightly tougher bristles that don't separate for applying eyeshadow (again invest in two or three to use with different colours). Wedge-shaped sponge applicators are excellent for blending powder shadow more easily — especially if you are mixing them with water. Also invaluable are a small toothbrush for tidying the eyebrows, and a flat, broad, pointed lip brush to both outline and fill in the lips. You may also need a large, soft chubby brush to flick off surplus powder and skim away flecks of eyeshadow that stray onto the face. If you like using block mascara choose the thickest mascara brush you can find for rapid and effective coverage.

Pencil sharpener

You'll need to use this regularly to keep kohl pencils, eye and lip crayons pointed.

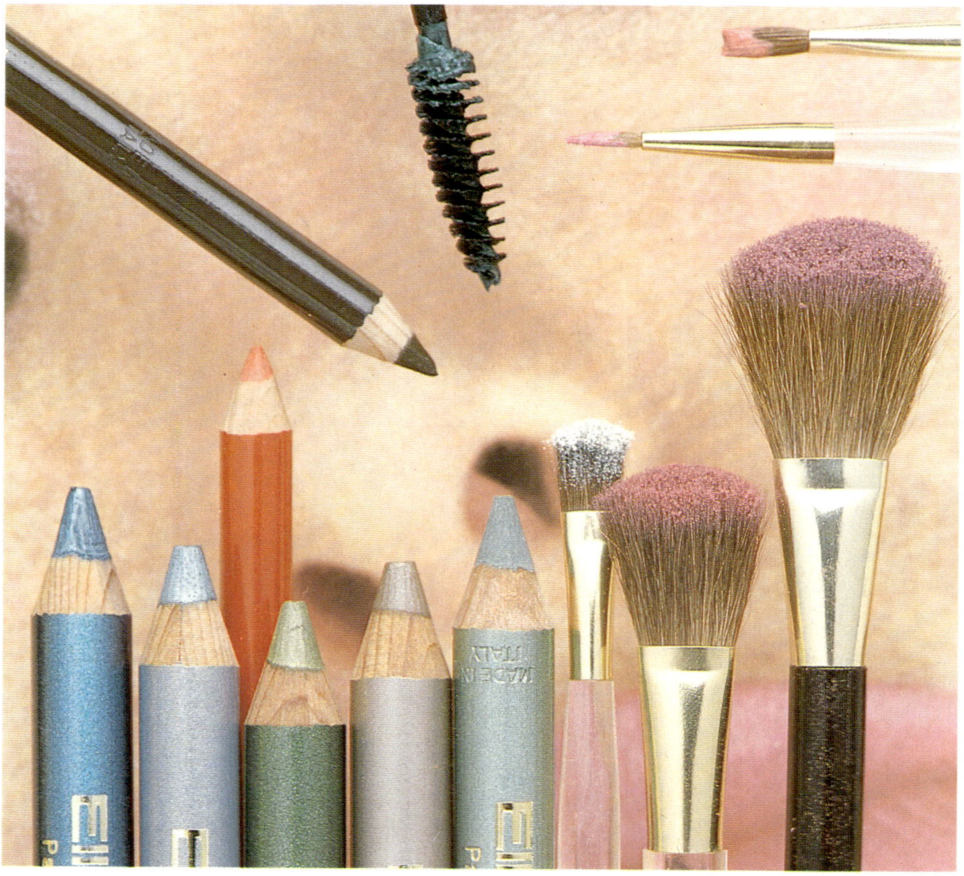

Ella Bache

Beautiful make-up is the sign of not only skilful application but also the use of proper 'tools'.

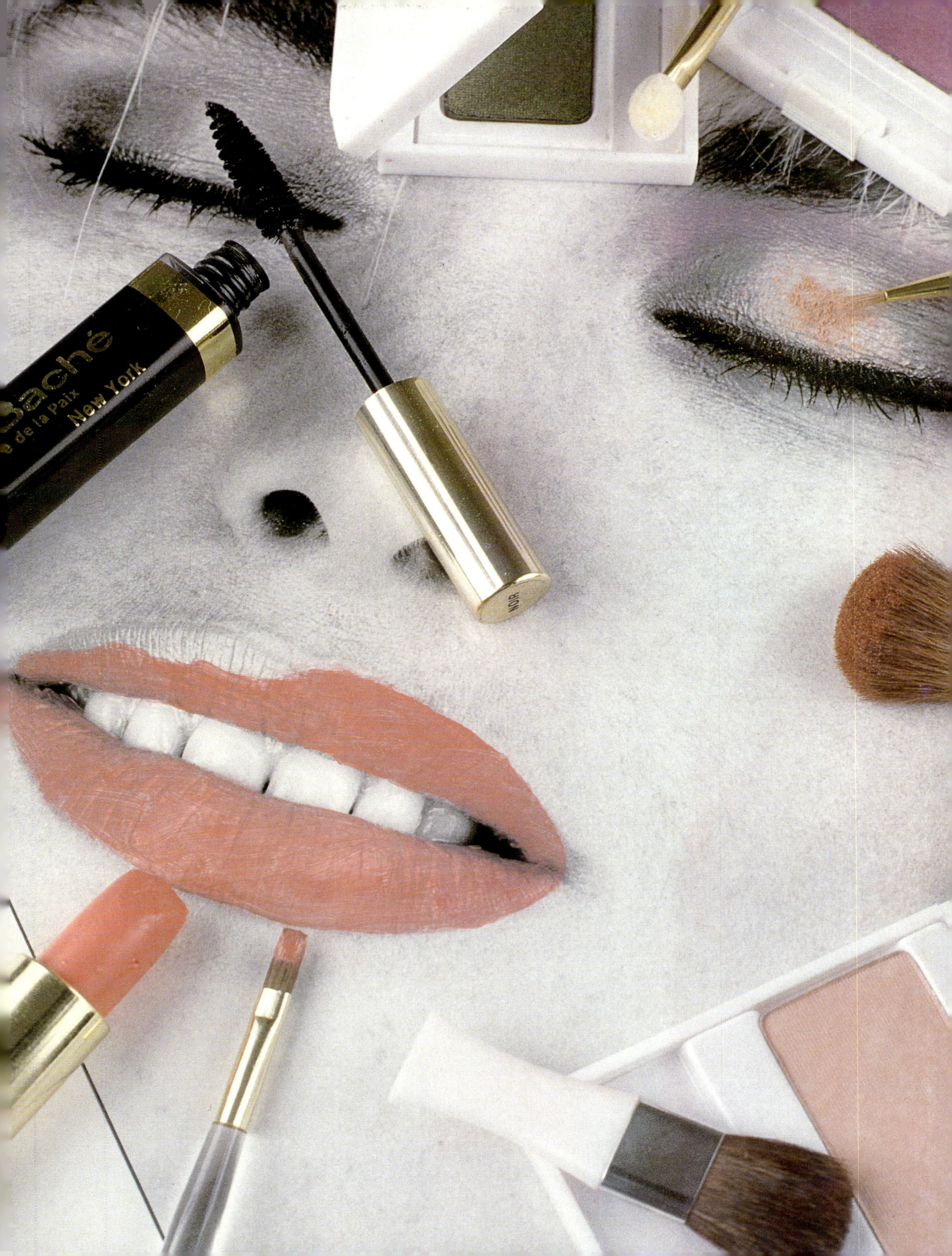
New York
NOIR

Sponges

A fine latex 'wedge' sponge is ideal for applying liquid foundation with a light touch so that you don't get a heavy or uneven streaky effect. Keep it clean by rinsing out after each application.

Cotton buds

Invaluable for mopping up smudged eyeliner or mascara especially beneath the lashes and for tidying up eye make-up.

SWEET SMELLS OF SUCCESS

Choosing a perfume is a complex business as there are literally hundreds of different types. As soon as you begin, you enter the mysterious and exotic world of the perfumers and the image makers. It is their business to capture imaginations with different blends and to give each perfume a character through packaging and marketing.

Of all the senses, smell is perhaps the most tantalising. Different scents affect us, sometimes in very obvious ways such as feeling hungry at the aroma of freshly ground coffee or of newly baked bread, or feeling happy at the heady scent of a bunch of fresh freesias.

We are also affected at a more subtle level by other scents, particularly our own body scents, known as pheromones. These are given out and received without conscious knowledge and are said to affect the way we react to each other. The same process is highly developed in animals who rely on scent for survival. Few of us need to rely on these scents in our everyday lives, but they are still there, working away and could be the reason why you are inexplicably attracted to or repelled by people.

Perfume is an extension of these body scents, which is why finding the right one is so much more than choosing a pretty fragrance. A perfume that 'works' blends perfectly with the skin to become an extension of self, complementing and underlining personality.

Capturing, bottling and marketing these elusive messages is a multimillion-dollar business and the result is a terrific choice of perfumes with something to suit almost every taste. It's just a question of isolating favourites from the huge range available.

Perfume families

The categories into which perfumes fall are determined by the ingredients and the blends used in their creation. One of the most recent examples of a successful perfume family has been the much publicised 'orientals'. These are the potent, heady scents such as *Opium* by Yves Saint Laurent, which are unmistakeably Eastern in influence, many containing spices and more than a hint of musk. Perfumers, known in the business as 'noses', blend many ingredients to make a single fragrance.

Joy by Jean Patou has always been marketed as the world's costliest perfume, containing no less than 100 different ingredients.

The oils used in perfume making are known as essential oils, extracted from the petals, stems and roots of flowers and from spices, fruits, trees and moss. Animal extracts which were traditionally used have been replaced largely by synthetic substitutes.

Floral oils are the main ingredients of most perfumes. Jasmine and rose are widely used along with extracts from almost every flower you can think of. To supply the perfume industry, it takes millions of blossoms grown in various parts of the world and selected for their quality.

Oakmoss is the type of moss commonly used in perfume making, usually to

add depth and staying power.
Patchouli is an Indian plant and the oil extracted from it is largely used in the exotic, oriental-style perfumes.
Sandalwood is the famous, exotically scented wood, so fragrant it has earned a place as a perfume in its own right as well as being a key ingredient in many favourite blends.
Vetiver is the name for the long, headily scented roots of an Indian grass. Its pungent quality is used in many perfumes.
Ylang-ylang comes from a Malaysian tree of the same name. It blends well with other ingredients, but is extremely pungent alone.

The right notes

A good perfume has different characteristics, rather like a good wine. At first there's a distinctive 'top note' which is apparent as soon as the perfume is applied to the skin. This fades to reveal a 'middle note' which is the centre of the perfume, strengthened by the heavier 'base note' which gives a perfume its depth and staying power, usually made from the mosses and musks. Since these changes do take place, it is essential to give yourself enough time to judge something new. The first impression on your skin may be too sharp, but left for a while the perfume may mellow, smelling warmer, sweeter or softer. A perfume which isn't right for you will continue to smell unpleasant to you. Try no more than two perfumes at a time to avoid confusing your senses. Pulse points at the wrist are best.

Since marketing plays a big part in perfume sales your first choices should be those you identify with from advertising. Make a list of those that appeal and work through until you find the ones you love.

Many chemists keep a book of perfume families — if they haven't got the one you ask for they can recommend others in the same 'family' to help narrow the choice.

Mood can affect perfume choice as well as your personality. Here's a quick guide with some perfume examples.

Extrovert, innovative — choose the lighter florals, fresh with a tang of citrus: *Barynia* (Helena Rubinstein), *Charlie* (Revlon), *Cristalle* (Chanel), *Diorissimo* (Dior), *First* (Van Cleef and Arpels), *Fidji* (Laroche), *K de Krizia* (Krizia), *Scoundrel* (Revlon).
Seductive, mysterious — choose the exotic, oriental perfumes: KL (Lagerfeld), *Opium* (Yves Saint Laurent), *Shalimar* (Guerlain), *Cinnabar* (Estee Lauder), *Pure Silk* (Yardley), *Serpent* (Covers).
Practical, worldly — choose warm perfumes, floral with a mixture of wood and spices: *Armani* (Giorgio Armani), *Cachet* (Matchabelli), *Epris* (Max Factor), *Ma Griffe* (Carven), *Miss Dior* (Dior), *White Satin* (Yardley).
Elegant, sophisticated — choose the classics, mostly floral with the smoky warmth of sandalwood, amber and musk: *Arpege* (Lanvin), *Chanel No 5* (Chanel), *Je Reviens* (Worth), *Mystere* (Rochas), *White Linen* (Estee Lauder), *Tweed* (Lentheric).
Calm, orderly — choose something floral with a hint of the exotic: *Forever Krystle* (Carrington Parfums), *Magie Noire* (Lancome), *Le Jardin* (Max Factor), *Youth Dew* (Estee Lauder).
Romantic, dreamy — choose the warm florals with ingredients such as gardenia and musk: *Anais Anais* (Cacharel), *Chamade* (Guerlain), *Fleurs de Fleurs* (Nina Ricci), *Beautiful* (Estee Lauder), *Lumiere* (Rochas), *Moonwind* (Avon), *Panache* (Lentheric), *Rive Gauche* (Yves Saint Laurent), *Soft Musk* (Avon).
Dare to be different? Choose the perfumes designed *not* to fit into particular categories: *Poison* (Dior) with its spicy, fruit qualities; *Alliage* (Estee Lauder) green and spicy; *Coco* (Chanel) orange and rose with frangipani, clove, mimosa and peach; *Vanderbilt* (Gloria Vanderbilt), fresh and fruity with a hint of warm spice.

Perfume is a very personal choice as it says a lot about your moods and personality. Find the scent that suits you.

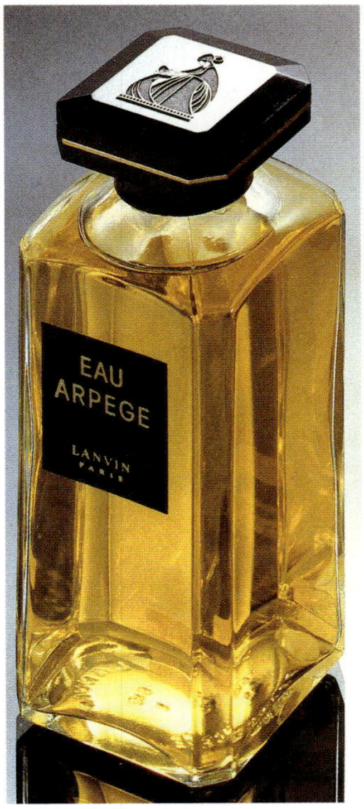

ageing gracefully

The term 'middle-aged' sounds strangely out of date nowadays, when styles in hair, clothes and make-up have reached the ultimate in easy-to-wear casual smartness that looks as good on someone of 20 as on someone of forty-five. Have you noticed also how so many women manage to look prettier, more confident and relaxed — more youthful even — than they did in their teens and twenties? Perhaps this is simply because self-assurance and knowing what suits you is something that can only develop over years of experiment to discover how to make the most of your colouring, skin type, figure and features. This of course doesn't mean wearing the same eyeshadow, blusher and lipstick at 40 as you did at twenty-two. In fact nothing is more ageing than wearing the same make-up as you did then or five years ago. Not only will those same colours and textures probably not suit you any longer — they'll also be out of fashion and look desperately dated!

Although the latest outrageous make-up gimmicks are not for you if you're much over 30 or 35, do keep an eye open for the newest colours and formulas which can enhance — not swamp — your own features. Nothing can beat well applied make-up to help you look your best as you get older. No matter how flawless or attractive a woman's face, good make-up can only make her look more attractive, radiant and probably younger.

Greater self-assurance and years of determining what does and doesn't suit gives many older woman a more attractive and radiant look.

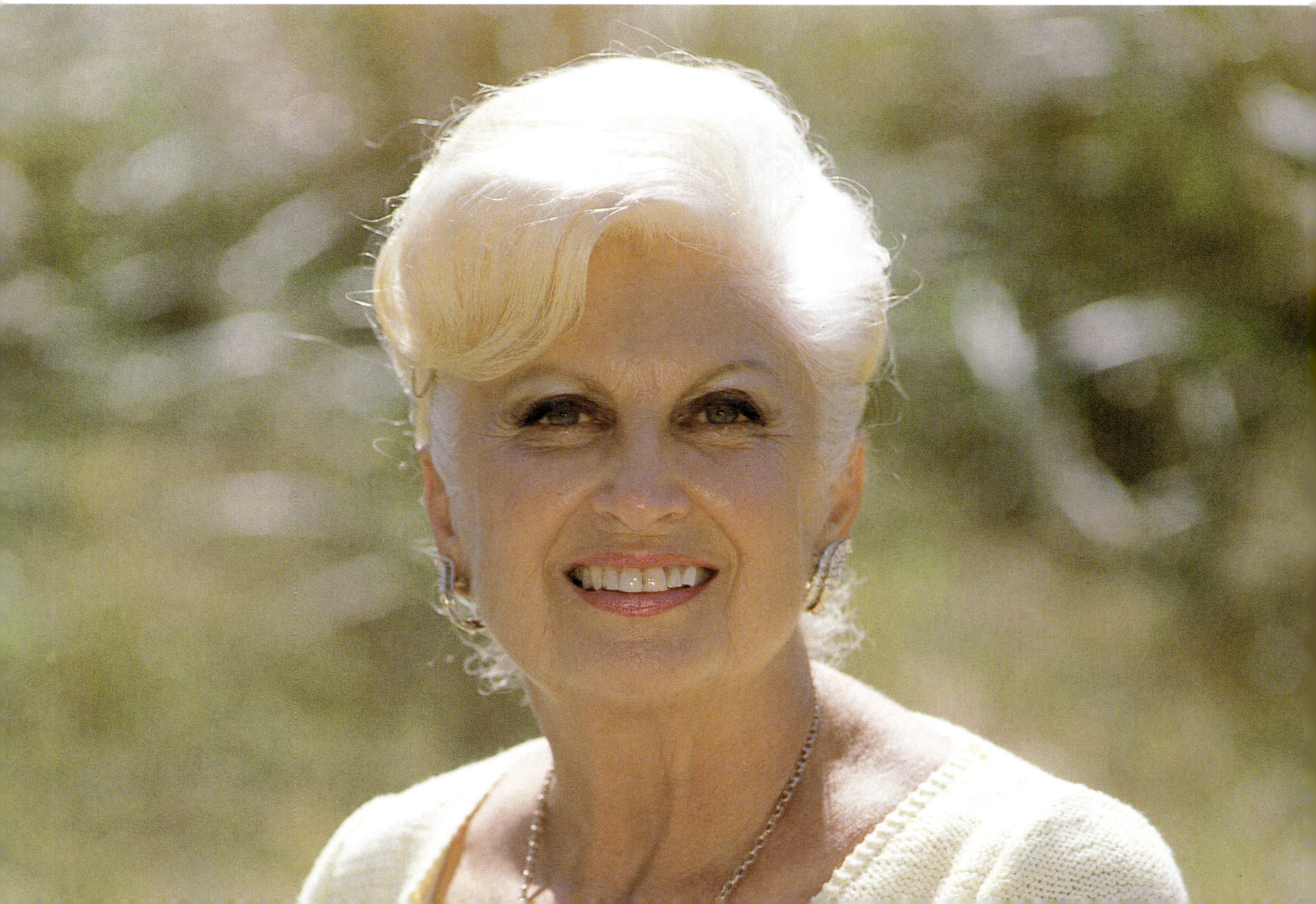

As you get older skin tone often gets sallower, greyer, more uneven and marred by patches of darker pigmentation, broken red veins and weathering. This is where a lightweight fluid, tinted foundation works wonders in evening out and brightening skin colour without giving a flat, matt, powdery effect. Choose a tint that's as similar as possible to your own skin tone and which blends in quickly to give a semi-opaque coverage: just enough to hide tiny flaws and blemishes and impart a healthy radiance to the skin. This doesn't mean lashing out on an expensive product. You can get very reasonably priced make-up these days that offers a wide range of shades and textures. Powder should always be colourless and translucent to avoid caking, settling into facial lines and creases, and altering your foundation tone.

For enlarging and defining the eyes, concentrate on the natural colour pigments such as grey, brown, taupe, beige, sage; tones that you'll find naturally in human skin under different lights. Bright, colourful eyeliners and shadows should be kept for parties and evening wear, when strong artificial lights drain the face of gentler colours. Upbeat purples, mauves, blues, greens and brick-browns tend to look hard and draw attention to lines and crepeyness around the eyes. Frosted powders also act as a rather cruel spotlight, focusing on wrinkles and slack skin, so it's best to stick to matt blushers, eyeshadows and highlighters after a certain age. Powder generally in all its different forms is easier to apply and gives a smoother, more long-lasting finish to make-up than the messier cream rouges and liquid eyeshadows, 'polishes' and highlighters that often give an uneven 'blobby' effect.

If you like to outline your eyes along the rim of the lashes you'll avoid any hard-edged definition by using a very soft, waxy kohl crayon or eye pencil that glides on in soft focus without pulling at the delicate skin around the eyes. Crayon gives a softly blurred line as opposed to liquid or cake liner which can look unduly severe. Very bright lipsticks can make even a young face look pinched, hard and garish — but on a more mature face or lips that are lined they look positively grotesque. Outline the mouth with a neutral-toned crayon — beige, dark brown, earthy red — then choose a sheer and creamy, slightly frosted tawny, beige pink, coral or peachy lipstick. Avoid so-called 'hot' pinks, 'dead' purply-browns and reds, pillarbox scarlet or blue-reds, which dry and stain the lips, add 10 years to virtually any face and drain it of colour.

SKIN CARE

The biggest bonus of getting older is that the skin often settles into a calm trouble-free period after the ups and downs of the teens and twenties. Acne, blackheads, excessive oiliness, pimples have generally run their course by the time you reach your early thirties. As you learn the method of skin care that is best suited to you, you're less likely to flounder around and will be more 'in charge' of the regular attention required by your skin type. Even though skin gets drier as the years go by, the basic rules of deep cleansing, toning, moisturising and nourishing still apply, although you may decide to change the type of products you use. Again, as with make-up, it's a mistake to think that spending more money on exotic or overpriced creams and lotions will prevent your skin from showing natural signs of age, because they won't — whatever the advertisements say!

Spending money at a beauty salon to have facials is only worthwhile if just for a change you want someone else to do for your skin what you should be doing for it yourself. However, if you lead a very active and busy life without much time to spend on home routines, a monthly facial will certainly help your skin to look fresher and better groomed — but probably no younger! This is because beauty therapists do use some extremely effective appliances to help them steam, deep cleanse, refine, brighten and soften the skin. For instance, a mild galvanic current (cathiordermie) helps creams and lotions penetrate the epidermis more effectively while rotating face brushes stimulate the circulation, and also encourage products to be absorbed by the skin.

As you get older you're bound to notice that certain areas of your face and body seem to age faster and in a different way to others — no matter how well you look after them. Being clued up and prepared for these gradual changes can help you cope with them more effectively and even slow down the rate at which they occur.

Upper lip

Tiny vertical creases that form along the upper lip sometimes creating a blurred or jagged lip line usually start to form sometime in the forties. These are often caused by puckering up the mouth or by smoking. Make sure you apply protective moisturiser at all times, and blend your foundation well into the lip line, and powder before outlining the mouth.

Eyes

The fine skin around the eyes can begin to show crow's feet, 'laughter lines', bags, dark circles and crepeyness as early as the mid- or late twenties. Avoid too much sunbathing, always protect the skin with a good sunscreen, use a lightweight eye cream at night and plenty of moisturiser under your make-up. Have your eyesight checked regularly to avoid screwing up the eyes and try to wear good sunglasses in bright, glaring light and sunny weather. Minimise dark lines and circles with a trace of buff-coloured concealer stick on top of your foundation, and make sure you get enough sleep so you don't cultivate shadows in the first place. Puffiness and 'bags' under the eyes can be caused by fluid retention — especially while you sleep — so use compresses soaked in ice-cold witch hazel, eyebright herbal tea, or an eye tonic to decongest the area and remember not to use too much eye cream at night as this can also puff up the skin.

Neck

The skin on the throat, neck and chest is often a prime giveaway of age, becoming rough, discoloured and marked with horizontal 'necklace' lines usually through poor posture, wearing rough polo-necked sweaters, too much sunbathing and lack of proper moisturising. Avoid this by carrying through *all* your usual facial treatments onto the neck area, particularly your moisturiser and night cream which should be extended right down to the collarbones to prevent crepeyness and lines from developing. A good clay-based mask used once or twice a month tightens and brightens the skin, counteracting dingy or yellow skin tones and refining the pores. From the age of 30 onwards a rich body cream or baby lotion smoothed in after bathing will help to keep the skin soft and supple.

Hands

The paper fine skin on the backs of the hands is particularly prone to dehydration and pigment problems from the mid- to late forties onwards. Keep the skin well cosseted by using hand cream every time you put your hands into water and by wearing an effective sunscreen when you go out into the sun. 'Liver spots', those dark mottled patches that appear after about the age of 50, are something of a mystery to dermatologists and unfortunately once they develop there's little you can do to shift them. A good bleaching cream may help to fade them slightly and a strong sunblock will prevent the sun from making them worse.

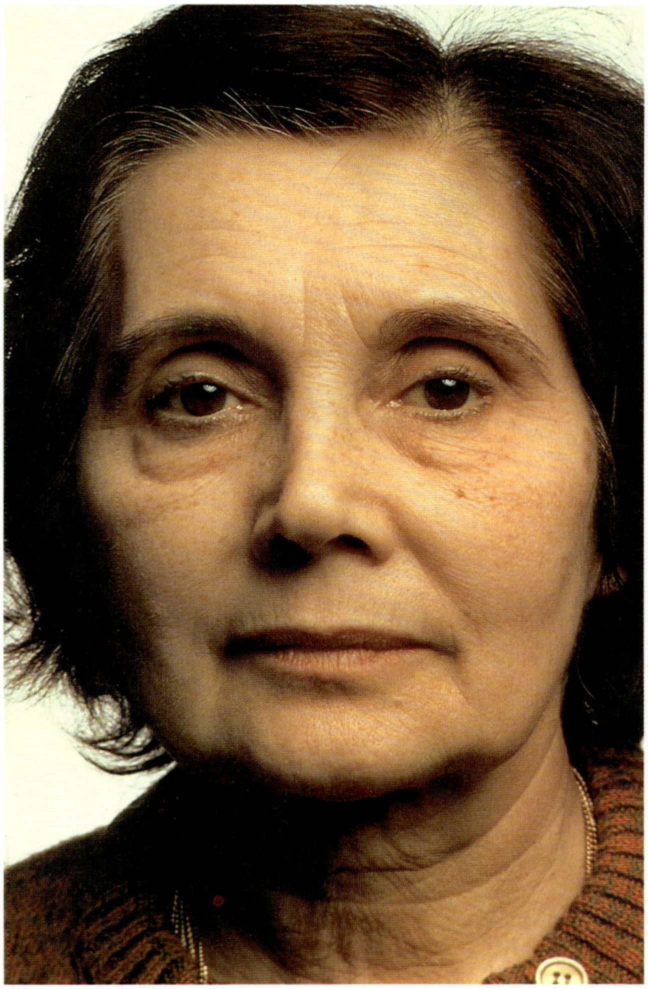

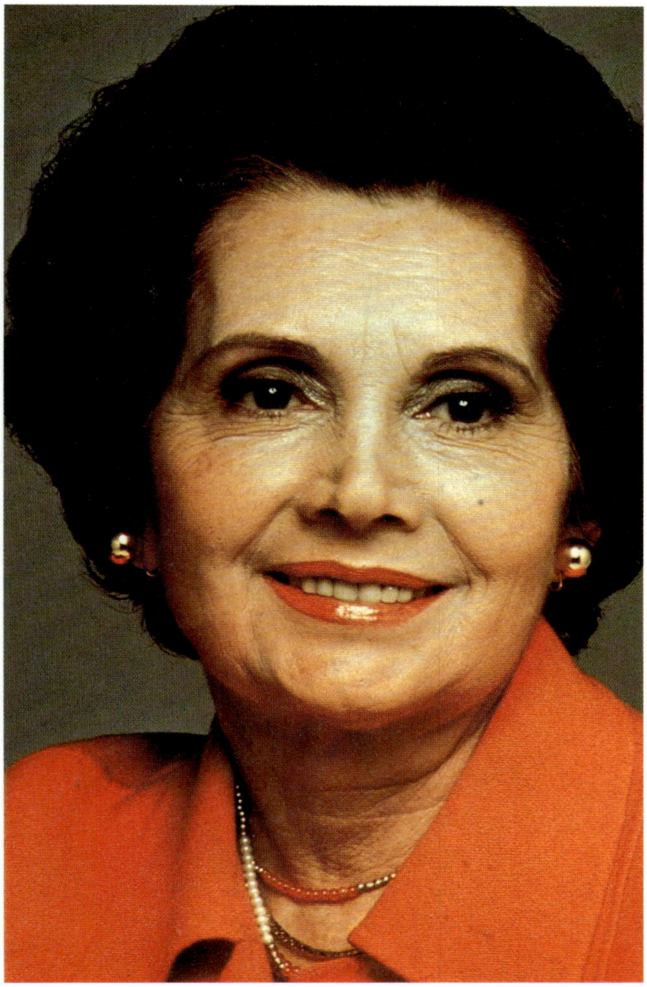

Make-up: Glenn Roberts (Elizabeth Arden)

Good make-up can take years off your face.

Stretch marks

One of the possible results of pregnancy (especially if you gain a lot of extra weight), is the appearance of fine white or silvery lines caused by overstretching and rupturing of the skin's surface. These can appear on the tummy, hips, thighs and breasts and cannot be removed once they've formed — so take care generally not to go through extreme yo-yo weight changes. Regular massage with a good body cream or oil helps keep the skin supple and conditioned during pregnancy.

Wrinkles and lines

A famous American beautician once said that a face without lines is like a book without words — and it's easy enough to appreciate her point, since few of us over the age of 25 would like a blank, vacuous, mask-like face, no matter how pretty it was. As we pass out of our teens, all of us inevitably develop a few lines and facial marks that distinguish individual character and personality. These are, after all, a natural and unavoidable side effect of the way we move and use our faces to talk, smile, eat, laugh and think; expression lines which start to etch themselves onto the face from the twenties on, and gradually become deeper and more pronounced over the years. The lines and wrinkles that you *should* try to prevent forming prematurely are those that result from skin damage. Too much sunbathing, very dry atmospheres, cold icy winds, smoking, drinking a lot of alcohol and crash dieting can all too easily lead to dehydrated, papery skin, the formation of deep wrinkles and creases on the cheeks, and a loss of elasticity and firm facial

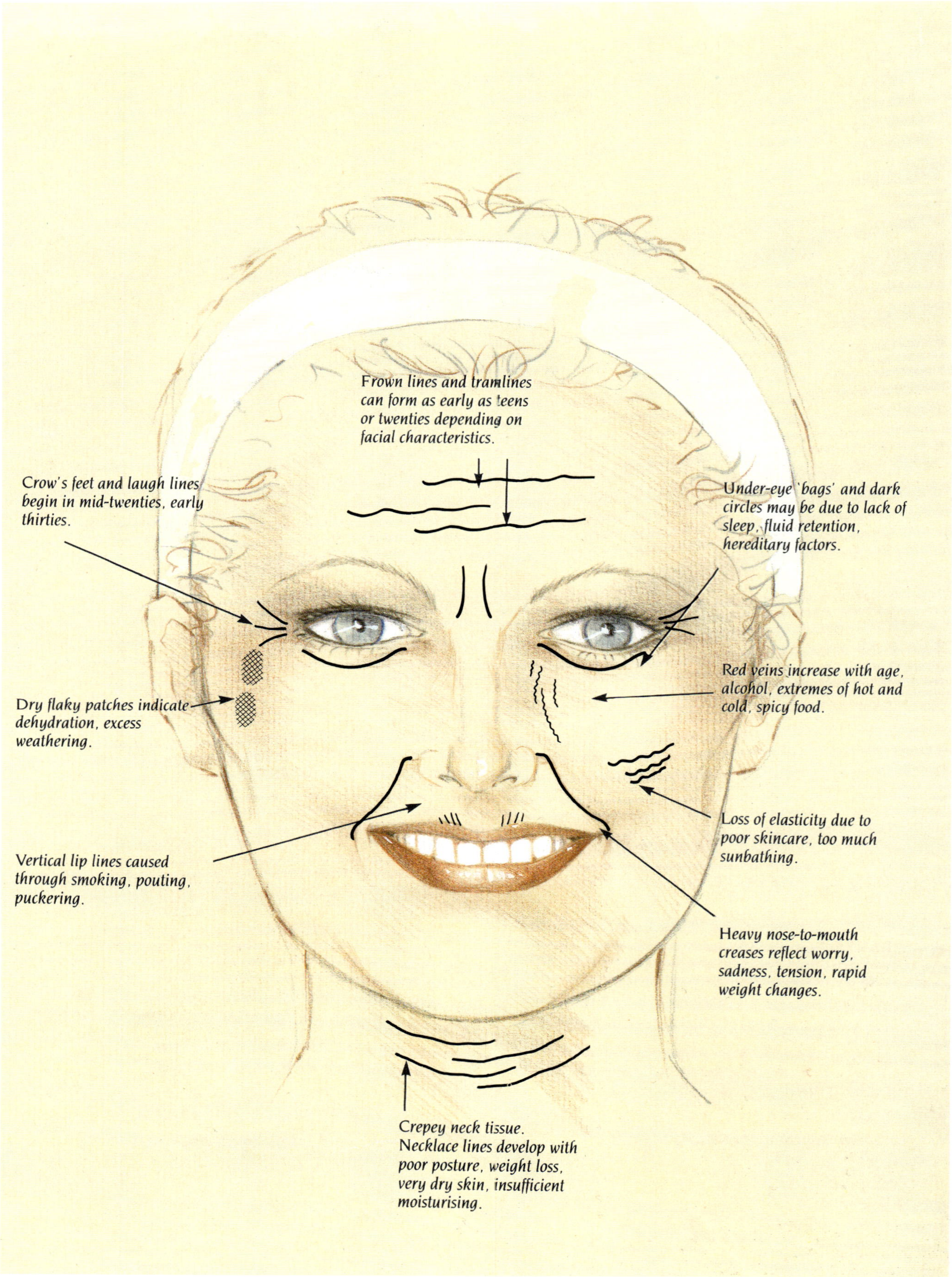
Frown lines and tramlines can form as early as teens or twenties depending on facial characteristics.
Crow's feet and laugh lines begin in mid-twenties, early thirties.
Under-eye 'bags' and dark circles may be due to lack of sleep, fluid retention, hereditary factors.
Red veins increase with age, alcohol, extremes of hot and cold, spicy food.
Dry flaky patches indicate dehydration, excess weathering.
Loss of elasticity due to poor skincare, too much sunbathing.
Vertical lip lines caused through smoking, pouting, puckering.
Heavy nose-to-mouth creases reflect worry, sadness, tension, rapid weight changes.
Crepey neck tissue. Necklace lines develop with poor posture, weight loss, very dry skin, insufficient moisturising.

contours. Caused by an excessive reduction in the skin's moisture level and the destruction of its collagen and elastic fibres, there is nothing you can do to remove these signs of age once they've appeared. They can, however, be minimised by using a rich daytime moisturiser under your make-up and massaging a deep-acting treatment cream into the face and neck at night. There are also some very effective so-called 'shock treatments' and 'cures' on the market, creams and serums designed to be used over a two- or three-week period to soften and smooth very dry skin and plump out lines. Deep-moisturising masks which can be applied all over the eye area also help to condition the skin, while, for the odd special occasion you can apply a temporary 'anti-wrinkle' gel or cream which subtly smoothes out wrinkles and tightens loose contours by covering the skin with a fine translucent film. It is very difficult to firm up the chin and cheek area and the skin around the mouth once the muscles have become slack and the skin has lost its resilience. Using a small electronic facial massage unit can help to tone lazy muscles and tighten the area — but only if you do this promptly and regularly. Exercising generally — particularly aerobics and dance classes — helps to keep facial contours firm and supple while increasing the supply of blood to the skin, giving the skin a healthier, less lined appearance.

Figure problems

Our general metabolism — the rate at which we burn up the food we eat — starts to slow down significantly from the age of 35 onwards, although to what degree depends on how far we allow our lifestyles to become less active and more sedentary. It's around this age that you should avoid gaining extra weight as it becomes increasingly difficult to shed the surplus kilograms you acquire in later years. Areas that are notoriously liable to 'fill out' are the waist, tummy, hips, thighs and buttocks, since women carry an extra layer of fatty tissue on these parts of the body. Try and trim your eating habits to suit your energy demands and remember that eating more food without compensating by taking extra physical activity to burn it up will most certainly mean that you put on weight where it isn't wanted. Resist the urge to indulge in snacks between meals and buns, chocolates, biscuits, sweets, ice-cream, sweet drinks and alcohol. Adopt a regular exercise programme that you enjoy to help firm the muscles, banish flab and burn up kilojoules. Specific problems such as a slack or drooping bustline, 'spare tyre' or wads of fat on thighs and hips can be improved by doing gym exercises that strengthen and whittle down those areas, going to a health club that offers 'spot reduction' treatments usually in the form of intensive massage, or attending aerobics classes which have a general effect.

RADICAL TREATMENTS FOR AGEING SKIN

Dermabrasion

This is one solution to facial lines, but it is not the answer for everyone. It involves removing the top layer of skin via an abrasive technique which must be carried out by a skin specialist or cosmetic surgeon. In some people, the after-effects may be long lasting, or even permanent, which is why it is vital to have advice from a medically qualified professional before going ahead.

The skin underneath the peeled layer is unattractively blemished for a couple of weeks after the process, but then the scabbing disappears and the skin adopts a pink hue which can last several weeks. This technique can be successfully accompanied by the threading of soluble vicryl into the lines under the skin. The body's defences mass to the area and, after the chemical has dissolved, fill the lines out and make the skin appear smoother. Some people suffer a marked difference in skin tone and pigmentation after dermabrasion.

Chemical peeling

This is a similar technique to dermabrasion, in that the top skin layer is removed, but in this case it is taken off through application of caustic chemicals. Again it is wise to seek advice from a medically qualified skin specialist before going ahead, as some people react badly to the chemical preparation used.

Cosmetic laser

This technique can be successfully carried out by trained beauticians and can go quite a long way towards improving lines and wrinkles, especially among middle-aged women with some skin elasticity. The wrinkles are treated with a concentrated beam of light and, while the results are less dramatic than those of a facelift, it is painless and less costly.

Collagen implants

Again, this technique should be carried out by a medically qualified skin specialist. Zyderm collagen is simply injected into lines and wrinkles with the use of fine needles, with the effect that they are immediately smoothed out. The process is costly and needs to be repeated fairly frequently, but is not suitable if a patient really needs a fairly radical facelift. Before going ahead, it is important to screen the patient to ensure there will be no reaction against the collagen.

Facelifting

Having a facelift is just one aspect of cosmetic surgery that can be used to arrest the ageing process. It must obviously be carried out by a surgeon who cuts the skin above the hairline to below the ear and behind the lobe, then takes away excess skin and lifts tissue and muscle beneath to form a firmer base. This tucking process will not provide the foundation of eternal youth, but will certainly do something for sagging facial skin. The ageing process does, of course, continue, so it may be necessary to repeat the procedure again in the future. Eyelifts, where either the upper lid is tucked to remove the hooding effect, or the lower lid operated upon to remove fat causing 'bagging', are also available.

Liposuction

Localised fat deposits can be removed via this technique and it can be applied to any part of the body. The fat is simply suctioned off via a tube which is inserted through a small incision made in a natural skin fold. As far as the face is concerned, liposuction has proved particularly successful in reducing fat beneath the chin, but should always be carried out by a medically qualified professional.

Acupuncture

If you hate the idea of surgery, or many of the scientifically based anti-ageing techniques, then acupuncture may be the answer. With the use of fine needles and a knowledge of this ancient skill, lines and wrinkles can be softened and skin sagginess firmed almost painlessly. Success varies from patient to patient, as does the length of treatment.

hair care

The condition and style of your hair can have a devastating effect not only on your general appearance, but also on your self-confidence and inner feeling of well-being. On a bad day the state of your hair can do as much to depress you and make you feel an unkempt mess, as on another it can make you feel glamorous and elated.

After all there are few things more demoralising than being caught out on a last-minute social event or business appointment with hair that's lost its style or needs a wash or trim. Ultimately our looks are judged by the quality and style of our hair. Fashionable clothes, jewellery, pretty make-up and chic accessories lose 80 per cent of their impact if they are teamed with hair

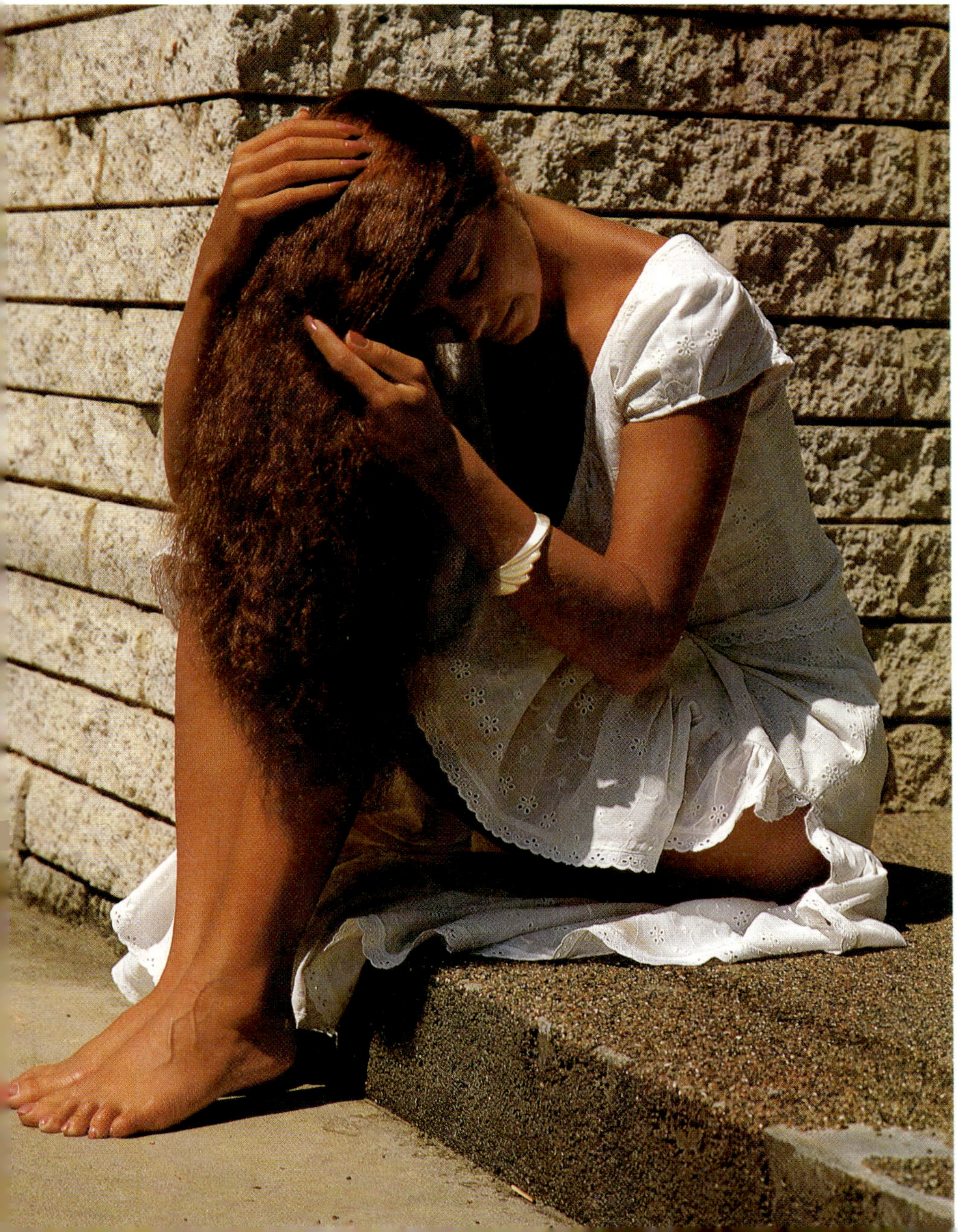

What has more overall impact than a head of beautiful, conditioned, healthy hair?

that's either in poor condition or badly styled. Over the past 10–15 years, there has of course been a phenomenal revolution both in hair care and styling, which has liberated us from gimmicky and elaborate hard-to-manage 'set' hairstyles and given more women the opportunity to state their individuality through the different ways in which they wear their hair. Almost any hairstyle is acceptable nowadays, as long as it suits your features, and never before has so much expert help been available when tackling hair and scalp problems or for altering the texture, colour and condition of hair itself.

HAIR TYPES

The texture and behaviour of hair (just like skin) determines both the way you need to treat it and how best to wear it. Since hair-care manufacturers nowadays produce special formulas for many different types of hair, it's important to identify yours.

Normal hair

Unfortunately rare it is usually delightfully well behaved, neither too dry nor too greasy. The effects of washing and styling may last anything between five and eight days. Whether straight or curly, it is easy to manage, and adapts to a selection of diverse styles. Try not to perm or colour it as you may encourage problems.

Dry hair

Generally it goes with a dry scalp which doesn't produce enough natural oils to keep the surface of the hair soft, smooth and shiny. Often rather fine and flyaway, it tends to lack lustre and reacts badly to perming, tinting and extreme heat. Prone to split ends and breaking, conditioning is all important to feed the scalp and moisturise the outer cuticle of the hair.

Greasy hair

It usually becomes lank, dull and dandruff-prone and loses its shape and bounce even a day or two after washing. Like an oily skin (which it often accompanies) it is due to overactive sebaceous glands (on the scalp) that coat the hair with an abundance of natural oils. Mild and frequent shampooing and a correct diet can help check oiliness.

SHAMPOOS

Conditioning comes before everything after that comes the cut, then the colour. But if you don't have hair that's in perfect condition the last two don't mean a thing. Strong words, but ones that underline today's all-out emphasis on an unstructured beauty that radiates health and fitness. Conditioning, more than a mere after-thought, begins the moment you wash your hair. These days this is a more subtle procedure than just shampooing up a storm of bubbles. To begin with, resist the urge to pick up any old jumbo-sized brand of cheap shampoo that catches your eye amongst the washing powders and scouring agents at the supermarket. Invest instead in protein-enriched, pH-balanced shampoos which cleanse hair and scalp gently instead of stripping them abrasively of oils and moisture.

Frequent shampooing with a harsh alkaline detergent product is the fastest way to loosen and rough up the outer scaly layer of your hair — the 'cuticle' — encouraging split ends and general dryness. Because all hair — whatever

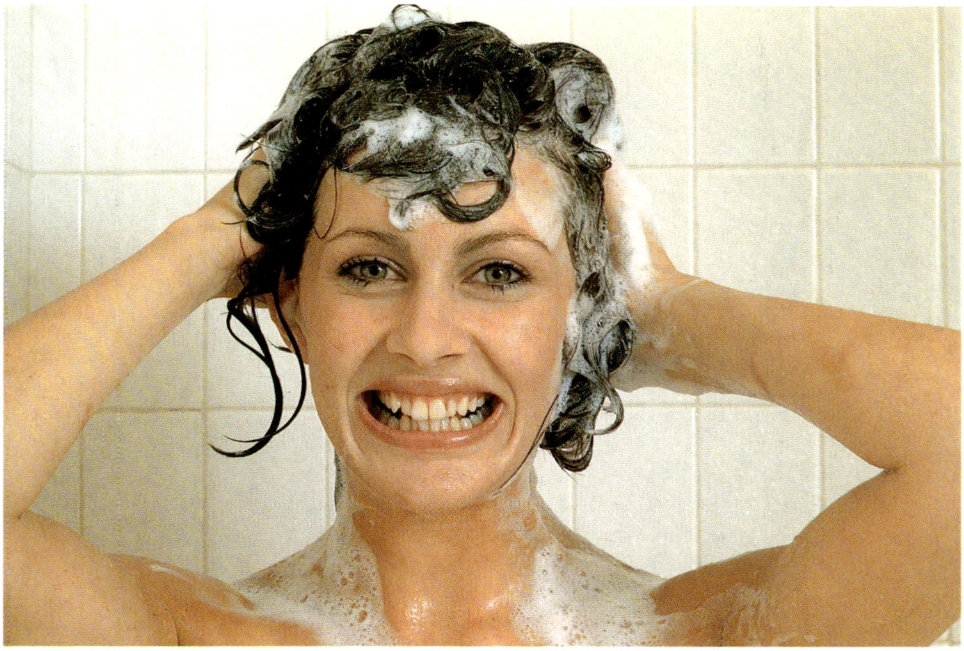

Treat your hair as you would your skin in so much as you wouldn't omit using a moisturiser, so why skimp on a hair conditioner? After shampooing, use a conditioner for protection and to repair dry and damaged hair.

its type — needs the tender touch, one really good shampoo can be used for every hair type. Just increase or decrease the frequency of washing, as well as the application, and work up less lather if you have greasy hair.

Resist the urge to let your hair wallow in suds; the more often you wash it, the more you should try and get by on only one application of shampoo — which is ample to dissolve and lift out grease, grime and general debris. However, if you suffer from a severely greasy scalp — with or without the added bane of dandruff — opt for a shampoo designed especially to combat and control the problem.

The way you treat your hair when it's wet also has lasting effects on its general condition. More damage is inflicted to hair through rough, hasty, slipshod towelling and combing prior to drying, than during actual styling. It's a pitfall you can come up against, even at an established and leading hairdresser, if the shampoo girl or boy happens to have climbed out of the wrong side of bed on a particular day! Squeeze and pat water out of your hair — don't rub it endlessly with a rough towel, and never use a brush or a cheap, spiky, fine-toothed comb on wet hair. Hair is at its most elastic, and therefore its weakest, when wet, so gently ease out irritating knots and tangles with a broad-toothed comb with round edges. If your hair is long, begin combing slowly at the bottom of the hair and work your way upwards to reduce stress on the hair fibres.

CONDITIONING

Just as you wouldn't cleanse and wash your face without protecting it afterwards with a moisturiser, you shouldn't ask for hair problems by skipping on conditioning and retexturising. Much like skincare products, conditioners work on different levels of the hair structure, depending on its degree of dryness and damage.

Instant *creme rinses*, fast and easy to use, act principally on the surface of the hair, coating it with a fine wax-like film that smoothes down the ruffled scales of the outer cuticle helping to make hair shiny as well as manageable, tangle-free and more able to hold its style. Protein *retexturising creams* and *moisturising treatments* should be left on the hair for 10–20 minutes as they help to correct damage caused by tinting, perming, bleaching, sunlight, central heating, seawater and chlorine as well as surface dehydration from hairdryers, tongs and heated rollers. They help to boost and strengthen the protein structure of damaged hair and should be used by anyone worried about brittle dry hair. Watch out for deeply nourishing and moisturising elements like avocado, peachnut oil, eggs, honey, camomile, henna, coconut oil, lemon, nettle and rosemary. All are renowned for restoring suppleness to hair of all types. *Treatment packs* are much thicker, creamier products, rich in extra oils, waxes and other emollients. Like a face pack they must be kept on the hair for 30 minutes or more, depending on the amount of abuse that has been meted out to your hair in the cause of fickleness and fashion! Anyone with tinted, bleached, permed, or continually tonged and heated hair needs to redress as many of the ill-effects as possible by applying monthly or even weekly packs. As the head is usually covered with a polythene hood or a towel to trap body heat and make the oils penetrate more deeply, there are plenty of things you can be getting on with in the home while your hair is being treated. Even applying warm olive or almond oil to the scalp and massaging it in well and wrapping it in warm towels can help to recondition dry, brittle hair. Very fine, extra dry or flyaway hair may need coaxing into order and style with a *hair thickener* or a *blow-dry lotion* which is not rinsed off. These merely bond with the hair's outer layer, providing an added protective coating which builds body and strength, adds shine, and protects hair from overcooking under the heat of the hairdryer. Blow-dry lotions are an excellent safeguard against damage if your style requires a lot of tugging, brushing and tweaking while you dry it.

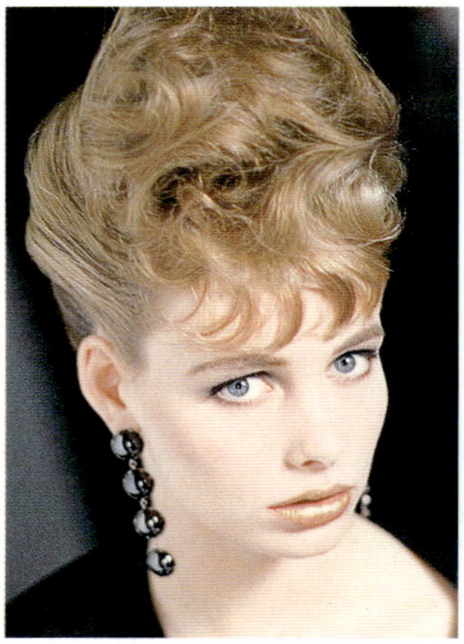

Hair by Sloanes of Paddington for Wella Australia

This set hair has shaped up to a stunning, elegant style.

SHAPING UP — SETTING AND DRYING

Women tend to forget the immense strain on the hair imposed by regular shampooing, setting and drying. Hair cannot handle even very mild and gentle shampooing without reacting adversely in some way — however small.

When you are drying hair the most important thing to remember is to keep the air warm, never hot. Hair, after all, burns as much, if not as dramatically, as skin.

Roller setting is pretty passe as far as today's free-and-easy unstructured styles go, as any leading hairdresser will vouch; towel and finger drying, the use of hairdryers and allowing the hair to dry naturally are all less aggressive ways of putting shape and movement into hair.

However, if you are determined to achieve a neatly 'set' look — or else if you have very long or thick hair — try and follow a few basic rules to achieve a professional effect with the minimum amount of damage.

1 Sprinkle damp hair with setting lotion that contains the very minimum of alcohol.

2 Section off small areas of hair with precise partings and the help of a tail comb. Roll these very carefully and not too tightly beginning at the crown, working towards the front and sides and then the back. Never put too much tension on the hair and avoid spiked rollers which can damage the hair and cause splitting and breaking.

3 When hair is completely dry, remove rollers gently and brush hair thoroughly in one direction, then the other to eliminate any roller or pin marks.

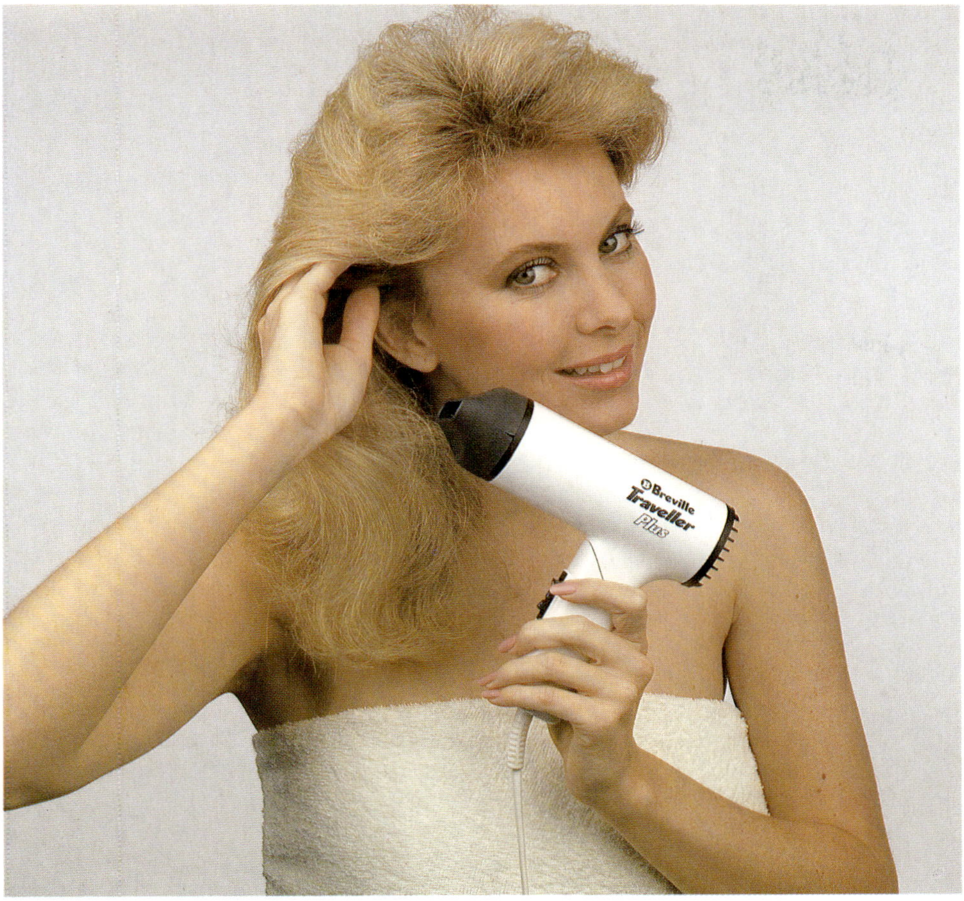

Breville/Cleo

Don't scorch your hair when using a dryer. Always keep the temperature down. Blow drying makes it possible to achieve a range of formal and informal styles.

BLOW DRYING

A good brush, an accurate eye and a deft wrist are all you need to create some of the most bouncy, smooth and natural-looking styles. Good blow drying gives long-lasting shape and volume to medium and long hair and is invaluable for adding swing and movement to hair of any length, plus giving that jaunty lift at the roots that stops hair looking flat and lank.

1 Blot hair dry with a towel, comb gently and apply blow-dry lotion if your hair is fine or prone to static electricity.

2 Hold dryer at least 15 centimetres from the hair and keep it moving. To begin with, ruffle the hair gently at the roots with the fingers to take out the dampness, then start to lift the base of different sections with your brush, drying the underneath of each section thoroughly.

3 To achieve last minute flicks or curves or to guide the style in a definite direction, wind sections of hair firmly over a round brush and direct the heat along the top of this for a moment or two, then unwind. Never 'grill' the hair.

4 Short, layered urchin cuts can be blow dried using just the finger to tweak and ruffle the hair casually into shape.

Your hairbrush

The size, shape and quality of the hairbrush you use is all important both to the condition as well as to the final result you want to achieve. Natural bristles are the gentlest, and ideal for very fine or frizzy hair, while nylon and bristle mixtures can be used on hair that's a bit thicker and coarser. Very long hair needs the support and even curve of a circular 'jumbo' brush, although it's easier to get under and around shorter, layered hair with a semicircular brush or one that's round but has a small circumference. Straight-as-a-die styles fall more evenly and fully if trained into place with a broad flat brush, preferably one shaped to the head with bristles set into a rubber cushion. Remember also to always keep brushes and combs immaculately clean.

STYLING

The style that's right for you flatters your face shape, is easy to manage *and* earns you compliments. The secret of great styling is in the mixture of your ideas and the expertise of your hairdresser in interpreting what you want and being able to follow it through. First you come up with the way you would like to see your hair based on your lifestyle and the image you have of yourself. Then your hairdresser considers how the look you love will work with your hair, head and face shape. Sometimes there has to be compromise, occasionally it's a straight 'no' when hair is too damaged to be permed or coloured. There's usually some alternative if you can't have what you want right away.

Your face

Its shape will dictate, to a large extent, which styles you can consider and those you should rule out. Draw your hair off your face and consider whether it is round, square, oval or heart-shaped and decide whether you have a long or short neck, as this can also affect styling.

Your features

Everyone has good points they wish to emphasise and others they prefer to disguise, and these can affect your choice of hairstyle as much as your face shape. For instance, particularly large and beautiful eyes can distract from a round and chubby face, while otherwise even and perfect features may need a little extra help from the hair if they also include a prominent nose. Assess your pros and cons — the strength of your bone structure and jawline together with the size of your nose, ears and eyes — by checking your face from all angles in the mirror.

Your style

Though you may be one of those lucky people who can successfully change their whole appearance at the drop of a hat, most of us feel more at home with a hairstyle that settles into our own established ideas of how we should look. Although we may be quite happy to lop centimetres off the length, or add some curls or colour, few of us are really happy with a style that makes us feel we've undergone a complete personality change — thus the punk rocker with the red and purple mohican cut will no more welcome the sleekly subtle blonde highlights adopted by the Princess of Wales than Her Royal Highness would opt for that outlandish look. It is also worth considering the time, effort and expense you're prepared to put into maintaining a hairstyle; there is no point in setting your heart on a look that requires endless blow-drying, gelling, tonging or teasing if you're the wash and wear type. Also, avoid cuts or colourings likely to need regular, costly touchings-up if you're on a limited budget.

Your shape

Do bear in mind your physical dimensions when choosing a hairstyle; for instance, a close crop may look out of proportion with a large or broad physique while a very dramatic style may overwhelm a very small figure.

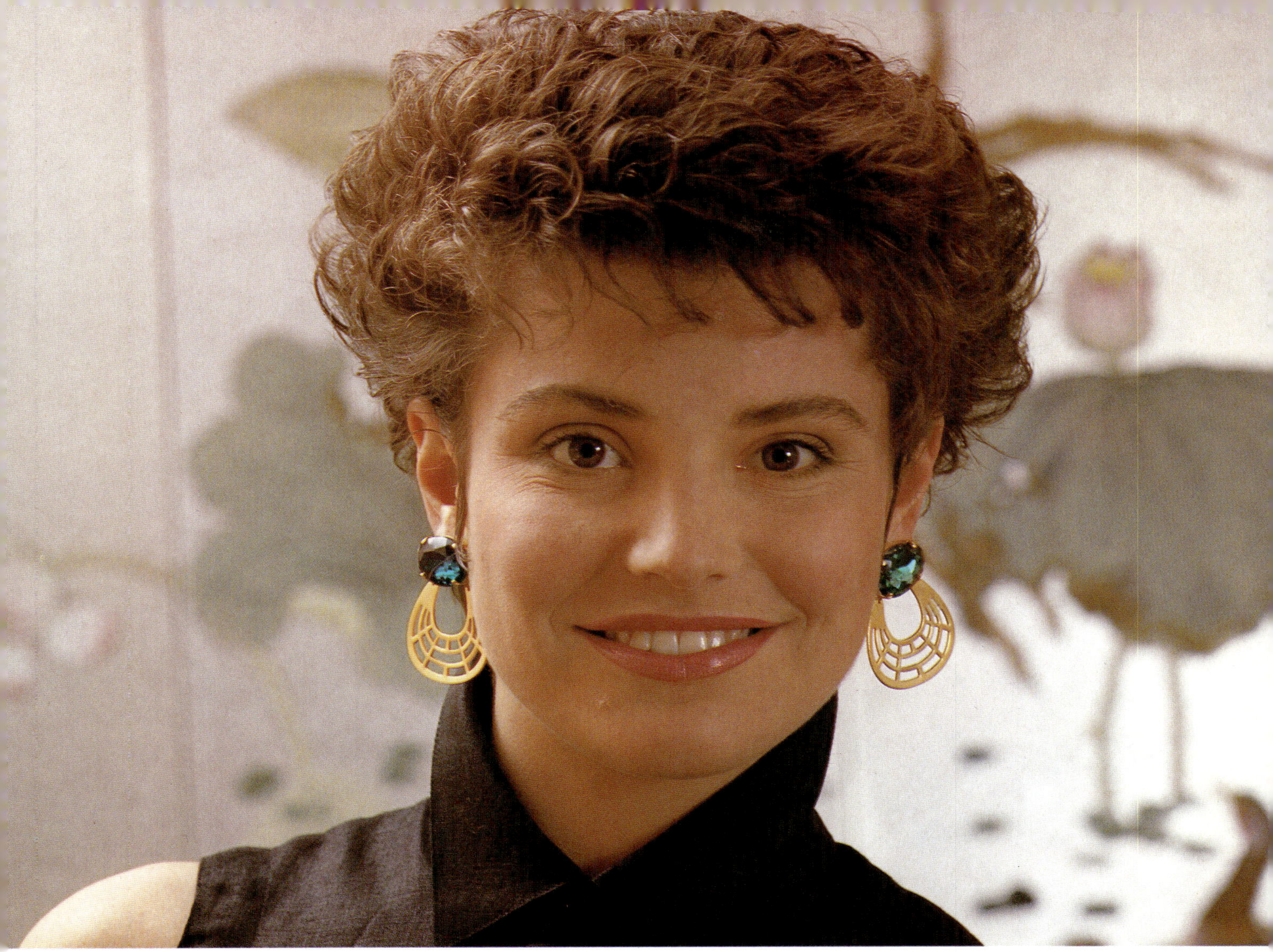

Choose a style that suits your shape, features and lifestyle. It is pointless getting a style which requires hours of blow drying, teasing or gelling if you're the wash and wear type.

Some tricks of the trade

Here are some guidelines used by hairdressers when assessing a client's hairstyling requirements:

Round face — to disguise a broad or chubby face, choose a style that gives height on top, while keeping fullness to a minimum at the sides.

Long face — to disguise length, create a style with fullness at the sides of the face and perhaps some hair around the forehead. Some faces may benefit from a fringe.

Square face — the solidity of a square face needs some softening, so it makes sense to break the line of the jaw, the cheeks or the forehead.

Low forehead — the slightly squat appearance created by a low forehead can be disguised with a style that conceals the hairline. Starting a fringe from the top of the head, near the crown, can also give the impression of a higher forehead beneath.

Large nose — a prominent nose can be minimised by adding fullness and fluffiness to the crown of the head, yet narrowing the way the hair falls onto the neck.

Flat crown — where hair flattens off the top of the head, more height can be artificially created by gelling or moussing it into a spiky style or leaving it longer and perming it for extra body. The rest of the hair is best kept short.

Fall-away chin — a flat crown and hair styled for fullness at the nape of the neck should go a long way towards disguising a receding chin.

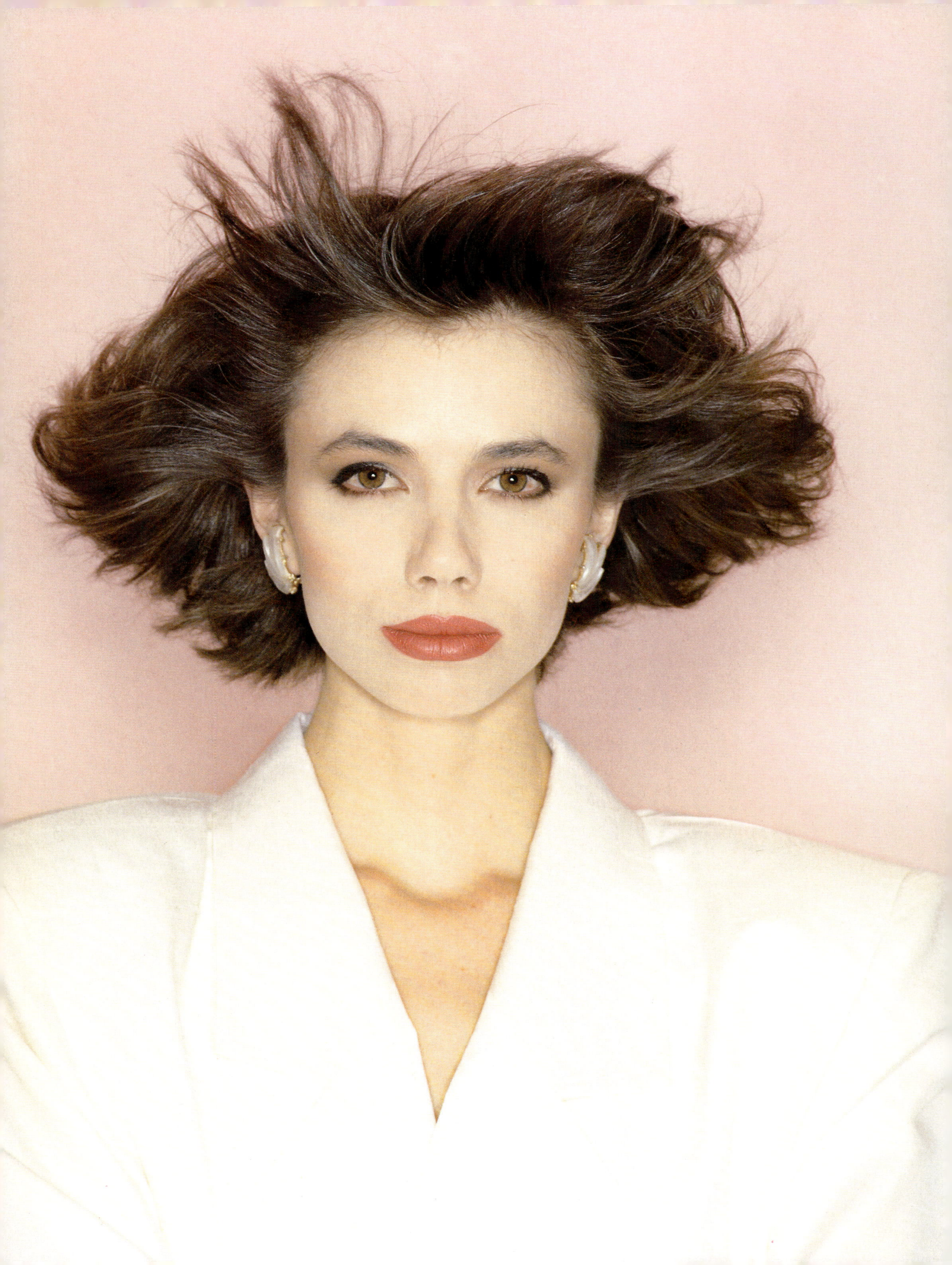

What's your hair type?

Though your features and face shape largely dictate what sort of look will best suit you, whether the style you want will work successfully will depend on two further factors — the thickness of your hair, and the amount of curl in it.

Fine hair — although long, fine, silken hair can look beautiful if lovingly maintained, too often it looks ratty and unkempt and therefore tends to suit short and simple styles rather better.

Straight hair looks marvellous if given a blunt cut, though hair with any degree of curling or wave tends to be improved by layering. Perming, highlighting or colouring should only be carried out on hair in tip-top condition as fine hair in particular will not stand up to the effects of strong chemicals if dry or listless.

Medium thick hair — this type of hair is especially versatile — it takes well to long or short styles, one length or layered and is also an excellent candidate for perming or colouring — so long as the condition is good. A hint of curl in the hair will be encouraged if it is layered and, similarly, this can be calmed down if it is styled in one length and carefully blow dried.

Thick hair — while it is often the envy of people with fine flyaway locks, thick hair can be hard to control and the range of styles may be limited, particularly when it is curly. However, if you hit on the right look, the effects can be stunning. Layering tends to be the best bet, as it saves the hair from looking over-heavy — particularly difficult if you have small features. A very short cut will necessitate a lot of thinning but the hair is generally strong enough to put up with the effects of colouring or perming.

STYLING TERMS — AND WHAT THEY MEAN

Asymmetric is a cut that is intentionally longer on one side than on the other. Ideally the difference should be quite marked for maximum impact.

Blunt cut is a straight, one-length cut, also called a bob.

Bulk refers to the actual thickness of the hair and the quantity of it. Often the sheer weight can make styling difficult, hair lies flat and won't move without expert cutting. Thinning, layering and razor cutting are all used to reduce bulk.

Channelling is when lines of hair are cut quite short to vary length and bulk, either throughout the hair or in certain sections. This is done to texturise and to add bulk.

Chipping in is a technique used to break up the straight edge of a section when a softer or more random finish is required. Very useful for fringes where the hairdresser will snip up at right angles to the straight edge.

Clipping means using clippers to achieve a graduated effect.

Dry cutting is used for very short clipper cuts. The hair may be wet, dried and re-cut several times until perfect.

Freehand cutting refers to hair combed then cut, section by section where it would fall naturally. The hair is not held during cutting. This technique is used for cutting the last sections of a bob — if hair here is cut wet and pulled taut it would spring up when dry and be too short.

Graduation is usually for styles which are short at the neck and sides, increasing in length until hair blends with longer lengths from the crown. Once a guideline is established, each subsequent section is lifted at a greater angle from the head before being cut.

Interior cutting is a description of techniques used to cut to reduce bulk

Feel glamorous and elated with beautifully conditioned and styled hair.

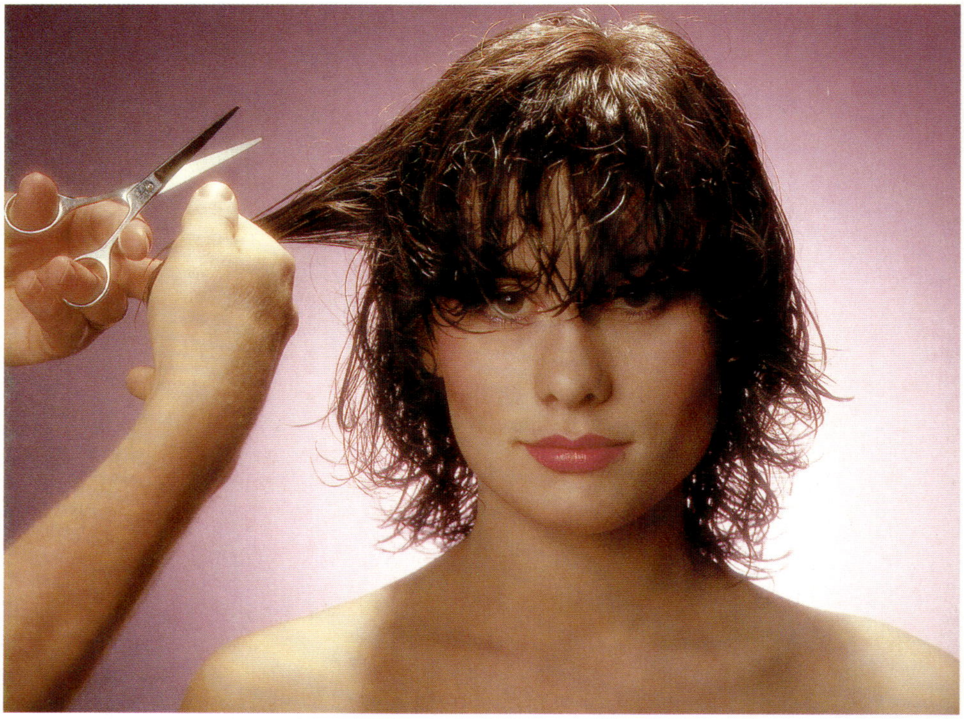

Have an idea of what style you want when next you visit your hairdresser. Different cutting styles suit different hair types.

without affecting the length of existing layers or finished overall length.
Knuckling is used to achieve shapes which could not be precision cut because of the angle — usually when the angle will not be parallel to the scalp. The section of hair is held in the fist so that the ends are splayed making cutting easier.
Layering means hair is held away from the head to be cut. Layers may be used to reduce bulk, add volume. The result is both versatile and bouncy.
Movement, applicably so-called when the direction of the hair is especially apparent. Clever cutting accentuates movement making hair look naturally suited to the style.
Pointing creates a thin, wispy look at the ends of the hair.
Precision cutting involves cutting hair in very small sections so that length is equal. This is displayed to superb advantage on the classic bob.
Razor cutting, mostly used to thin hair makes hair easier to manage because it removes any that isn't essential to the finished look. Useful for making the ends of neatly cut sections look more random without destroying proportion and shape. When razor cut, shorter hair springs up to support longer ones, creating natural volume.
Shattering disguises the fact that hair has just been cut. Sections are cut into at angles to break up the neat regularity which would detract from many casual styles.
Slicing refers to small sections of hair which are cut much shorter at intervals throughout the hair to thin it and to create texture.
Texturing is a cutting technique to create movement from the roots.
Volume describes the fullness of the hair when styled.

STYLE IDEAS

Plan to take ideas with you for your next appointment so you can be positive about the way you want to look. If you haven't got a hairdresser at the moment, find a good one by asking around and reading magazines to tell

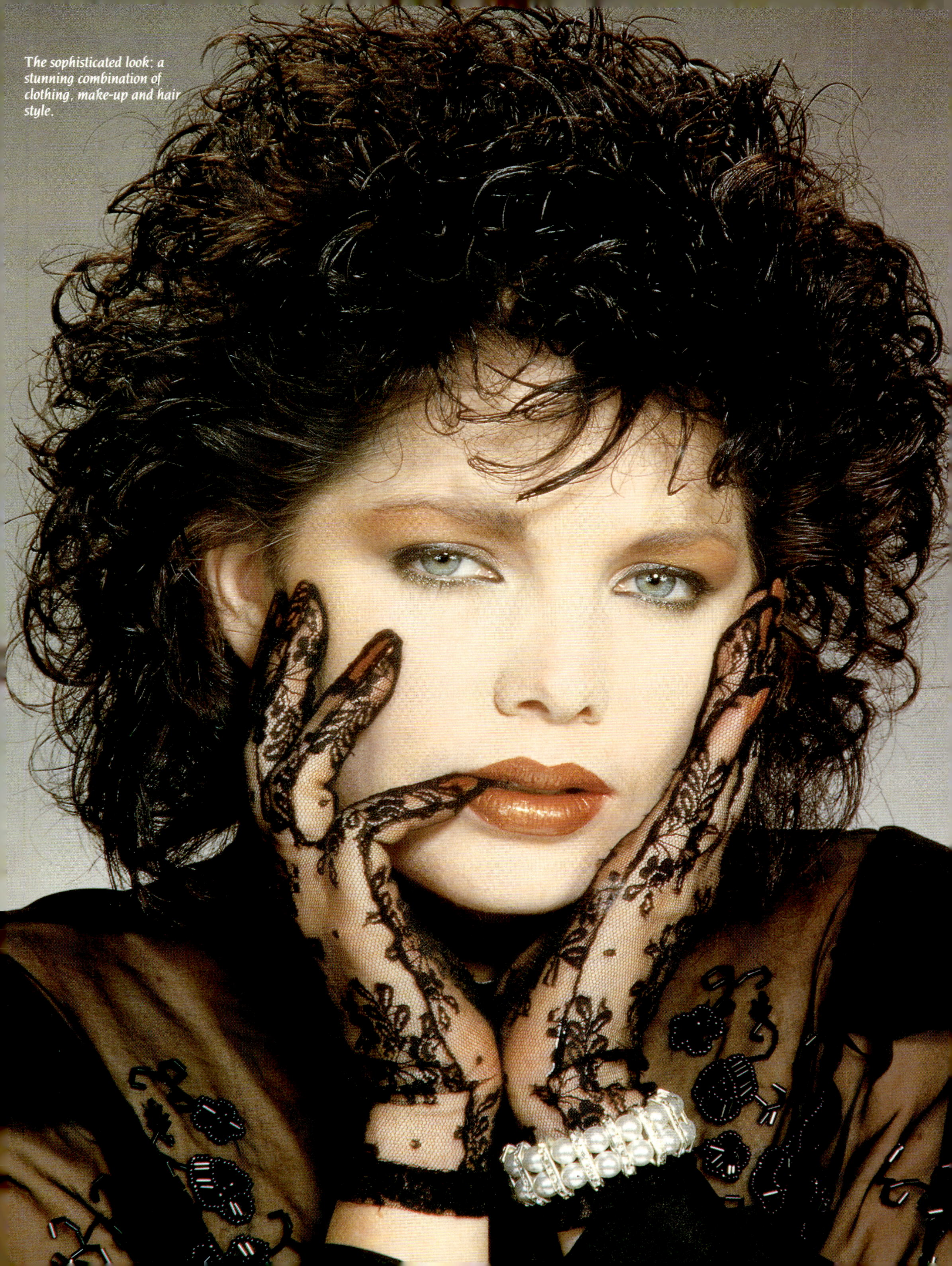

The sophisticated look: a stunning combination of clothing, make-up and hair style.

you who is cutting good styles. Approach people with hair you admire and ask who cut it — you need the name of the actual stylist responsible, not just the salon. Deciding on a look is exciting and gives you a chance to take a good look at yourself, while drifting through books and magazines for looks you love. Remember that hair can be young and spunky whatever your age — or it can be smooth and chic and with so many good perms and colourants around it's easy to achieve an astonishing variety of looks, even with hair you thought impossible to manage. Here are just some ideas:

Keep the length but change the overall look with a trim of just a few centimetres. One-length hair can be changed by feathering the ends, snipping up into the fringe so hair is shaped around the face. This keeps the length, but is lighter than the blunt cut.

Layers can lift dull hair, but be guided by your hairdresser as, perversely, layers can make fine hair floppy and impossible to control.

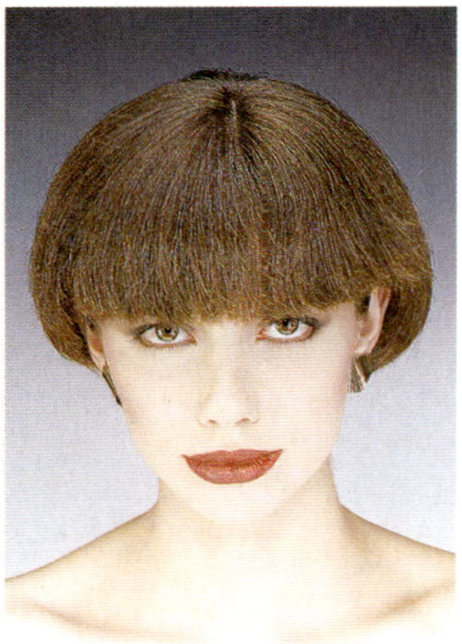

The classic bob cut — extremely attractive on the right person.

Change the line of a straight cut. Have it snipped shorter at the back, left longer at the front, or have it cut really short still retaining the bob shape.

Trim a fringe making an existing one lighter by shattering (thinning) the ends. This makes it easier to style in the direction you want. Alternatively, blend a fringe in with side hair for a different look so face is framed all round. Fringes need constant trimming to keep them correct, about every three weeks or less if hair grows fast.

Long to short is a major step. Think carefully — short hair will be easier to manage but your visits to the hairdresser will be more frequent. The hair you may have been hiding behind will be gone, exposing features — you will be especially conscious of jawline and head shape. Having hair cut gradually might be the answer if you do have doubts as there are all sorts of styles you can enjoy in between very long and very short hair.

Bring back the shine — sometimes it isn't the cut that's spoiling your hair, it's the condition. Perming, sun damage and improper washing can all leave hair dull and in need of a good conditioning treatment. Consult your hairdresser for the best way to condition, using the best of the treatments around.

Give it a body boost — fine, floppy hair looks thicker when it is all one length but it still doesn't style as well as thicker hair. The answer? A body perm to make it manageable. It might give your hair a slight wave but this can be styled out when you dry.

Root perms for short cuts — hair that's short and layered can be root permed at the base so it stands up and appears to have lots of natural body.

Natural waves for longer layers — a soft perm will make longer, layered hair more manageable and make it nicely wavy. The effect is achieved by perming hair on large rollers.

Perms for curls may be the answer for you if your hair is quite curly but unruly or if you need a style that's easy to control — or maybe you just fancy curls. There are many different types of perm for different effects and different hair types. Hairdressers now work with computers to gauge processing time on your particular hair so you get the result you want. Hair will need to be cut and layered before it is permed. Newly permed hair is always a bit too curly but relax — your perm will too in just a short time!

Lighter cut for curly hair — consider having naturally curly hair cut short at the nape of the neck, left longer on the top. Ends can be softer, too, to soften the bulk of the hair.

Perming longer hair — lovely long curls are a romantic thought and it *is* possible to have long hair permed. However, there are problems such as the time and expense involved (check with your hairdresser before making the appointment), and also with the life of the perm. Long hair will simply pull the curl out after a short time, especially if hair is long and heavy. Ask your hairdresser's advice *before* you opt for perming, so you know what to expect.

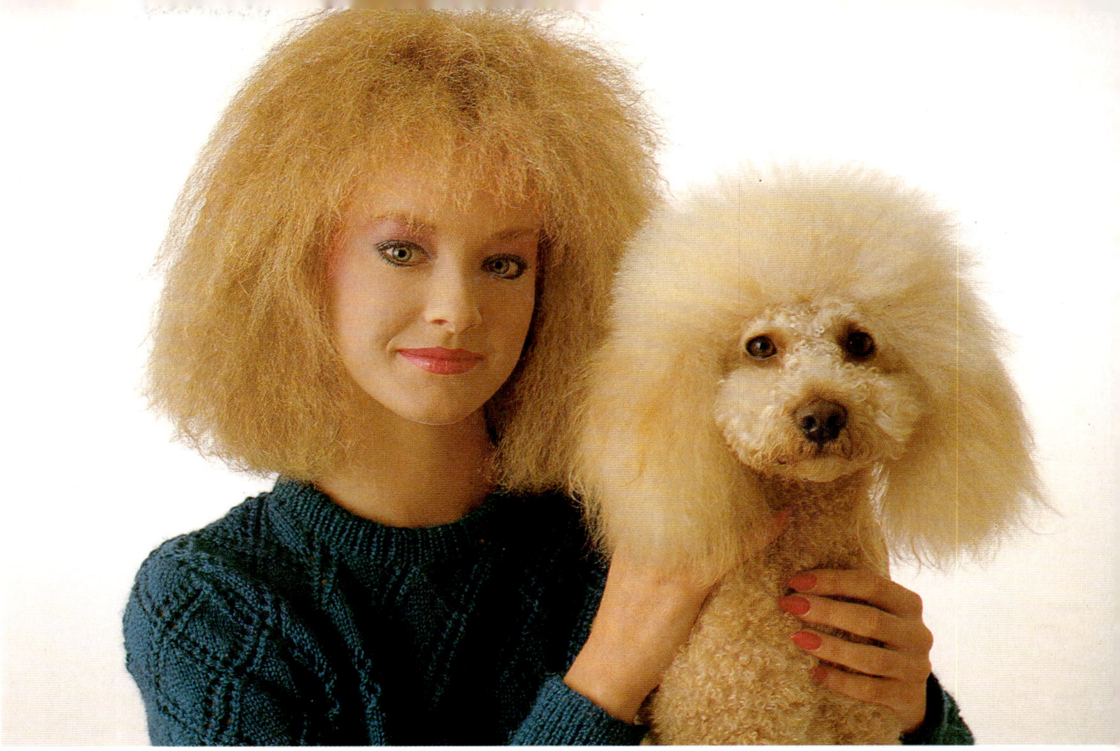

For someone who may love curls, a perm could be the answer.

Long hair can be waved with a number of styling aids including the bendy sponge rods which are simple to use.

Trimming a perm — long or short, trimming will help keep a perm in place. Most perms on shorter hair last about three months but curl will appear to drop before that, in which case a trim will put back some life. You may find that your perm will be revived two or three times before hair needs to be re-permed.

Wear it up — if you haven't tried it before you might find that an upswept style is perfect and could be the answer while you decide what to do with hair that is growing out of a shorter cut. Twists, plaits and chignons can be very successful, use bows and clips for decoration.

COLOURING

Although the opportunities to change hair colour have never been greater, safer, or given such authentic effects it seems many women still have largely unrealistic expectations when it comes to transforming their hair shade. Too much enterprise, however, especially if you are using a home product, can often end in disaster.

There are no problems with today's over-the-counter colourants — they are all safe and well formulated. Mistakes lie in the hands of the user. People shouldn't fight their natural pigmentation, as you can't expect to go ash blonde successfuly if you're very dark, say with typical Mediterranean colouring. Whatever your colouring, you should only go two or three shades lighter than your natural colour and never attempt to go darker. This is why no reputable hairdresser today likes to bleach hair as it's an extreme process and gives a flat, uniform 'dead' look that's unnatural and looks obviously 'dyed'.

Tinting comprises as much as 50 per cent of all hair treatments carried out, but today's effects are so subtle and natural that it's virtually impossible to tell if a woman has had her hair tinted — or at any rate that's the ultimate goal of any good colourist! More and more popular are tints that change the tone rather than the shade of the hair. Most effective are the honey gold and

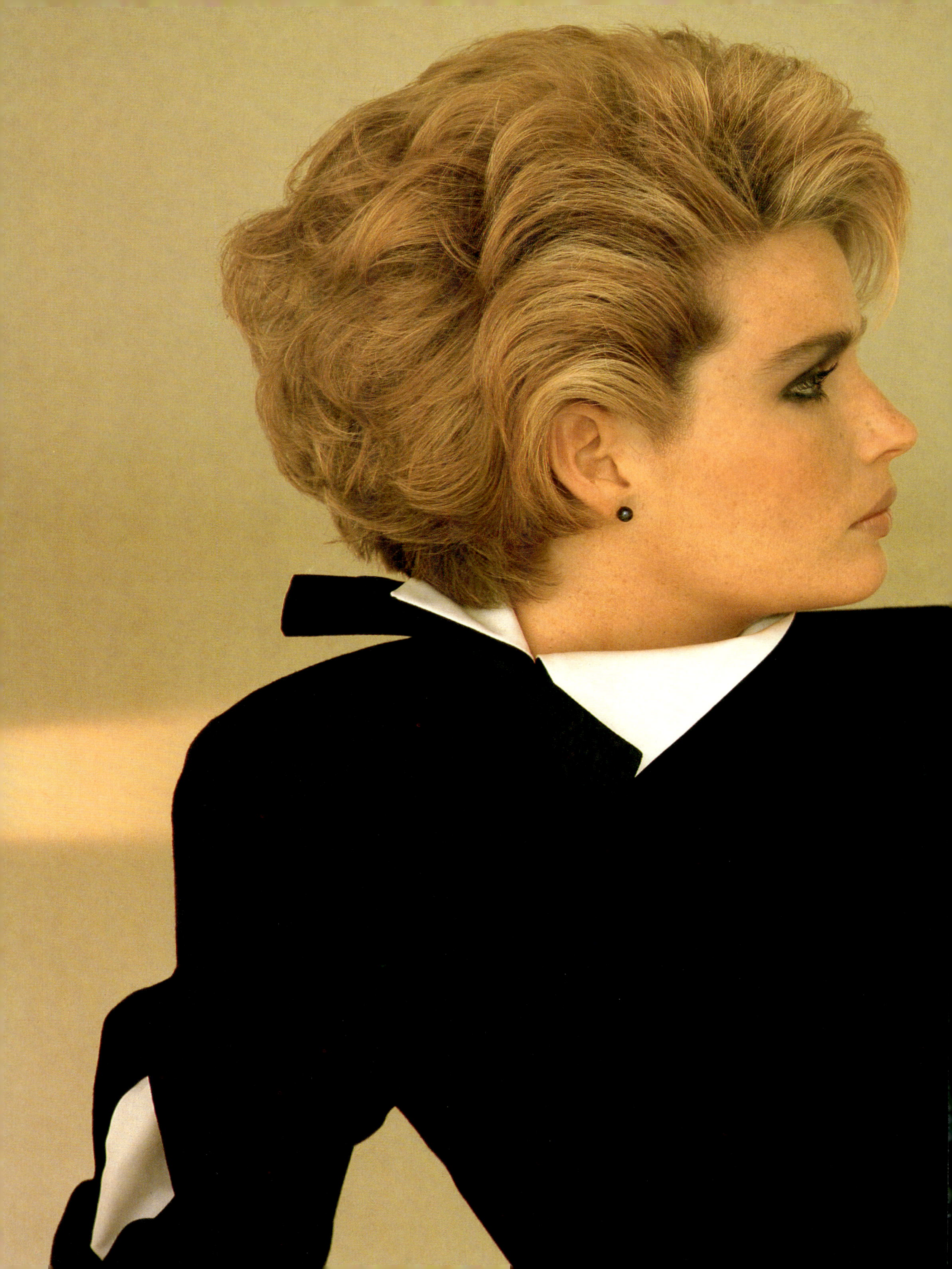

hazel blondes, the rich russety red-browns and chestnut shades, and the warm deep sherry and burgundy browns that add sparkle and dimension to brunette hair. Nor need colour changes be drastically irreversible or involve a three-act drama. Nowadays there is a wide range of very different products to choose from, most of which have been perfected to take the terror out of tinting.

Water rinses

These are the most superficial and temporary of treatments, designed merely to add colour to the outer cuticle of the hair and wash out with your next shampoo. These can be used to tone in the odd patch of grey or white hair, or to cool brassy blonde tones. Dark shades, however, may come off on clothes and bed linen.

Semi-permanent tints

These have a toning, not a lightening, effect, although the minute molecules of colour do penetrate the inner cuticle temporarily, gradually fading out after three or four weeks. These are excellent for first-time home tinters and anyone not used to colouring. They add particular richness to brown, red and chestnut tones and liven up dull, mousy brown shades. Semi-permanents are also extremely effective for refreshing the basic colour of hair that's dry and porous, since they enhance the quality and add extra sheen.

Permanent tints

These are mixed with hydrogen peroxide which activates their small colour molecules, allowing them to penetrate right into the hair cuticle and there react with the hydrogen peroxide — expanding and becoming locked into the body of the hair. These are the most versatile of all tints, since they can darken or lift natural colour and tone it at the same time. Over-the-counter permanents are effective if you choose a product which will lighten your hair one or two shades — no more.

Highlighting

Increasingly popular in recent years, it offers the most natural-looking effect that can be achieved with colouring. Highlighting emphasises the multiplicity and nuances of shade that we all have whatever the basic colour of our hair — often between two and six tones on one head of hair. Any natural hair colour can be improved by using one or more different types of high or low lights, scattering them as densely or as sparsely as you wish. Streaks can be merely tinted — especially on mousy or brown shades — lowlighted with a mild bleach, or highlighted with a stronger bleach. These can also be concentrated on just one section of hair, say the fringe, or just the tips of the hair. The great bonus is that there's no need for the prompt retouching necessary when you use an overall tint, since highlights generally only need 'filling in' after three to four months' regrowth, depending on the style of your hair. The main drawback? Highlighting is a complex, refined and expensive procedure, and can only be carried out by an expert hair colourist at a salon. Never attempt to put highlights in yourself at home, unless you want to end up with hair tones that match the subtlety of a zebra skin.

HAIR PROBLEMS

Streaks of pale blonde and warm red . . . a cut above the rest.

Human hair — along with skin and nails — is like litmus paper. It keeps constant and accurate tabs on our inner health, reflecting the ups and downs on our general well-being, the food we eat and the drugs we take. Each individual hair, and there are about 100 000 of these on the average adult head, depends for its strength and overall condition on the cell activity and nourishment it receives at root level within the scalp. These tissues are rich in nerve endings and blood vessels which fuel each growing hair with all the nutrition necessary for maintaining shine and strength. Anything therefore that interferes with the flow of blood to the scalp, or alters its quota of nutrients, is eventually bound to alter both the rate and quality of growth. Stress, illness, emotional shock, taking drugs, hormonal changes, crash diets, can all impair circulation and clutter up the blood supply with poisonous wastes which, just as they make your skin look grey and sallow, affect the basic condition of your hair.

Excessive hair loss

This can be triggered by conditions as diverse as anaemia, thyroid problems, coming off the pill, childbirth, taking a long course of antibiotics or prolonged emotional upheaval. If you think you may be losing more than your fair share of hair over a certain period make sure you consult either your doctor or a trichologist to check up on your general health. But don't panic unnecessarily. Most of us lose between 50 and a 100 hairs every day, with slight seasonal fluctuations when this can become either more or less pronounced. It is absolutely no indication that you are heading for baldness — so relax! Hair grows in very definite cycles which include a resting and growing phase, fast summer growth and slower winter growth. Very often nature

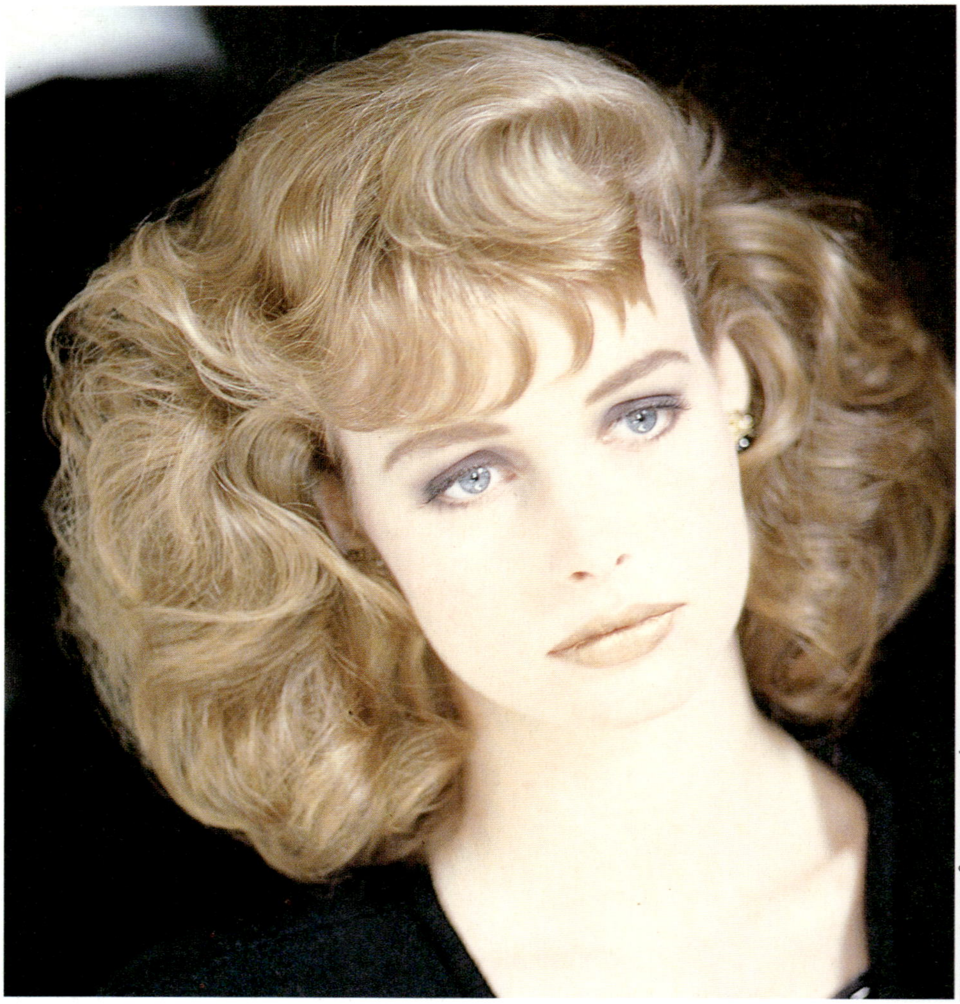

Hair by Sloanes of Paddington for Wella Australia

Thick hair beautifully cut and styled.

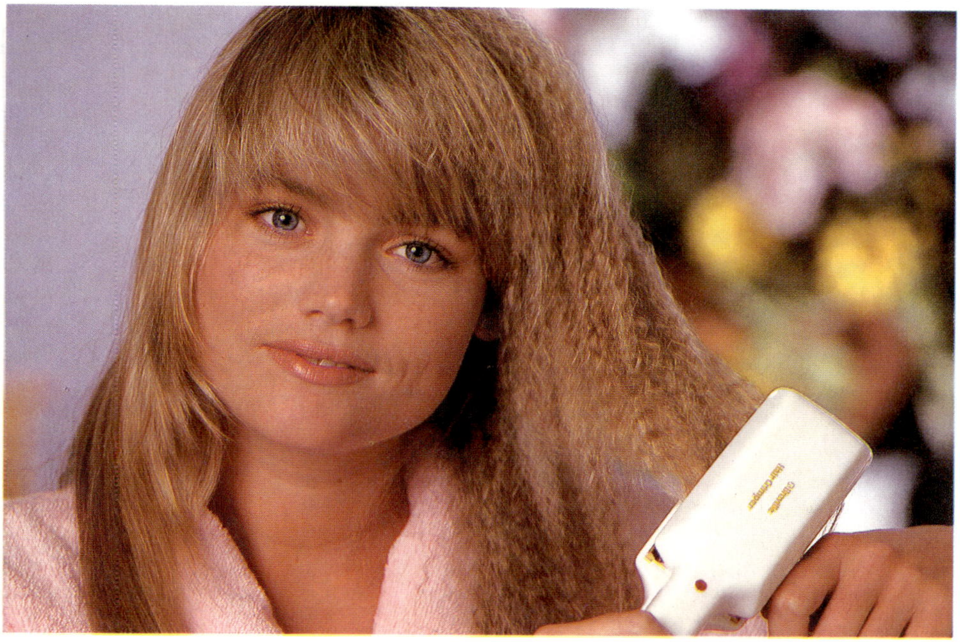

Breville/Cleo

Crimping hair for that quick, hi-tech style.

tends to get out of rhythm and these cycles overlap, causing hair loss to be temporarily more noticeable — rather like a moulting cat or dog! Nervous tension, by making the muscles at the back of the neck and scalp rigid and knotted, can also starve the scalp of its regular blood supply, so try and keep the area relaxed by massaging the scalp gently with the fingertips, moving it in circular motion over the entire head to keep it flexible and the blood vessels unconstricted. Hair is about 95 per cent protein, and as such shows up unbalanced or outright sloppy eating habits. Fresh fruit, salads, vegetables, fish, dairy produce and wholemeal foods are essential for cultivating lustrous hair. On the other hand, consuming too many sweet foods, salt, smoking and drinking too much alcohol can rapidly lead to excessive oiliness or just boring, lacklustre hair. If you suspect your diet may be lacking in a lot of basic nutrients, try taking a 'tonic' course of wheatgerm and brewer's yeast — both rich in the B complex vitamins essential for healthy nerve tissue and beautiful strong hair.

Split ends

These are nearly always caused by over-zealous brushing (usually with a cheap, nylon brush), tugging your way through knots and tangles, using a cheap alkaline shampoo and a very hot hairdryer or heated rollers, or too much perming or tinting with insufficient conditioning. Like the edges of a frayed robe, these must be trimmed regularly to stop the split from creeping up the hair shaft and making the effect appear worse. Dry and delicate hair is more liable to split, so make sure you treat it carefully; use a good conditioner and invest in a twice-monthly hair pack.

Dandruff

This is undoubtedly the commonest scourge to affect both scalp and hair. There are few people who haven't suffered the disorder in one form or another at some point in their lives. Dandruff is often mistakenly classified as a problem that goes hand in hand with overactive sebaceous glands and an oily scalp. Unfortunately it isn't as simple as all that. Exactly what causes dandruff still remains a mystery. Skin is continuously shedding its upper layer in the form of microscopic dead cells, which are normally brushed and washed away so that there's never any build-up or residue. The scalp, however, seems to be particularly sensitive to chemical changes in the body and, as metabolism changes, the surface of the scalp loses large flakes and scaly particles instead of the normal powder-like substance.

Certainly, teenage dandruff is commonly a result of hormonal changes that begin at puberty and make the oil glands work overtime — the cause of acne as well as greasy hair and dandruff. This can carry on into your twenties and is relatively easy to control once you've found a good antiseptic shampoo which successfully controls oiliness, as well as dandruff.

HAIR ACCESSORIES — THE FINAL TOUCH

Mousse

A vital aid to practically every hairstyle these days, you simply massage in a palm-full of hair mousse from an aerosol — they come in soft, medium and firm hold — and use it to give your hair extra body and bounce. Coax it into shape by finger drying or using a hairdryer and the effects should last until the next day at least, depending on the weight and style of your hair.

Gel

Though you use this in pretty much the same way as mousse, the effects are more dramatic and tend to give hair a more spiky, sculptured look. Many also give the fashionable 'wet' look.

Fake hair

Hair pieces and wigs are just as popular today as ever — the difference is that they are used far more flamboyantly than before. While they can be used to extend or enhance your natural hair, more and more frequently we are turning to neon-coloured wigs and switches to make a determined and indiscreet fashion statement — shocking pink punk wigs to complement extravagant evening wear

Curling tongs and brushes

These are ideal if you favour a straight style that needs a little taming — the ends turned under, for instance — or are trying to create gentle curls or ringlets. Tongs can be used on long or short hair and are a useful aid to blow drying that falls a little short of the style you are aiming to achieve.

Heated rollers

Though they do just the same job as ordinary rollers, the heated versions create a hairstyle that will hold far faster. Styles can be varied according to the roller sizes used and many of the sets on the market these days can be used in conjunction with their own conditioners, preventing the drying effects on the hair that can otherwise be a problem with frequent use.

Crimpers

For those with ambitions to wear a really hi-tech, 21st century look, crimping sets are a tremendous answer. You simply heat them up then crimp the hair into style, section by section. It generally looks best on hair that is cut to one length, though there's no telling what a real maestro may be able to achieve.

Body builder/styler

A different type of styling brush with thermo-loop heated bristles which helps create a soft, curly look and is also ideal for giving fine hair more body and life.

Glorious hair lovingly and beautifully cared for.

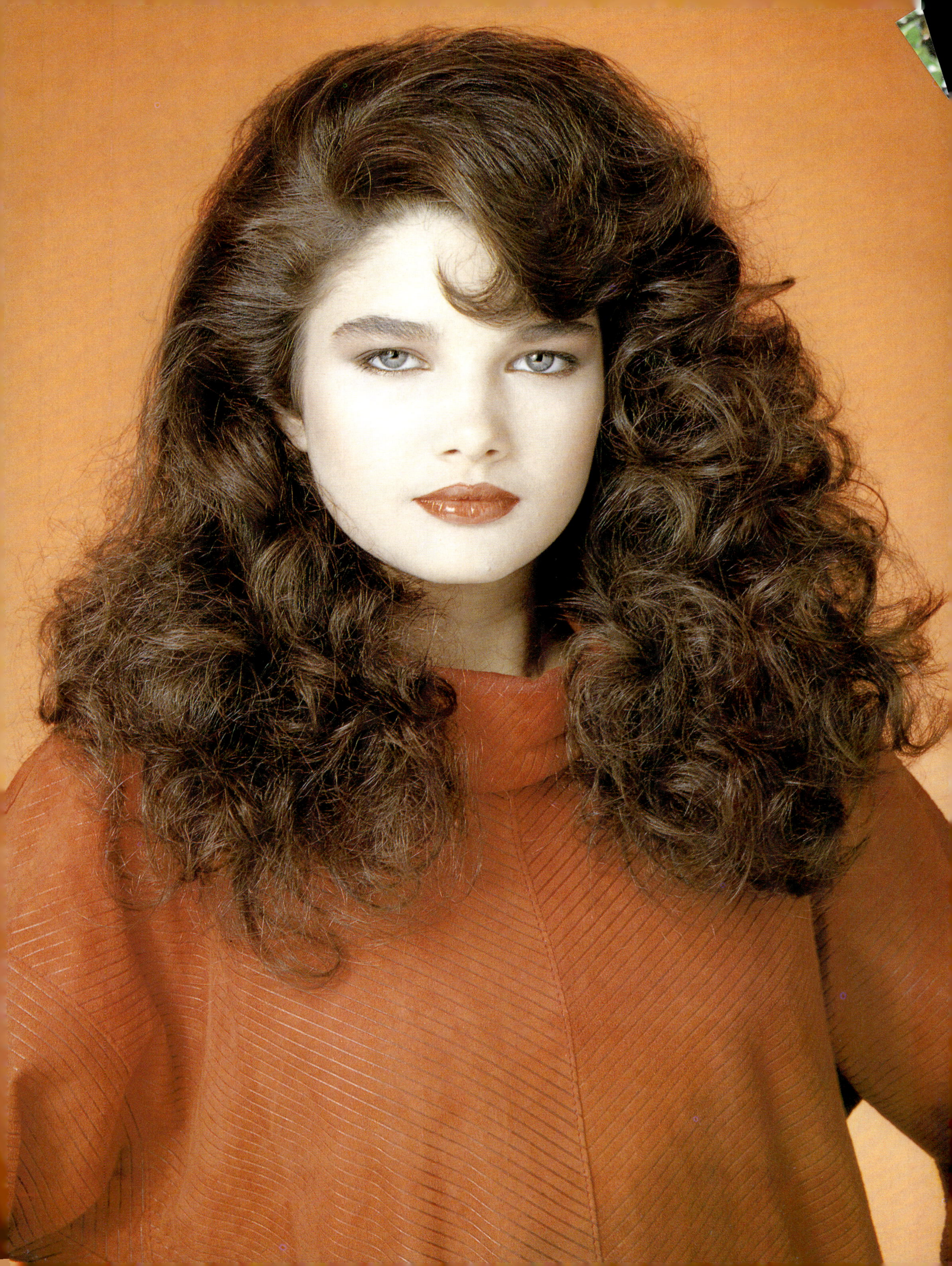

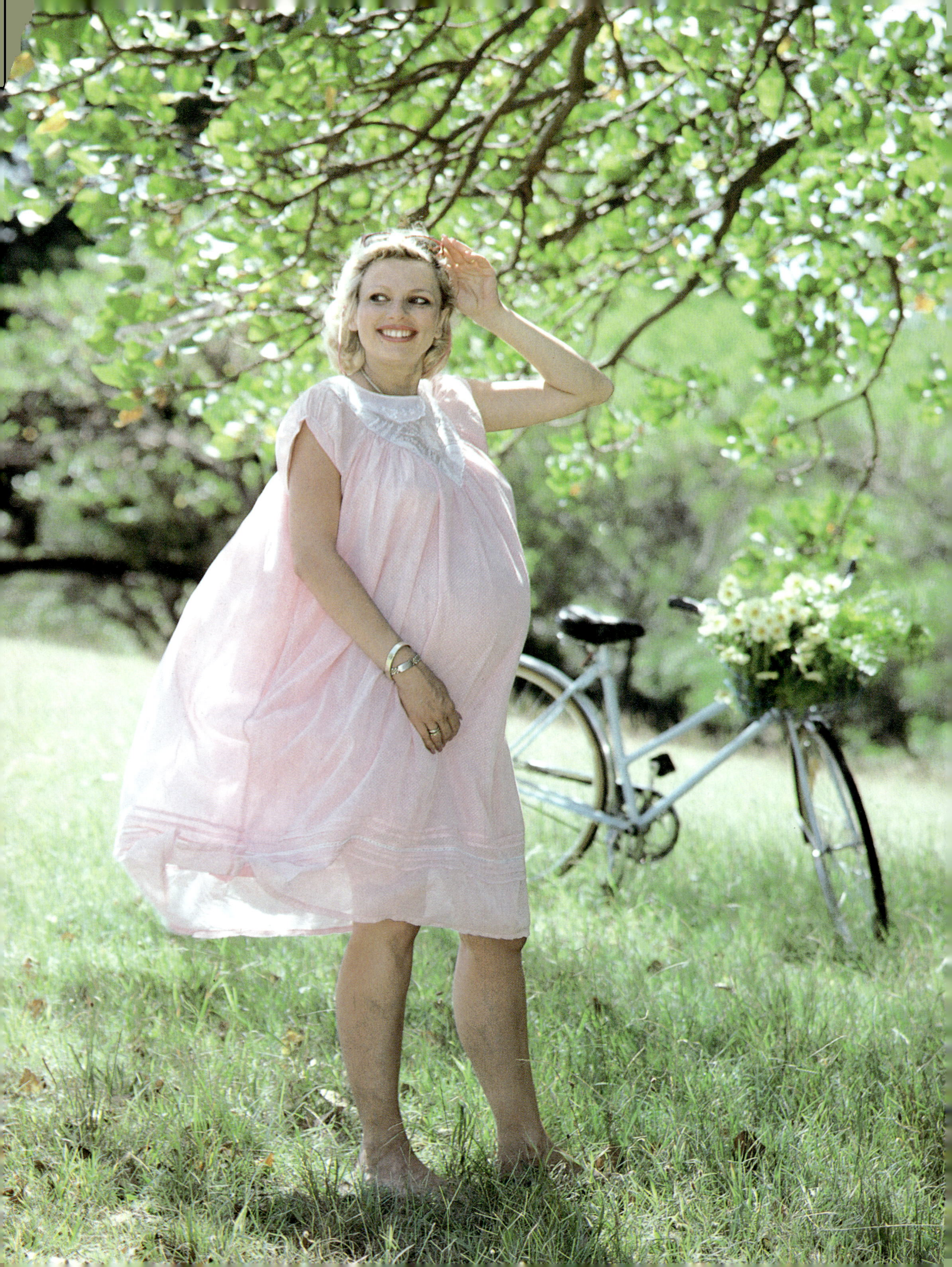

A HAPPY PREGNANCY

Pregnancy can be an immensely rewarding experience as you prepare for the birth of your child. It is a time of great change in your psychological and physical make-up. The mother-to-be must recognise that new demands are being made on her and adjust normal routines accordingly.

There is much you can do to minimise the negative effects of the massive hormonal upheavals — and changes in shape — while accentuating the positive benefits to your appearance that pregnancy brings. Following a careful body routine will ease the transition to normality after the birth and make it easier for the mother to cope with the myriad demands which will be made on her. Taking good care of yourself will also help you to handle the emotional swings — a guaranteed part of the package — and enhance your self-esteem.

During pregnancy special attention must be paid to nutrition but this does not mean doubling your food intake. Exercise programmes should be continued and breathing techniques to promote relaxation should be included. Skin care is a must with allowances made for the changing nature of your skin; make-up can enhance the newly acquired 'bloom'. A touch of resourcefulness and awareness of basic style rules works wonders as an ever-expanding girth demands larger fittings in clothing.

The need for rest is greatest during the first three months. The sudden surge in hormones and increased outpouring of the sebaceous glands will result in oilier skin and hair and will need to be counteracted.

A great sense of physical and emotional well-being is common during the middle three months. Now is the time to think about making the most of your appearance as you prepare for future changes.

Both the highs and lows of pregnancy are an immensely rewarding experience, especially if you look after yourself during the nine months, eating properly and following an exercise routine.

Experiencing great changes physically and psychologically, it is important not to fall into a morass of self-pity and remain cooped up at home.

The last months of pregnancy can be difficult as fatigue, breathlessness and occasional dizziness take their toll. It is most important to continue breathing exercises, take things quietly and remain calm. Adhere carefully to the sensible body and skin-care routines outlined in the following pages and you will enjoy a beautiful pregnancy.

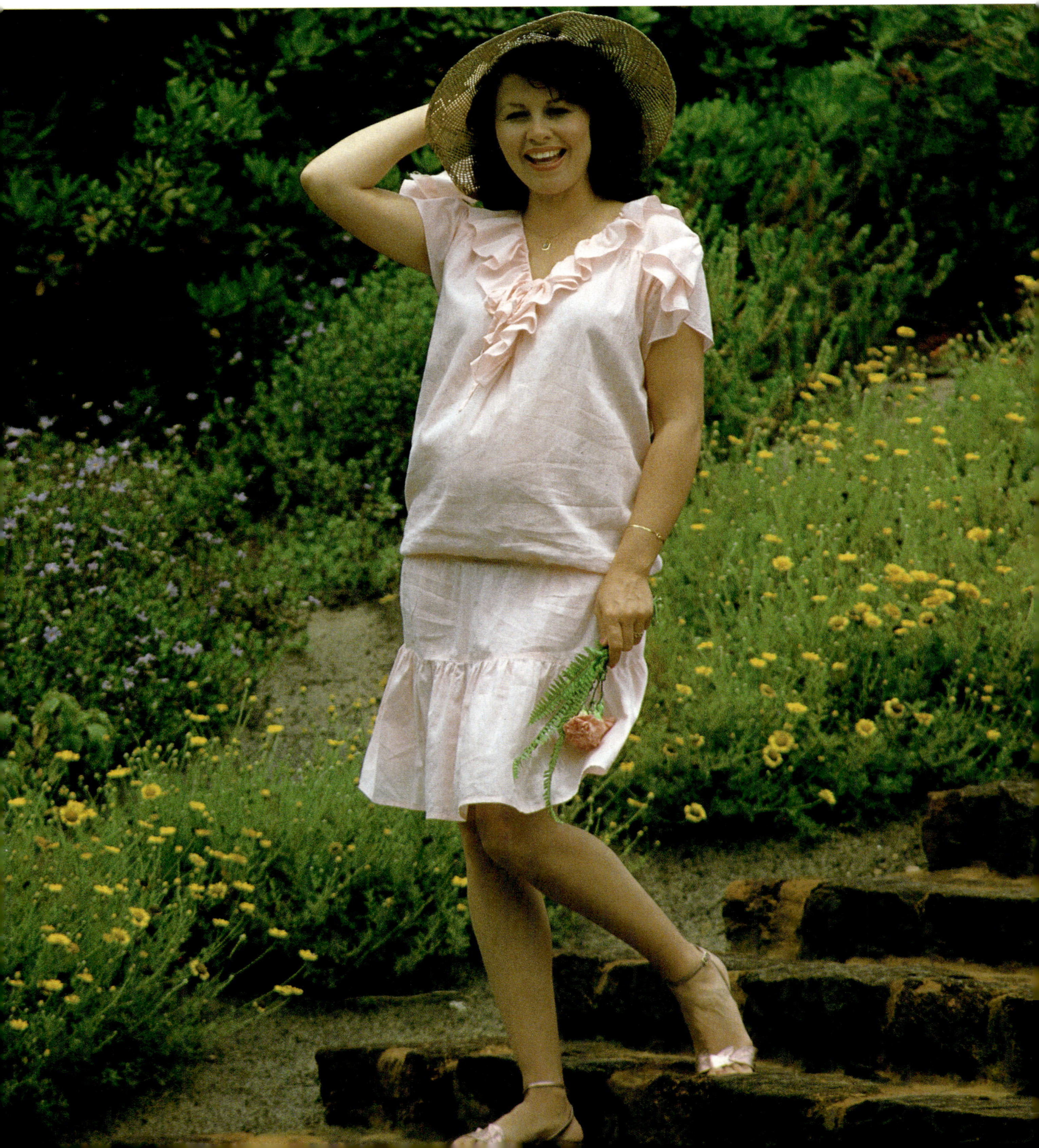

feeling pregnant

While everyone expects you to be happy, radiant and content as a mother-to-be, there may well be times when you feel depressed, anxious, irritable, even suddenly and inexplicably in tears, no matter how delighted you are with yourself and your growing baby. Such down-in-the-dumps feelings can last five minutes, or might continue all day, but usually they disappear as suddenly as they arrived. Anything may set you off; a chance remark about your looks or mood, or any one of the little things that can go wrong at home. Your forgetfulness, overwhelming tiredness and sudden anxieties about the future can all depress you. But while you and all those around you should be prepared for some uncharacteristic changes of mood, you don't have any excuse to be permanently bad-tempered. It's unlikely that you will feel depressed for any length of time — but if you do don't be afraid to seek medical advice.

Women commonly experience emotional 'lows' during puberty, the menopause and just before a period, due to the rising and falling of hormone levels in the body. Some women taking the birth control pill report similar reactions from time to time. Similarly, in pregnancy the exceptionally rapid increase of certain hormones, particularly the major female hormones oestrogen and progesterone, can be emotionally unsettling. Progesterone, especially, is produced in large quantities at the onset of pregnancy and is the cause of the earlier symptoms, notably the enlargement of the breasts and sensations of nausea during the first weeks.

During the first three months of pregnancy your body is going through its most drastic upheaval — a single fertilised cell is growing minute by minute into a human being. By the end of 12 weeks your baby will be fully formed and swimming in the surrounding fluid. All that has to happen now is for the baby to mature, develop and grow bigger and stronger. Once this initial phenomenon has happened hormone levels settle down, and as nausea and tiredness recede and your appetite returns, together with the blooming good looks characteristic of pregnant women, you should find that you feel emotionally more settled too. Irritability, outbursts of temper and sudden emotional changes from high to low and back should be much less frequent.

Your circumstances as well as the physical changes may affect the way you feel. If the pregnancy is unexpected or unwanted, and you have had to make a difficult decision to go ahead and have the child, you will almost certainly experience sharp fluctuations of mood. Looking after small children can make you feel emotionally drained especially if you are suffering from nausea and sickness during the first 14 weeks. One hundred milligrams of pyridoxine, or Vitamin B6, taken each night and morning, is helpful and for more troublesome cases there are safe and effective drugs available.

Understanding from those around you is a definite bonus — of course you need sympathy and comfort — but at the same time you don't want an overdose of indulgence. Everyone has bad days and even though you may feel especially sensitive, try not to fall into a morass of self-pity. Don't neglect yourself or remain cooped up at home brooding, instead make an effort to get out and seek the company of others you can talk to — friends with small children have been through it all before and can be of invaluable help.

a growing concern

The old saying 'eating for two' is definitely out of date and anyone who suggests that this is what you should be doing can be politely ignored. It used to be thought that a fat, bouncing baby was a healthy baby. Now we know that fat children often become fat adults and that obesity can lead to heart disease. However, there will be a natural increase in your appetite during pregnancy, which you should not deny providing you don't satisfy it with too many refined and processed foods. A well-balanced diet is important throughout life, but particularly so during pregnancy when you have to satisfy your baby's nutritional requirements as well as your own. So make sure you are eating wisely and well.

It is not healthy for anyone to be overweight — or underweight — and the importance of keeping your weight under control cannot be overstressed. A large weight gain during pregnancy may give rise to high blood pressure, swelling of the feet and ankles and undue strain on the heart. It can also be very hard to lose the excess fat after the birth.

Most doctors these days watch weight gain keenly. Every time you attend the prenatal clinic you will be weighed and if the doctor feels you are gaining too rapidly, you will be advised to cut down on starchy foods. If there is concern about the amount of weight you have put on, a strict diet plan which is sensible to follow will be recommended.

On average, a woman on a well-balanced diet will put on around 10–13 kilograms during her pregnancy (although some women may put on a lot more or less than this). The gain is due to the combined weight of the baby, placenta, increasing blood supply to the uterus (which at full term is about 25 per cent of the total body circulation), amniotic fluid around the baby, water retention, plus a natural increase in fat reserves and the enlargement of various organs such as the breasts and the uterus.

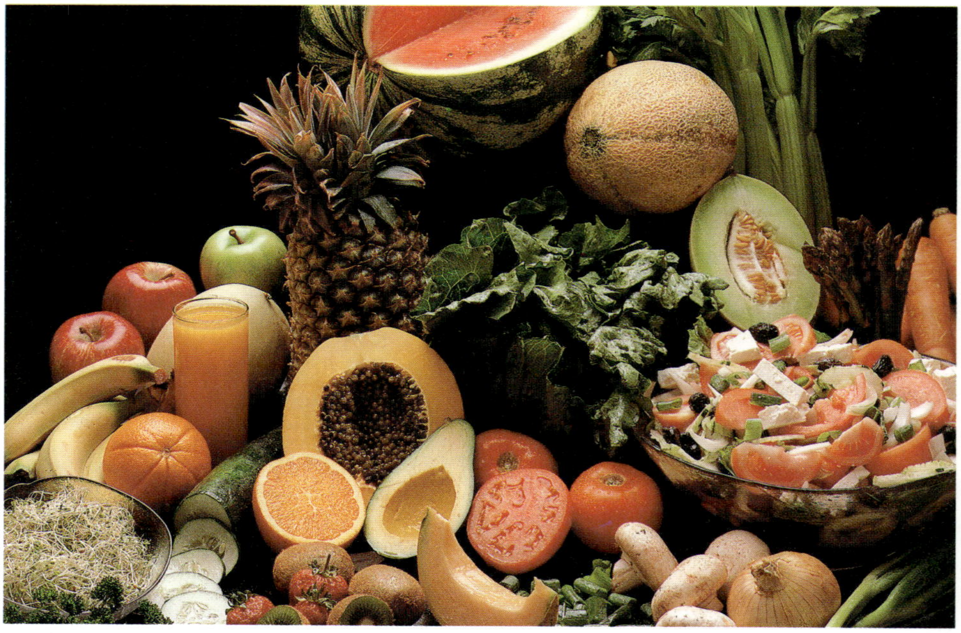

High in vitamins and fibres, fruits and vegetables are an important component of a balanced diet.

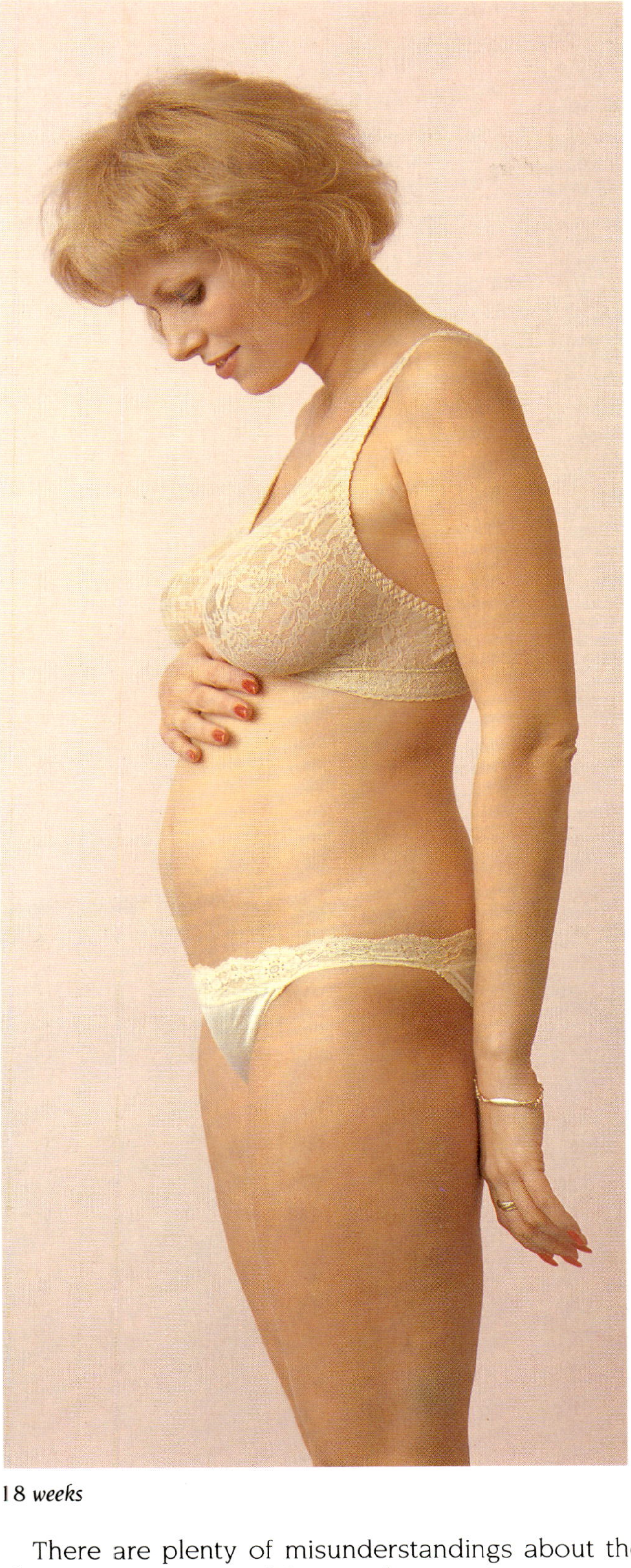

18 *weeks*

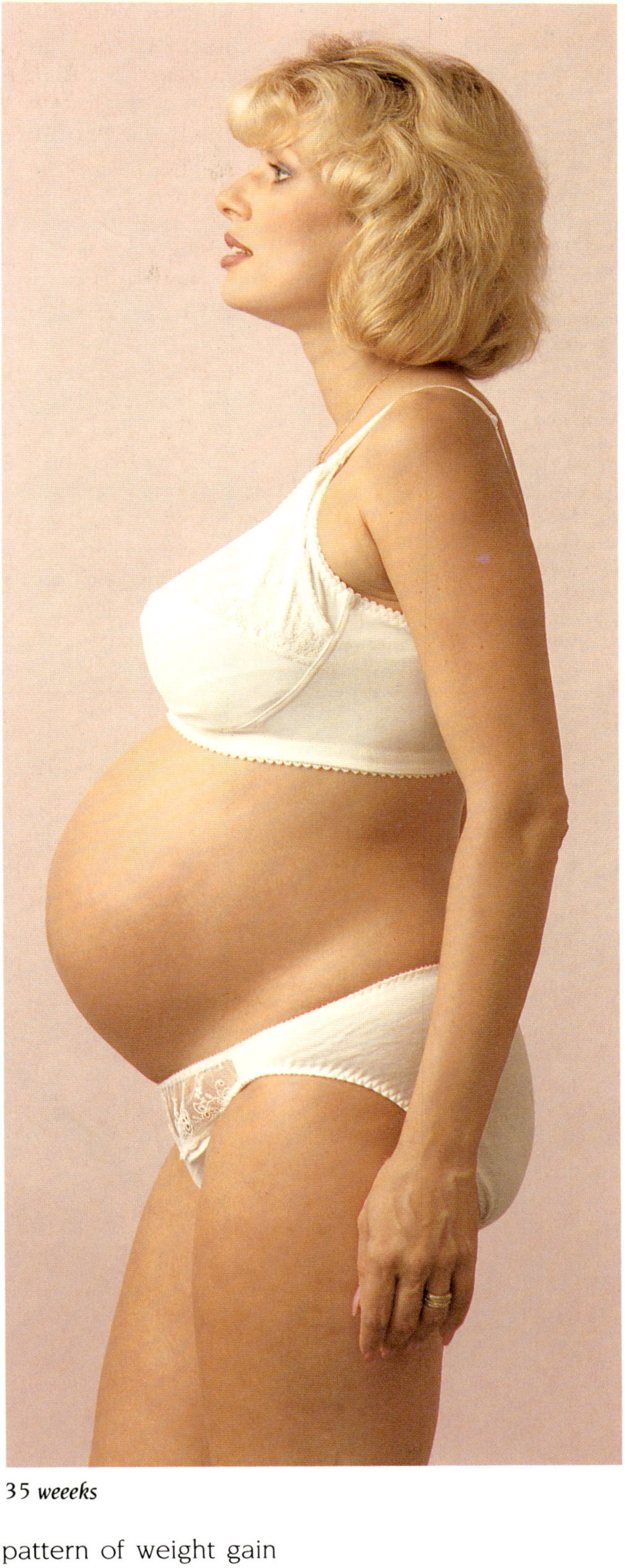

35 *weeeks*

There are plenty of misunderstandings about the pattern of weight gain during pregnancy and for weight-conscious women this can be a source of worry. You will notice a difference in your general shape apart from the obvious 'tummy'. The face tends to get fuller especially around the cheeks, jowls and neck, and the shoulders thicken, as does the waistline. A little extra padding may be noticeable around the lower back, thighs and bottom. This increase in stored fat is quite normal and is laid down as an energy deposit in preparation for breastfeeding. It is easy to feel despondent as your clothes get tighter and tighter in places you hadn't expected, but don't fight this natural weight increase. Going on crash or fad diets while pregnant can certainly be harmful to both you and the baby. Diets with less than 6300 kilojoules per day are particularly undesirable.

Patterns of weight gain can vary enormously, even for healthy normal pregnancies. So while many women put on weight more or less steadily throughout the nine months (red line), some may actually lose a few kilograms initially (yellow line) due to morning sickness, catching up again later, while others may begin well, but then lose weight towards the end of term when the baby puts on a sudden spurt of growth and uses up the mother's reserves (blue line).

Everyone is different and whereas some people don't start putting on weight until about 14 weeks or so, others find the scales shoot up immediately. Often it is the thinner women who put on most weight and fairly early on, whereas women who are overweight to start with gain comparatively little throughout their pregnancy.

You may like to check your own weight every week to chart your gain. Aim at 1.5–2 kilograms during the first three months, then on average about 1.5–2 kilograms each month. But if you do seem to be putting on too much too soon — it should average between a quarter and half a kilogram a week — don't panic. Think about your diet. Are you eating too much refined food? If so, cut out fattening cakes and if you feel hungry between meals, nibble fruit and raw vegetables such as carrots or celery. A plain biscuit or slice of lightly buttered toast won't make much difference but frequent chocolate bars or jam doughnuts will.

Sensible planning of your meals throughout the day will ensure that you and your baby get all the vitamins, minerals and nutrients needed.

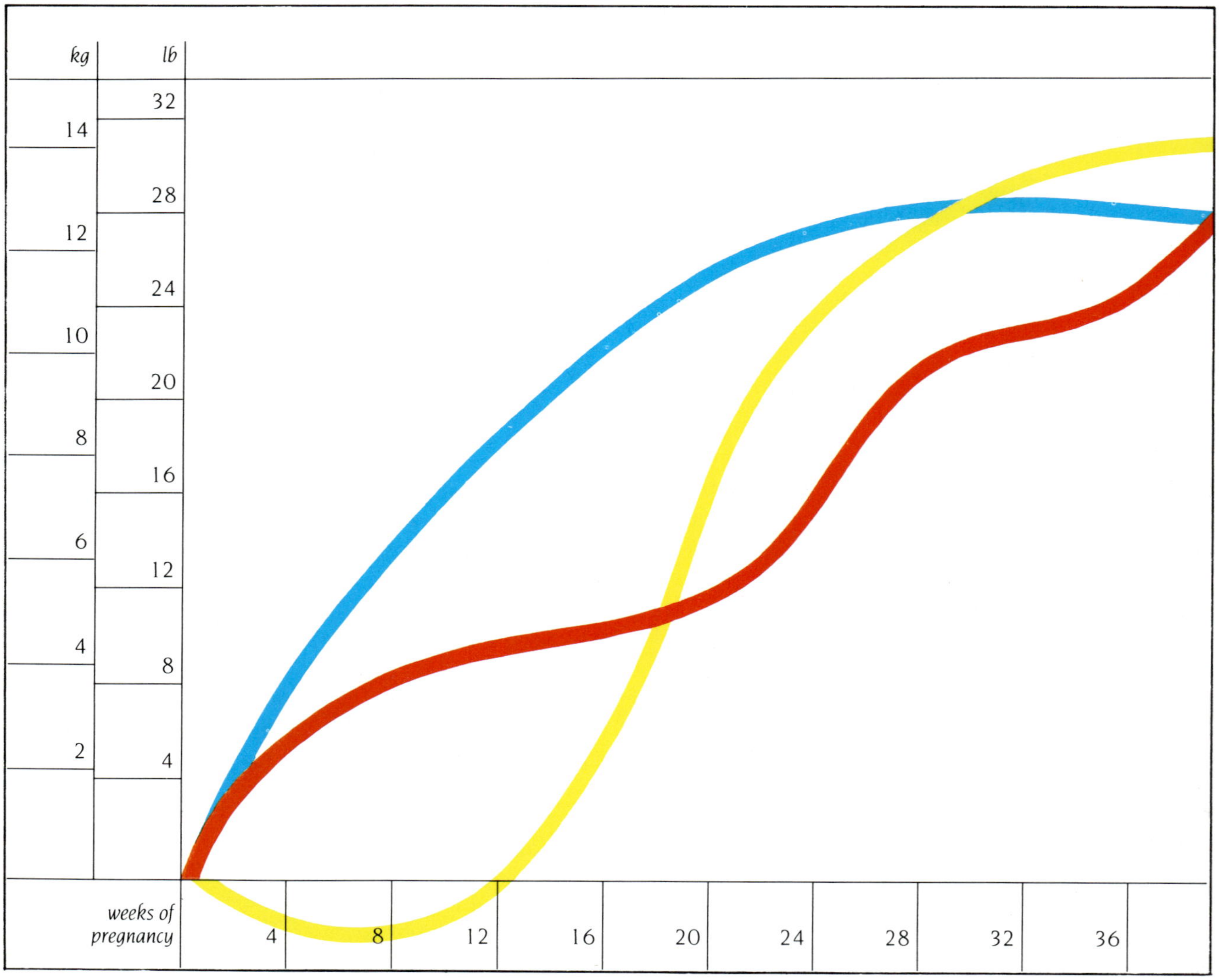

HOW TO KEEP A BALANCED DIET

The important thing in maintaining a well-balanced diet is not to eat too much of any one type of food: you need variety in order to get adequate supplies of essential protein, minerals and vitamins. Try to keep the same kind of balance of these in your diet as before you were pregnant — about 10 500 kilojoules daily should be sufficient for your energy needs. If you eat too many refined carbohydrates, found for example in cakes, sweets, and soft drinks, your kilojoule intake will become excessive and the body's metabolism simply won't be able to burn them up fast enough.

You can make sure of getting all the necessary nutrients by planning your daily meals from the following five basic groups. Try to eat as many fresh and untreated foods as possible, as the processing and heat treatments used to produce 'convenience' foods considerably reduce their nutritional value.

Dairy products

Milk is the best dairy product, as it is high in protein and calcium. Skimmed milk is less nutritious as it has lost essential fatty acids, which are important as vitamins. However, there is one skimmed milk product now being recommended to pregnant women. 'Shape' or its Victorian equivalent 'REV' is a specially modified skimmed milk which contains vitamins and extra calcium but not the fat found in whole milk. So if you are worried about your weight, drink this milk or drink less whole milk rather than substituting skimmed milk. Cheese is fairly rich in protein and calcium and contains vitamins A and D, but is also high in fat. Cottage cheese is a nutritious alternative. If you have a small appetite or don't like drinking milk, a good quality dairy ice-cream is rich in calcium, carbohydrate and fats, so a small portion would make an ideal dessert. Avoid the commercial varieties described as non-dairy produce, as they contain dubious fats rather than milk, plus chemicals and additives. Cream is high in calcium and protein — and fat. For those who dislike milk, natural yoghurt makes a good nutritional substitute, as it is high in calcium.

Suggested daily intake:
600 to 900 mL *Note*: Teenage pregnancy 900 mL
30 g hard cheese = 200 mL milk
200 g yoghurt = 250 mL milk.

Meat, fish, poultry, eggs and legumes

Offal (liver, kidneys and heart) is an excellent source of protein, iron and B vitamins. It is especially good for you if you are anaemic and essential if, for any reason, you are not taking iron tablets. Red meats (beef, lamb and pure beef hamburgers) also contain a lot of protein and iron. Poultry (chicken and turkey) has a high protein content, and roasting is a good way to cook the meat without losing the goodness. White fish (cod, gemfish, ling, flake, etc.) are similar in nutritional value to poultry. Tinned fish (pilchards, sardines, tuna and herring) are rich in calcium, iron, vitamin A and protein, but they tend to be oily so their calorie content is higher. Eggs too, are a good source of protein, calcium, fat and vitamins A and D. Legumes (beans, peas and pulses — dried beans and peas — such as lentils, chick peas, etc) are an ideal source of protein and dietary fibre.

Suggested daily intake:
2 to 3 servings. Include 1 of these foods at 2 or 3 of your meals each day.
1 average serving is: 75 g to 100 g meat, fish, poultry, cheese, or, 1 or 2 eggs, or ½ cup cooked legumes.

Bread and cereals

All bread contains calcium, carbohydrate, iron and protein. However processed bread contains 'empty kilojoules' which means that you are getting more stodge and fewer nutrients than you will in wholemeal bread — which is also a good source of roughage. Whole cereals contain similar nutrients to wholemeal bread. Pasta and rice products contain carbohydrates, calcium

A scene many doctors recommend to pregnant women; relaxing.

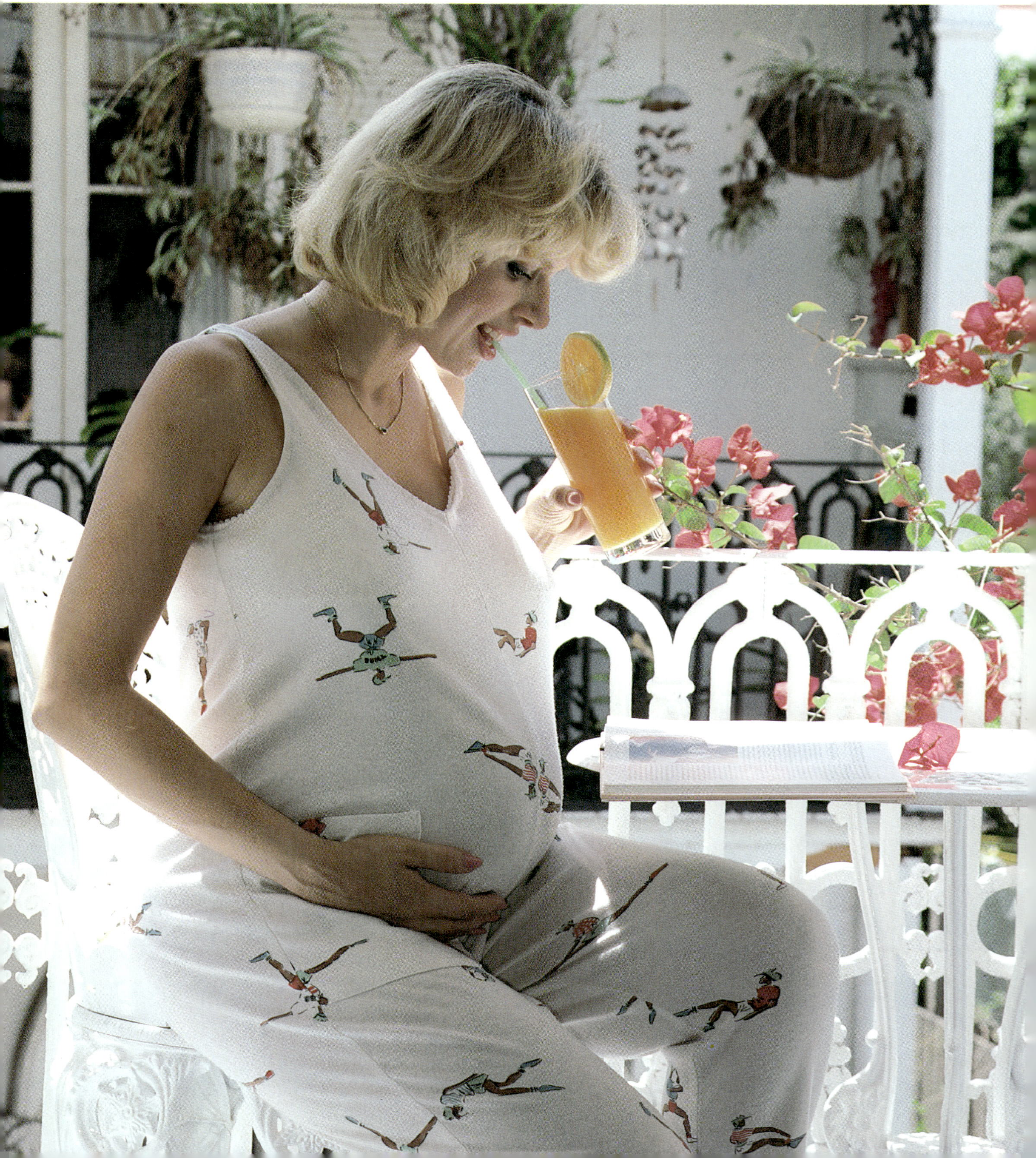

and iron, and are not as fattening as is generally assumed — it's the rich sauces served with the pasta and the creamy milk in the rice puddings that do the damage. Again brown rice and pasta are better for you than white.

Suggested daily intake:
4 servings or more. 1 serving is: 1 slice bread, or ½ cup cooked rice, spaghetti, macaroni, noodles, rolled oats, or ¾ cup breakfast cereal, or 2 crispbread.

Vegetables and fruit

Dried beans and peas are a cheap source of protein. Green vegetables and potatoes are high in vitamin C and a major source of dietary fibre. Vegetables are best eaten raw or steamed to avoid nutrient losses during cooking, and potatoes are most nourishing cooked and eaten in their jackets. Spinach haricot beans and lentils are high in calcium and iron. Carrots are a valuable source of vitamin A. Blackcurrants, oranges, lemons and grapefruit are rich in vitamin C. Try to eat some of the pith of citrus fruits, too, as this is exceptionally high in vitamin content. 'Fleshy' fruits such as bananas and mangoes are less plentiful in vitamins but contain carbohydrate. Dried fruits such as currants, sultanas and dates contain concentrated sugar and are a valuable source of energy.

Suggested daily intake:
4 servings or more. Include 1 vitamin C fruit or vegetable daily: citrus fruit, berry fruit, raw tomato, raw capsicum, fresh pineapple, mango, rockmelon, pawpaw, Brussels sprouts, broccoli and juices from these fruits and vegetables.

Include green vegetables daily. Include yellow vegetables and fruits regularly: carrot, pumpkin, apricot, rockmelon, pawpaw.

Butter, margarine and other fats and oils

Butter and table margarine are rich sources of vitamins A and D. All these foods are very high in kilojoules.

Suggested daily intake:
Use in moderation.

VEGETARIAN DIETS

A vegetarian diet during pregnancy is acceptable as long as an adequate supply of protein, iron and energy is included. Protein foods such as eggs, cheese, legumes, nuts, seeds and fish should be a constant feature of your diet. Extra bread and cereal can also help. Total vegetarians will require a vitamin B_{12} supplement.

If milk, cheese and yoghurt are excluded from the diet, a calcium supplement should be taken. All vegetarians are strongly urged to take iron supplements.

WHAT YOU NEED

It is particularly important when you are pregnant to include in your diet adequate amounts of all the essential nutrients, vitamins and minerals. These are listed here together with their chief functions and main food sources.

PROTEIN is tissue-building and therefore essential for your baby's growth, a healthy placenta and uterus. It also keeps your blood sugar level high which will help prevent depression. Main sources: meat, fish, eggs, milk, cheese, soy beans, nuts, pulses.

IRON increases the number of red cells in the blood and will stop you becoming anaemic as your blood increases in volume and therefore tends to thin. It will also stand you in good stead if you lose blood during delivery. Main sources: liver, beef, kidney, cocoa powder, green vegetables, watercress, dried fruit, wholemeal bread. Your doctor will probably also prescribe iron tablets.

FOLIC ACID helps fight anaemia, which can arise in pregnancy from a deficiency of folic acid. Main sources: offal, raw dark green leafy vegetables, pulses, wholemeal bread, oranges, bananas. Your doctor may prescribe folic acid in tablet form.

VITAMIN A builds up your resistance to infection and will also help relieve allergies and maintain healthy skin. Main sources: liver, halibut liver oil, carrots, spinach, also milk and butter.

B VITAMINS are important for many different body functions. They are essential for a healthy skin, for mental stability, and for the proper functioning of the digestive system. After the birth they increase the production of milk for breastfeeding. Main sources: meat, liver, milk, eggs, wholemeal bread, wheatgerm, fish, yeast extract.

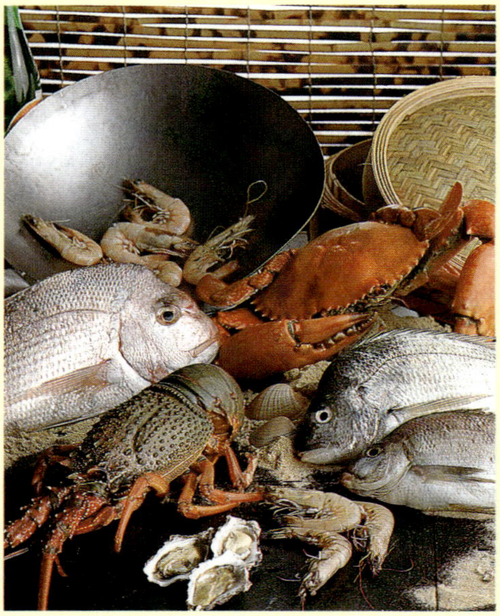

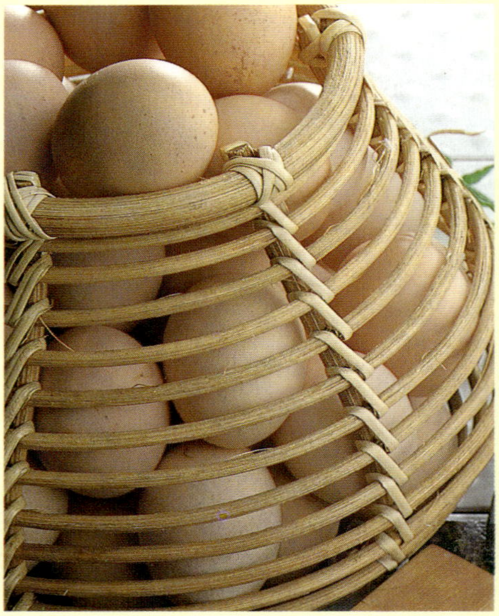

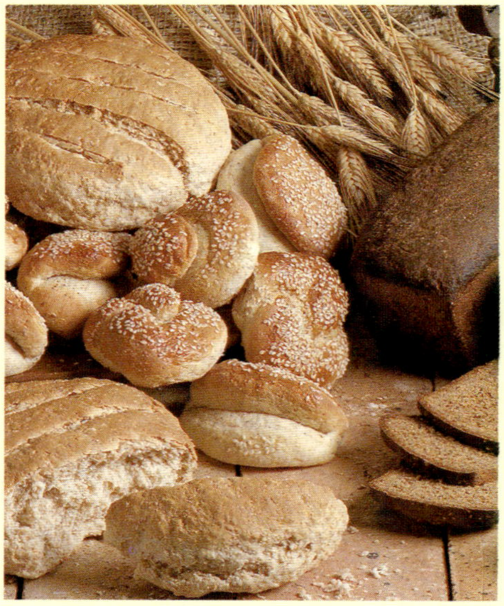

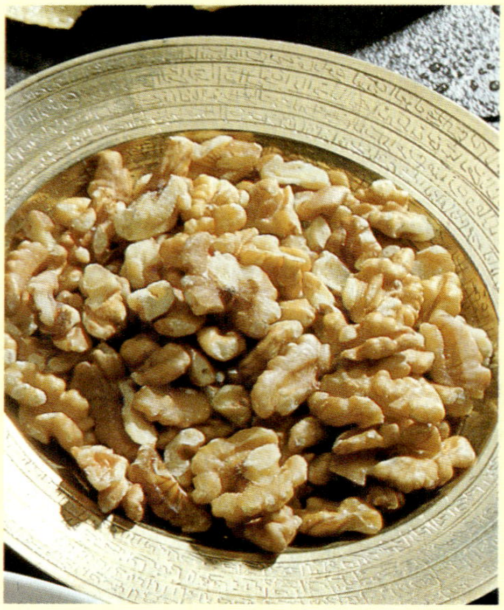

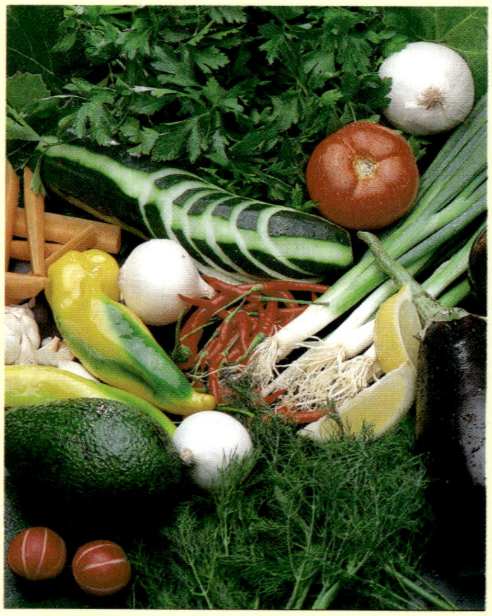

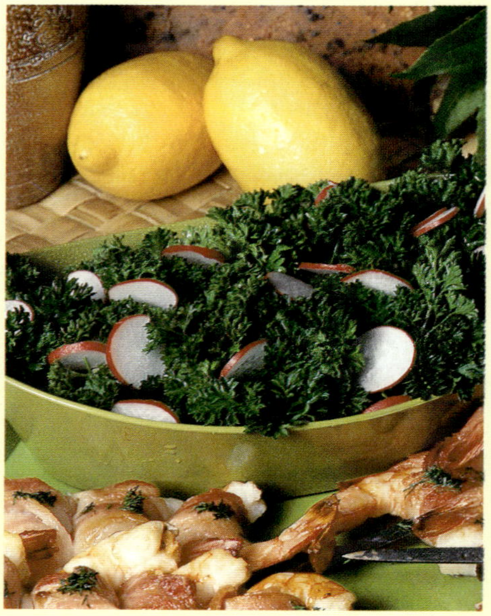

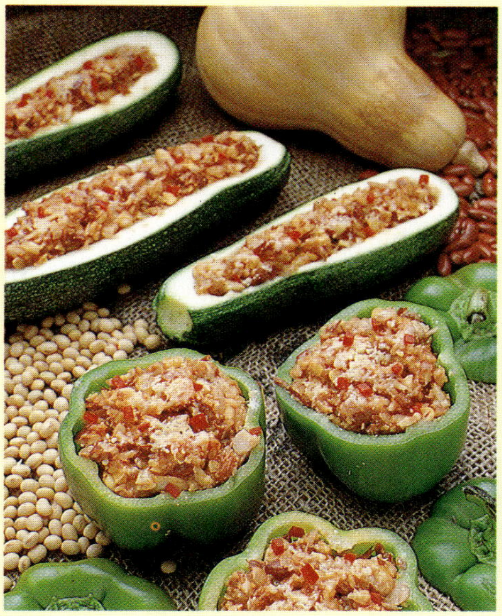

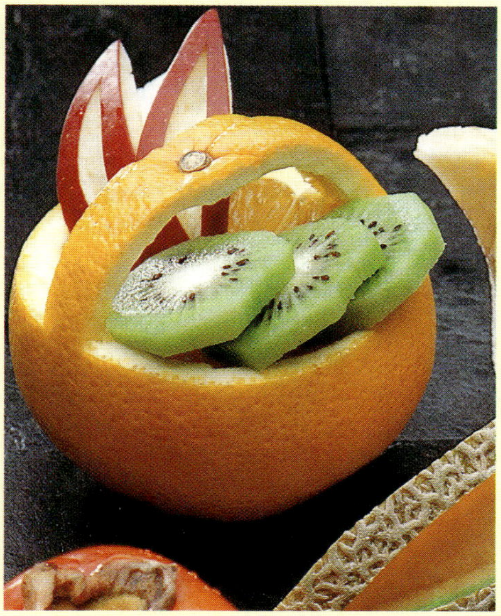

VITAMIN C helps the body absorb iron and keeps the tissues strong and healthy. Main sources: citrus fruit, green vegetables.

VITAMIN D aids the body in maintaining the level of calcium and phosphorus in the blood. Main sources: fatty fish, eggs, butter, margarine. It is also produced when the body is exposed to sunlight.

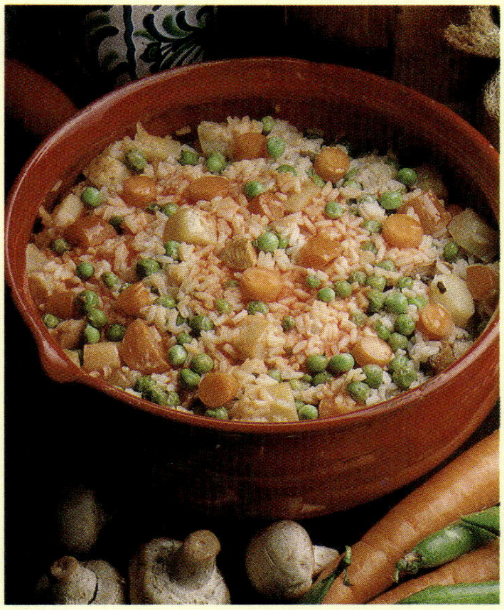

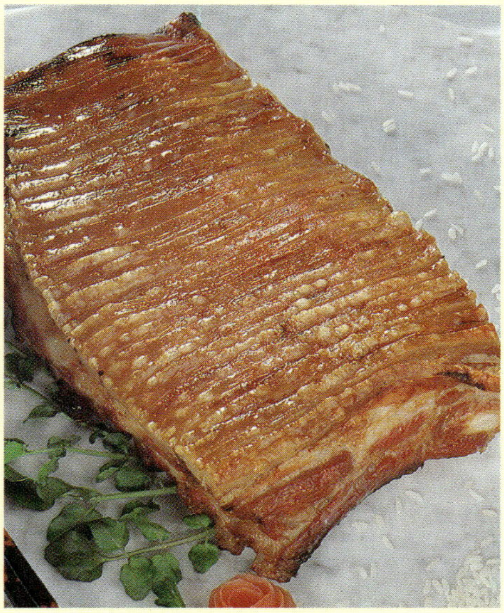

VITAMIN E can help strengthen the foetus and placenta, and improve the circulation thus preventing varicose veins and piles. Main sources: eggs, dairy products, unpolished rice, wholemeal bread, vegetable oils. Vitamin E supplement (wheatgerm oil) can be bought from a chemist or health food shop. You should never take vitamin E and iron together as the effectiveness of vitamin E is destroyed by iron — a 12-hour gap between them is necessary to avoid this.

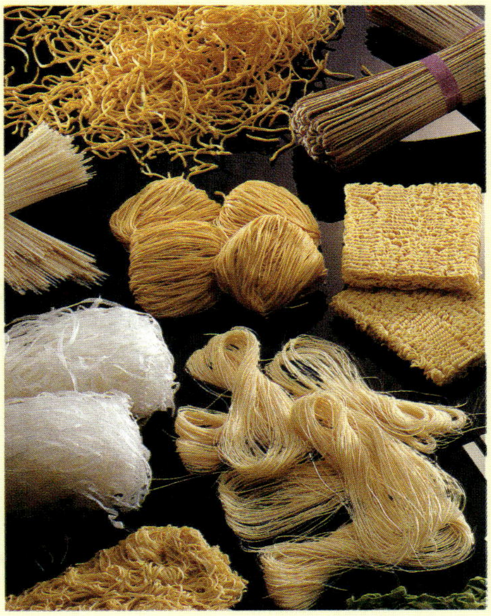

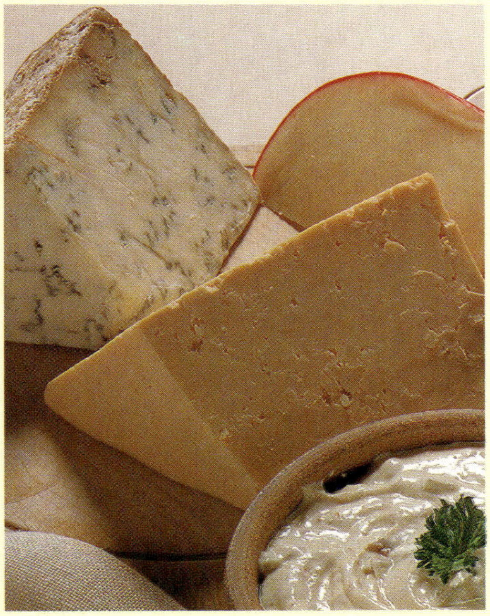

FATS AND CARBOHYDRATES provide energy and build up reserves of body fat. They also contain fat-soluble vitamins and minerals. Main sources of fats: butter, margarine, fatty meat and oily fish, dairy products. Main sources of unrefined carbohydrates: wholemeal bread, cereals, pasta, brown rice, potatoes, fruit. These are an essential part of a balanced diet. Main sources of refined carbohydrates (not good for you): sugar, cakes, biscuits, sweets, jam, soft drinks and alcohol.

CALCIUM is important for the development of your baby's teeth and bones. Main sources: milk, cheese, bones of tinned little fish, ie, sardines, pilchards.

body briefing

Your skin and muscles are stretched quite radically during pregnancy and labour, and if you allow yourself to become out of condition may take some time to return to normal afterwards. A little care and regular exercise can do a lot towards keeping you fit and supple while you are pregnant, and help to restore your figure after the birth.

Pregnancy inevitably brings about all kinds of minor changes to the body apart from the obvious bulge. The important thing is not to worry about these, but to understand what is happening and why. Every woman and every pregnancy is totally different and you may sail through your pregnancy with little or no inconvenient side effects. However, it is just as well to be aware of what changes can happen so that you know how to cope with them should they arise.

BREASTS

The breasts do not contain muscle and once they are allowed to sag no amount of exercise will ever revive them. So a good supporting bra as you enlarge during pregnancy is absolutely essential.

You should make sure that your breasts are firmly supported at about the 10th week, by which time they will probably be noticeably larger. Check their size again at the 20th week — often there is another noticeable increase by this stage. Your breasts should then remain the same size until delivery, but make sure that your bra has several alteration hooks at the back as the chest wall expands by 6–12 centimetres towards the end of pregnancy due to the ligaments relaxing.

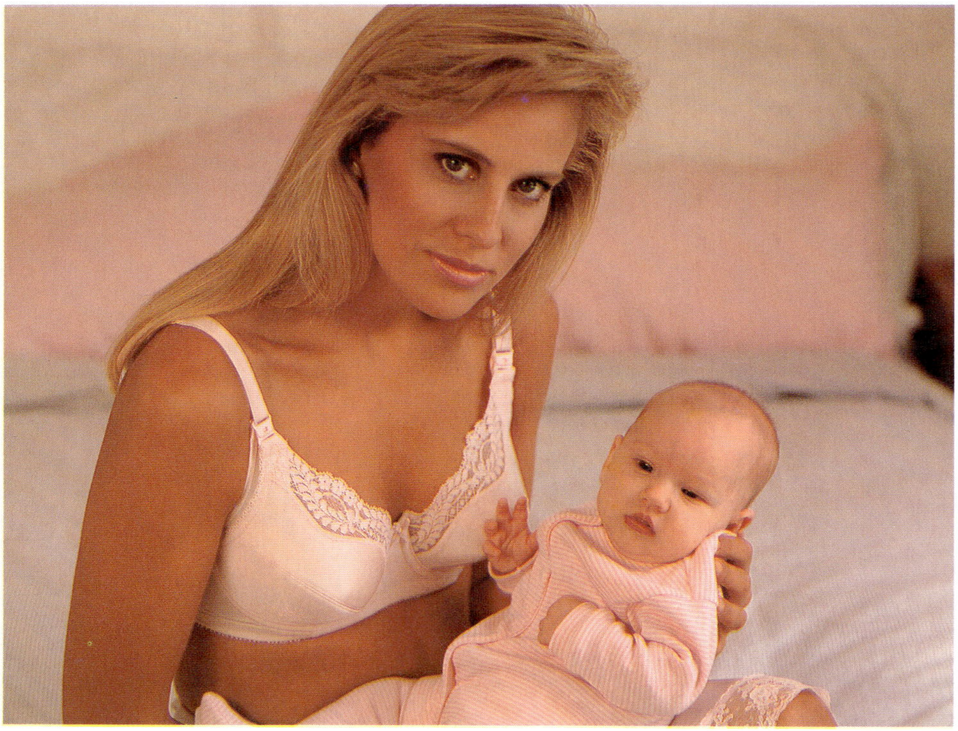

Berlei

Once your breasts sag, no amount of exercise will revive them. Throughout your pregnancy and while breast feeding, it is imperative to wear a firm support bra.

For a lot of women, the improved bust that pregnancy brings is a welcome bonus and a look at some of the bulky, unflattering maternity bras available could well be depressing. Don't despair — there are plenty of pretty, fashionable bras on the market that will give you perfectly adequate support. As long as the bra has strong, fairly wide shoulder straps (narrow elastic is not sufficiently supportive), good uplift underneath and a wide adjustable back, you can choose anything from fresh broderie anglaise to sexy black lace. If you find that your breasts feel heavy at night a light unribbed sleeping bra may be advisable.

To find your correct size, measure directly under the bust next to the skin and round this figure up to the nearest standard bra size. To get the correct cup size — which is the measurement most likely to increase — measure the fullest part of the bust and shoulder blades. If the difference between the two measurements you have taken is under 15 centimetres, then you need a B cup; if it is over 15 centimetres you want a C cup; and if even greater, try a D cup.

Don't buy a nursing bra — that is one that opens at the front to enable you to breastfeed — until the last month of pregnancy when you have a good idea of the size your breasts will be after the birth. Again, make sure the bra you choose has adjustable hooks at the back to cope with changes in breast size after the milk arrives.

Wash your breasts daily when you take your regular bath or shower, but be sparing with the soap as this can be drying. To keep the nipples supple in preparation for breastfeeding, massage them gently every day with a little oil, lanolin or nipple cream.

ABDOMEN

If you have never worn a girdle and haven't put on an excessive amount of weight there is really no need to wear one now — with care and exercise your muscles will return to normal soon after you have had your baby. However, some women do find that midway through pregnancy they have a certain amount of aching in the lower abdomen; a feeling of dragging down. If you feel this kind of muscular discomfort or your abdomen becomes very large, a lightweight maternity girdle will help. If you normally wear a girdle then, of course, you must not discard it during pregnancy as your muscles will not be able to cope. As long as it is still comfortable, wear your normal girdle, which will stretch as you get bigger, or buy a maternity girdle, which gives particular support to the lower abdominal muscles. When you find you are growing out of a girdle, replace it with another straightaway — don't give the muscles a chance to sag. It's an old wives' tale that support underwear can damage the baby in the uterus — so don't fear that you may be squashing the baby; the thick walls of the womb protect the child. It's your own comfort that's the important thing here. When choosing a girdle, always measure the widest part of the hips, about 20 centimetres below the waist.

BACKACHE AND POSTURE

The best way to prevent backache is to make sure your posture is correct. The hormone progesterone causes the tendons and ligaments of the body to soften and stretch, especially in the back and pelvis, and the strain caused by the weight of the baby on the lower joints of the spine can cause a nagging, uncomfortable ache. A firm bed, massage and an electric pad or a hot water bottle wrapped in a cover and placed on the back will all help, but if you stand as upright as possible and avoid the pregnancy slouch (the classic droop of the shoulders and relaxation of the stomach) you will improve your posture and be less prone to backache. To check your posture, stand with your back against a wall, balance your weight evenly between the heels and balls of your feet, pull your abdomen in and make yourself as tall as possible. Try and keep this straight stance whether standing still or walking.

Strain on the back can of course be caused by bending or lifting badly. When you pick anything up, always bend your knees and keep your back straight. Never try bending from the waist, which will pull the muscles in your back. Remember this when picking up a small child or pet. If you have a lot of shopping to carry, never pile it all into one bag, spread the load evenly between two bags and carry one in each hand. But don't attempt to carry more than you can comfortably manage.

Housework can also cause posture problems. Try to sit at the sink or ironing board rather than stand; kneel to make the bed rather than bend; kneel by the side of the bath to clean it.

THE PELVIC FLOOR

The softening of the joints and ligaments during pregnancy is necessary because the pelvis needs to be as flexible as possible for the birth. For the same reason it is important to keep the pelvic floor — the larger muscle that supports your pelvic organs — toned up in preparation for labour. If you practise these simple exercises now, they will also help you after your baby is born in getting your muscles back into shape.

1 Tighten and relax the ring of muscles immediately around the anus (back passage), keeping your stomach and buttock muscles relaxed.
2 Tense and relax the muscles that surround openings of the bladder and vagina — as if stopping yourself passing urine. In fact, this is a good time to practise pelvic floor exercises — a few minutes stream-stopping every day will do a lot towards toning you up.
3 Now pull up the whole of the pelvic floor by contracting both sets of muscles together. You can do these exercises anywhere — while driving the car, standing at the bus stop — whenever you have a spare minute and remember.

STRETCH MARKS

Stretch marks are thin red scar-like lines that appear very suddenly during pregnancy where the skin stretches on the abdomen, breasts, or thighs. After the birth they gradually fade to silvery marks, but never disappear completely. Some women seem to be more prone to them than others and are likely to get them if they put on too much weight. Apart from watching your weight gain there is no way of preventing stretch marks and creaming or oiling the skin with exorbitantly priced 'wonder preparations' will not be effective. However as the skin often becomes dry during pregnancy creaming will certainly help to keep it supple. Prenatal cream, vitamin E oil or a little baby oil in the bath will all make your skin feel softer.

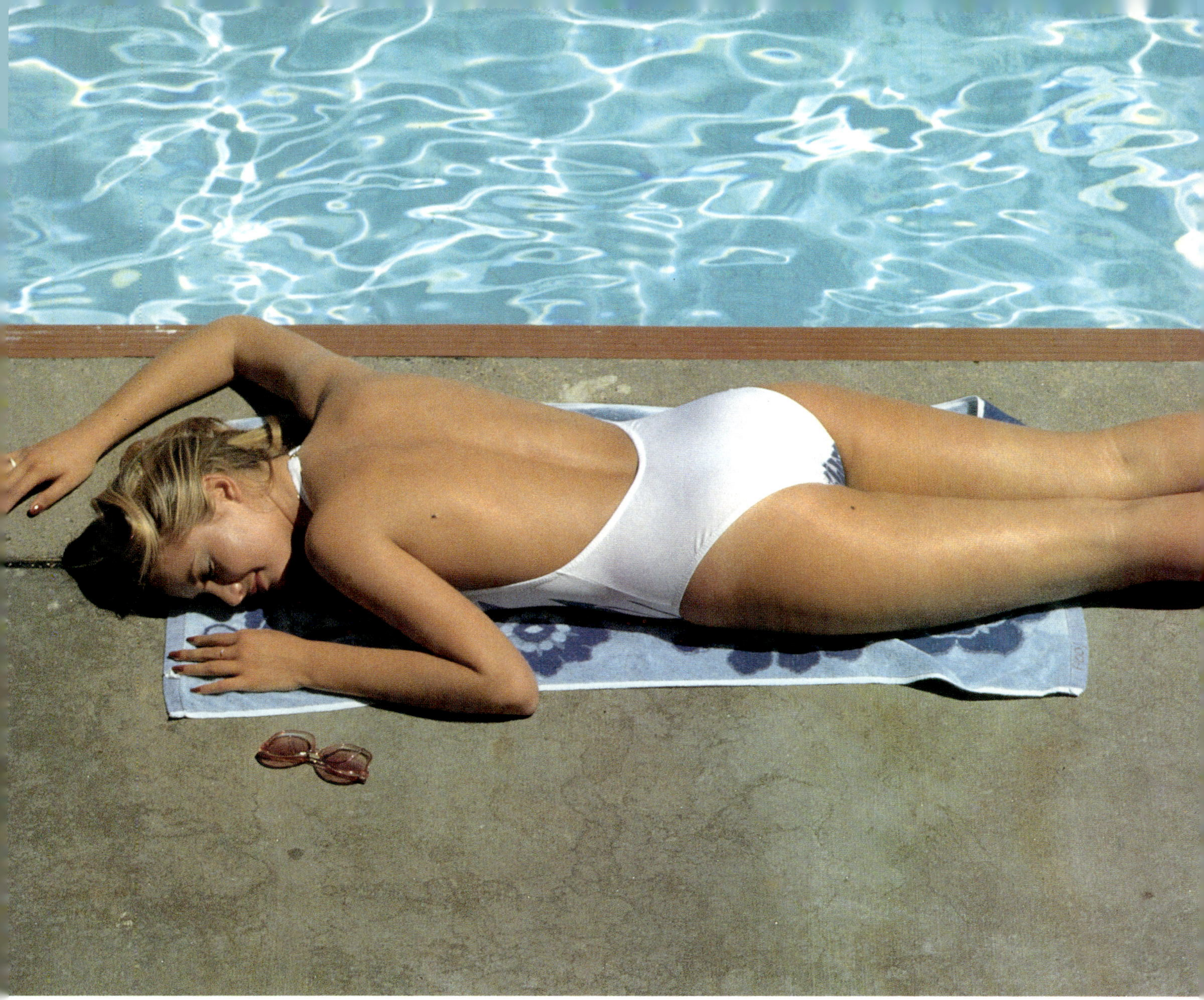

PIGMENTATION AND SUNBATHING

Before rushing out to boost your tan, beware of skin pigmentation brought on by pregnancy and highlighted by sunlight. However if you don't have any skin pigmentation and can tan, it is a great way to build up vitamin D supplies. Remember though pregnant women are more susceptible to sunstroke.

There is usually an increase in pigmentation of the skin during pregnancy, which brunettes find most noticeable — freckles, birth-marks, moles and some scars seem to get much darker, especially if they are exposed to the sun. The nipples and areola — the area of delicate skin around the nipple — change colour at around the 14th week of pregnancy either changing from pink to brown or simply becoming darker. Again, this is far more marked in dark-haired women than in women with fair skin who have very little pigmentation of the breasts. A dark line called the *linea nigra* develops down the middle of the abdomen at about the same time. The line can stretch from the pubic hair to the lower ribs, but often only extends as far as the umbilicus (which can also pigment and flatten towards the end of pregnancy). It usually fades a few weeks after delivery.

If you are very fair-haired, you may suddenly notice a light down on your face — especially around the jawline — or abdomen, and even fairish hair on your arms and legs that you never thought you had. In fact this is not excess hair developing, it's just a darkening of the existing hair and will return to normal after the birth of your baby.

Occasionally a freckly, butterfly-shaped 'mask' known as *chloasma* spreads over the face in late pregnancy and can be brought out if exposed to the sun or a solarium. If you sunbathe and notice a distinctive pattern — like a tea stain — forming from the nose, over your cheeks and on your forehead, it's as well to cover up straightaway with a hat and keep your face completely shaded. The mask will fade with your tan but if established may never completely disappear.

However, not all women get this type of pigmentation during pregnancy (darker women are again more prone), and one of the advantages of sunbathing — apart from the psychological boost of a suntan — is that the action of sunlight on the skin helps to form vitamin D in the body. But if you do sunbathe don't allow yourself to become too hot. Because of the increase in metabolic activity pregnant women tend to feel the heat more than usual and can be more susceptible to sunstroke, which is unpleasant under any circumstances.

FEET AND ANKLES

During pregnancy a great strain is placed on the feet, again due to the softening and stretching of ligaments combined with your weight increase, and it's important to pay extra attention to them. Sit with your feet up whenever you can and never stand still for too long — this will cause your ankles and feet to swell as the blood gets down to them easily but has a lot of trouble getting back. The following exercises will help to keep the blood flowing freely. Ease aching feet by soaking them for 10–15 minutes in a bowl of salted tepid water.

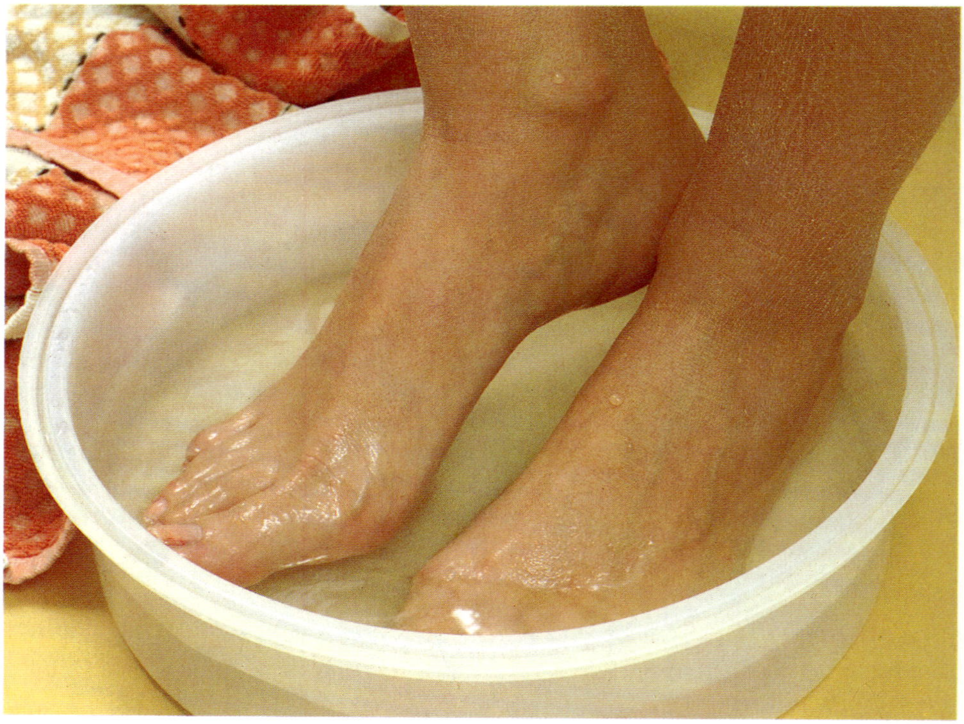

Feet need special attention during pregnancy. Soaking feet in salted tepid water will ease the aches and pains.

Foot massage

1 Sit comfortably on a chair with your back straight. Place the balls of your feet on a rolling pin, press them down and roll the pin backwards and forward — on a carpet is best.
2 Next tie your big toes together with a piece of tape (not too tight) then try to pull the feet apart. These are good exercises to do while watching television!
3 Still sitting — or else lying on the floor or in bed — rotate each foot in a circular motion, first to the left, then to the right. Take hold of each toe separately and wiggle it up and down as far as possible and then in a circular direction. These exercises help to loosen the joints as well as improving the circulation in the legs.

As care of the feet is so important, a visit to a chiropodist every two months is a good idea, and more often than this towards the end of pregnancy. When manicuring your feet yourself, always cut the nails straight across and then round off the edges with a nail file. Your nails grow faster during pregnancy than at any other time, and if you cut down the sides or leave jagged corners you may find you have ingrowing toenails before too long. Massage dry and scaly skin regularly with an unperfumed hand or body lotion and use a pumice stone to rub off hard skin on the soles. Your feet will probably sweat more towards the end of pregnancy; if they do and the skin seems to be getting slightly soggy, make a habit of wiping in between the toes with a little surgical spirit to prevent this. Dusting with talc is *not* a good idea as it will just clog up the pores and make you sweat more than ever.

VARICOSE VEINS

Varicose veins can develop at any stage during pregnancy and are caused by the pressure of the enlarging uterus on the veins in the pelvis constricting the upward flow of blood from the legs to the heart. The veins in the legs may dilate and stretch if the strain becomes too great and become painfully hard with a blue, lumpy appearance. There are usually warning signs before the veins appear: aching legs, cramp in the calves at night, swelling in the lower leg and around the ankle. Long hours of standing or sitting still (especially with the legs crossed), wearing elastic-topped socks or stockings or boots that are too tight, being overweight, and hereditary factors, can all contribute towards getting them.

Support tights worn from an early stage are the best way to ease or help to prevent varicose veins, but make sure they are not so tight that they cramp your feet. In some cases your doctor may prescribe support hose, but the medical varieties are usually rather drab and thick and guaranteed to make you feel dowdy. You can buy lightweight tights in flattering colours which will look every bit as attractive as your normal tights or stockings. Put them on first thing in the morning, preferably even before you get out of bed or immediately after a bath, and wear them all day.

Varicose veins usually disappear after pregnancy when the weight is removed from the legs, but once you have suffered from them they will inevitably return with subsequent pregnancies. Try to avoid the problem by always sitting with your legs straight and uncrossed, if you cannot put them up. Don't sit for a long time in the same position — move your feet up or down — or stand in the same stance. Walk whenever possible — this will help maintain a steady flow of blood around the body. Also, watch your weight. The less bulk your legs have to carry, the less strain on the veins.

VAGINAL DISCHARGES

There is an increase in mucus discharged from the vagina throughout pregnancy which, although you may find it annoying, is perfectly normal. Its occurrence is due to altered hormone levels and an increase in blood supply to the pelvis. However, if it begins to make you itch or causes an offensive smell, tell your doctor. You have probably developed a common fungus infection called thrush, which can be dealt with promptly. Hygiene is important, so take as many baths as you like — it is very rare for water to actually enter the vagina and even if it did it would certainly not infect it. Keep the area surrounding the vagina scrupulously clean during pregnancy, but always make sure you rinse away the soap. Wear cotton underwear, and when washing it take care that everything is well rinsed and no traces of soap powder have been left to cause irritation.

TEETH

It is very important to keep your teeth particularly clean during pregnancy. Extra hormones in the circulation make the gums much softer and unless you meticulously remove all the debris from between the teeth, the gums easily become damaged and then infected. This inflammation of the gums is called gingivitis. Gingivitis is common among non-pregnant people too but your gums are far more susceptible to infection at this time. If you notice that they bleed when you clean your teeth, it's likely that you have developed gingivitis. If you don't visit your dentist and have this remedied by thorough cleansing, your teeth will be more prone to decay than ever.

Cleanliness is the most important thing. Follow a strict regime of cleaning and dental flossing and visit your dentist for regular check-ups. Brush your teeth after every meal if possible with a medium or soft brush. Use dental floss daily to help remove food particles from between the teeth. If your gums do bleed, don't stop brushing them. Gentle friction will stimulate the gums and help release any trapped particles. Use a mouthwash to rinse these away.

NAILS

Although their growth rate is invariably speeded up during pregnancy, nails may tend to become dry and brittle and split easily. Rub olive or baby oil into the base of the nails at night and massage — this should help to stimulate a stronger growth.

EYES

Wearers of contact lenses may find that these become uncomfortable during pregnancy. This is because the shape of your eyeballs may change very slightly as a result of fluid retention. If they do then it is probably best to revert to wearing glasses until the eyes return to normal.

There is no reason why your eyesight should change during pregnancy. But if you do seem to be growing a little more short- or long-sighted than usual, don't change your lenses until after your baby is born.

Baby or olive oil for nails and a moisturising cream for hands will keep them in great shape during pregnancy.

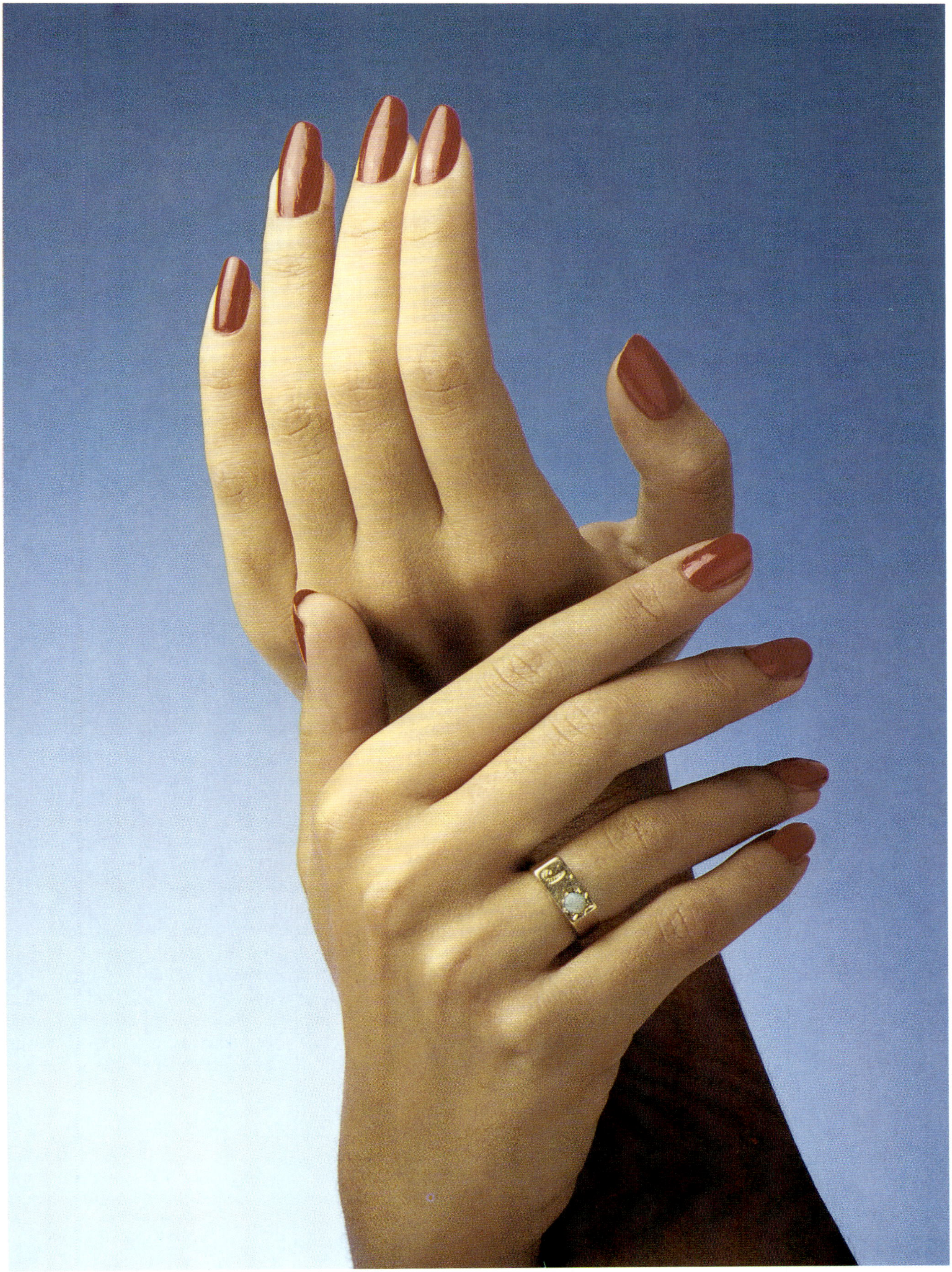

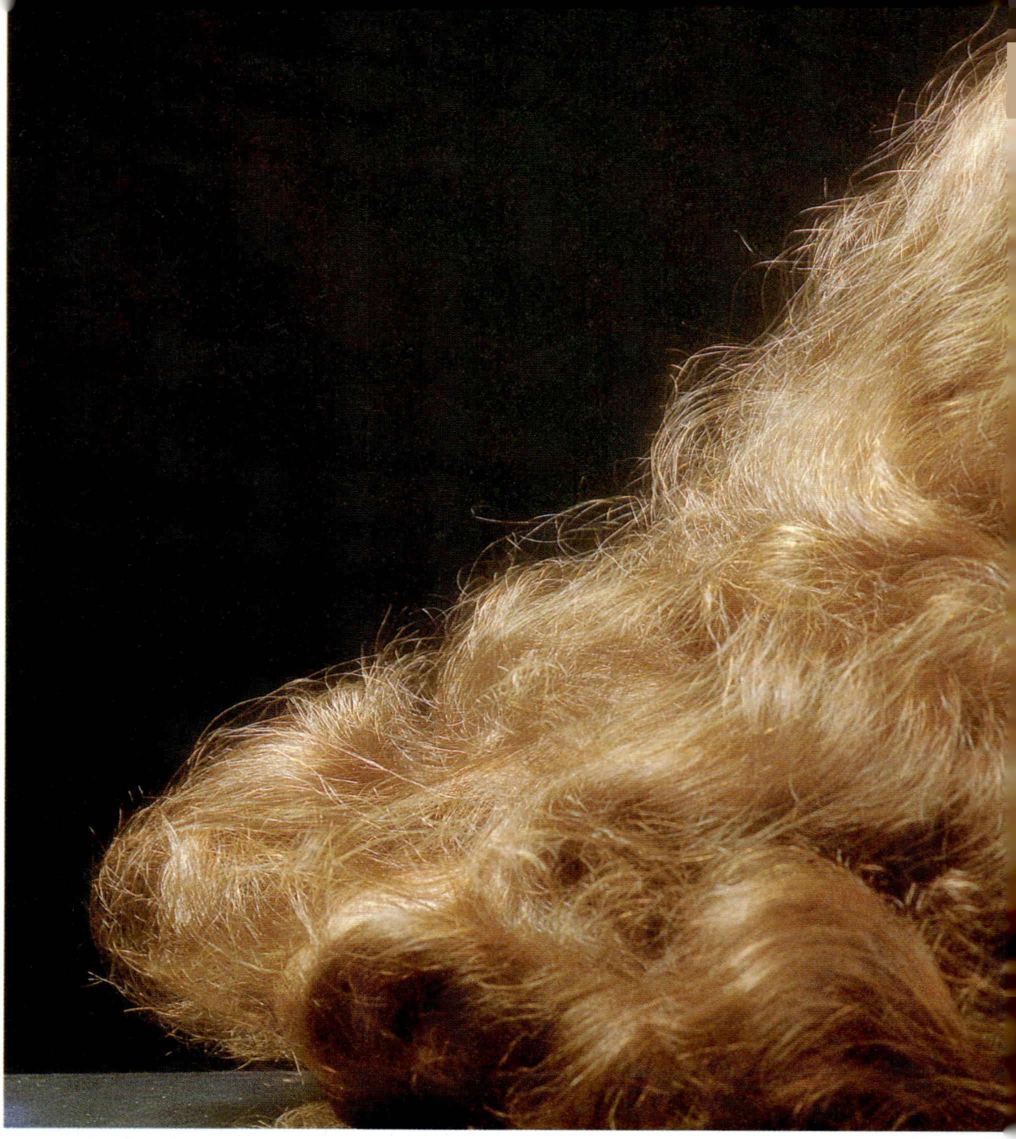

HAIR

With all the upheavals going on in your body it is inevitable that the condition of your hair will change to some extent — whether for better or for worse. But while the re-balancing of hormones is the reason for this, the state of your health has a lot to do with it and some trichologists (hair-care specialists) feel that the best hair tonic of all comes from a pregnant woman's own effort and well-being. For instance, you are probably taking more interest in your diet, making sure you get the right vitamins and so on. You may have stopped smoking or at least cut down. You probably don't drink as much alcohol as before. You are possibly taking life a little slower and sitting with your feet up more often and are therefore more relaxed. So, although nature plays a large part in your appearance during pregnancy, so does the way you look after yourself.

Many women find that their hair in fact changes for the better during pregnancy even though it does tend to become a little greasier. This is because the body is producing extra sebum (or oil) which protects the elasticity and prevents the hair from splitting. You may need to wash your hair more often but if you use a mild shampoo you should have a healthy, shining head of hair.

If, on the other hand, your hair seems to have become drier (less sebum) take extra care. It may break more easily and because of this more may fall

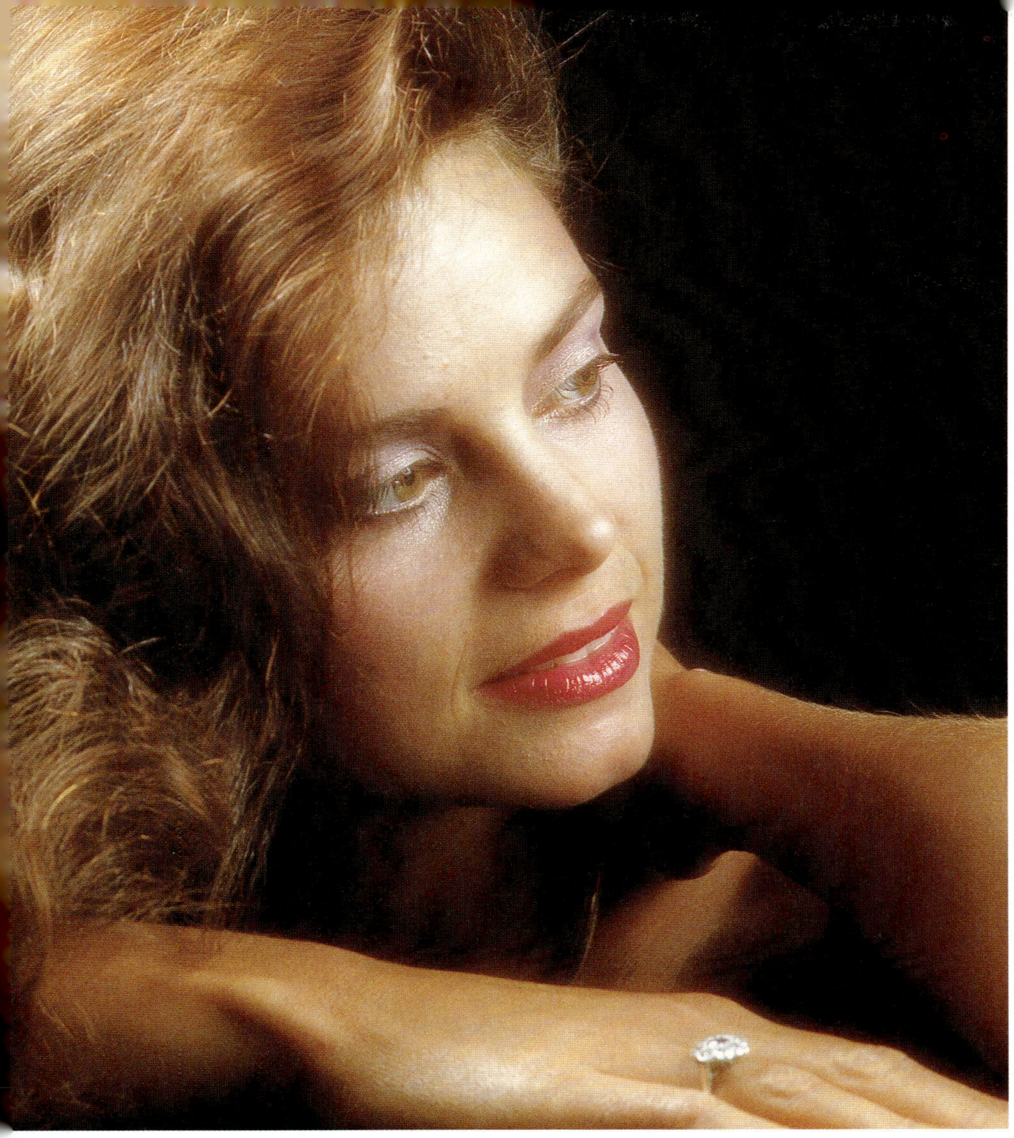

In many instances, hair changes for the better during pregnancy.

out than usual. In this case, use a very mild shampoo and be careful not to brush or comb your hair harshly or to use too much heat on it when drying — rather let it dry naturally. If the condition of your hair has not improved after the first 12 weeks or so — or indeed has deteriorated — it is probably not the fault of your pregnancy at all. Perhaps you are not in particularly good health. Try to include more fresh fruit and vegetables in your diet and see your doctor if you feel very run down. You may be worrying or feeling tense or may not be getting enough rest. If you have tried to remedy your hair problem without success think about how you feel in yourself and don't be afraid to discuss this with your doctor.

The increase in metabolic activity during pregnancy causes a greater amount of blood than usual to reach the skin and you may find that you often feel hot and sweaty. Because you sweat more frequently your hair may well become lank towards the end of pregnancy. The only answer here is frequent washing to keep it looking fresh and clean. This will not do your hair any harm, but always use a mild baby shampoo or a herbal shampoo to avoid stripping off the natural oils.

Hair grows much faster during pregnancy than at any other time but this rapid growth rate slows down after birth. Some women find that a considerable amount of hair actually falls out after delivery, which can be worrying. However, this is a perfectly normal thing to happen and it will certainly not lead to baldness — new hair begins to grow almost immediately to replace the hair that has been lost.

limbering up

Pregnancy is not an illness or a handicap, so there is no need to wrap yourself in cotton wool. On the whole, a sensible rule is to follow your habits rather than change them, but it's a pretty sure bet that if you make some attempt to keep your body exercised you'll feel much better for it — less lumpy and awkward — and find it easier to get back in trim after you have had the baby.

The kind of exercise you can do while pregnant depends very much on the sort of physical activity you have been used to before. If you have not previously played active games of tennis or squash, or attended aerobics classes, this is hardly the time to start. The work of the heart may increase by as much as 40 per cent by the 28th week. In fact, the heart itself enlarges with the increased load so don't give it extra, unnecessary work to do. Rest comes before exercise during pregnancy. If you have a home and other children to look after, you will automatically be kept fairly active. Washing floors, vacuuming and making beds are all vigorous duties and you should be careful not to over-tire yourself just with everyday housework.

However, if you are used to participating regularly in sports, there is no reason why you shouldn't continue throughout the first half of pregnancy — providing everything is progressing normally and your doctor agrees. There are obvious exceptions: water-skiing, snow-skiing, skin-diving and horse-riding are out since there is always a risk of injury. Cycling is fine as long as you are extremely careful not to tire yourself or to lose balance. In early pregnancy an accident could result in miscarriage and during the last few months the sheer bulk of the abdomen makes balancing precarious. By this stage it is very unlikely that any blow to the abdomen would actually harm the baby, but there is always a chance that the shock might bring on miscarriage or early labour. There is absolutely no excuse for not walking. Obviously mountaineering, cross-country runs and hiking are not advisable, but walking short distances — getting to and from work, for example — rather than taking the bus or driving, can only help you keep fit so long as you don't exhaust yourself. The same is true of dancing — it's good for you providing it's not too acrobatic. The amount of energy involved in your dancing will depend entirely on how you feel, and of course, your weight will dictate how late into your pregnancy you wish to continue. It is unlikely that you will feel much like leaping around in a disco during the last two or three months.

Swimming is fine — so long as you don't allow yourself to become out of breath and over-tired. But if you are not used to swimming you should avoid it during the first three months. Never swim in very cold water as you are more likely to get cramp, and don't try any high diving. Only experienced divers should even attempt to dive and then only from heights of under one metre, as the sudden change in your blood pressure could affect the baby's circulation. Check with your doctor before embarking on an exercise programme — if you have a history of miscarriage your doctor may not advise it. The exercises on the following pages are simple and medically approved, and will gently tone up your body during pregnancy whether you have exercised before or not. Don't be complacent and leave it all until after the birth — it might be too late then. Aim to go into labour with your body supple and trim.

Work out on a blanket or heavy towel if the floor is too hard, and wear

Pregnancy is not an illness or handicap. Being pregnant does not mean avoiding all exercise. If you do exercise of some sort, you will feel better and will find it easier to trim down after having the baby.

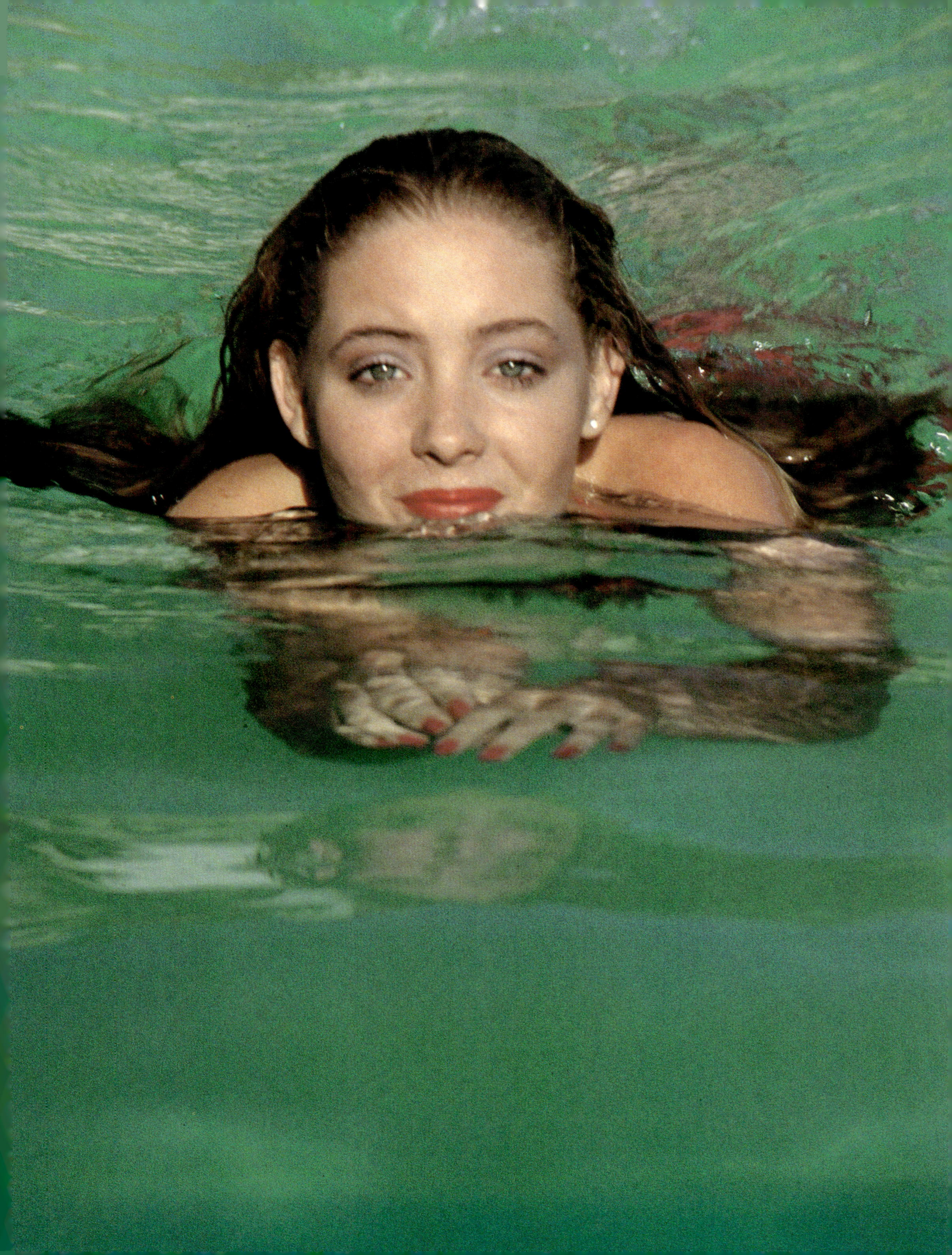

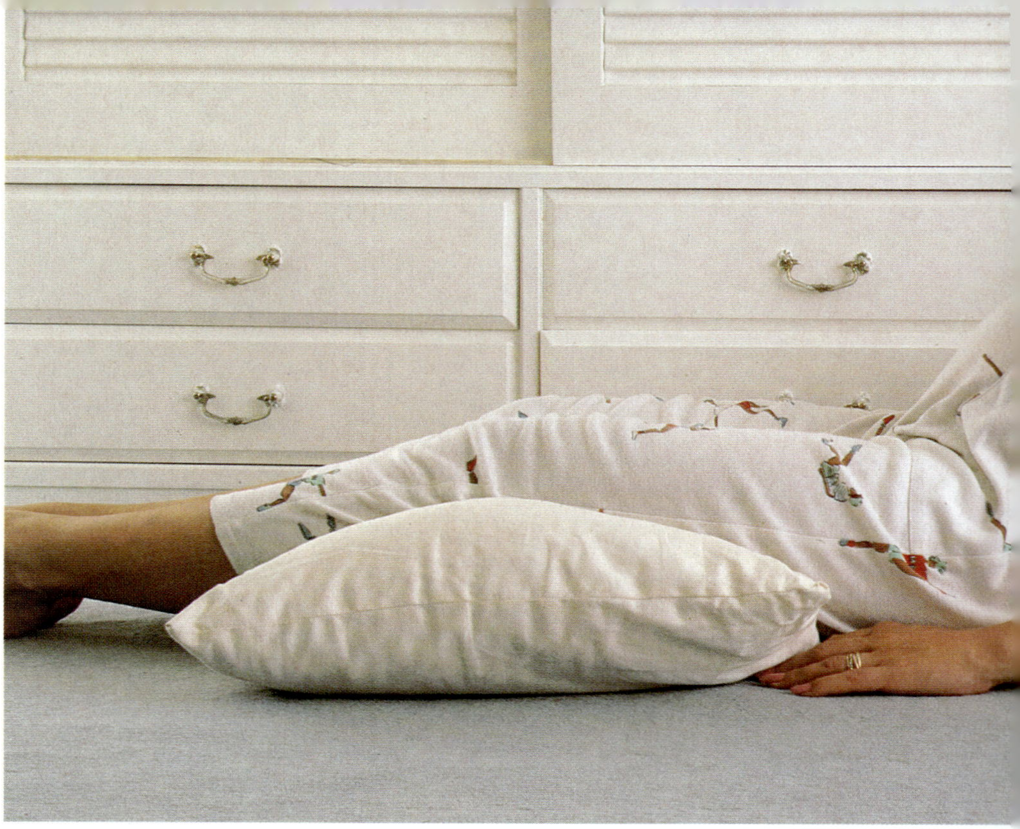

loose-fitting garments — a leotard is all right if it stretches enough but don't wear one if it's constricting. All these exercises are safe to do throughout pregnancy, but stop at once if a position becomes uncomfortable or hurts, and take particular care in the first few weeks.

RELAXATION EXERCISES

Begin your programme with these simple breathing exercises for relaxation, especially if you have never exercised before. Remember whenever you get up off the floor to roll onto your side first.

Hand press

Stand straight with your hands together in a prayer position in front of your chest, shoulders dropped and elbows lifted outwards. Breathe in (slightly slower than normal breathing), expanding your stomach. Then breathe out, pulling your stomach in and pressing the palms of your hands together as hard as possible. Repeat 10–20 times. Apart from being relaxing, this exercise is good for your stomach muscles, breasts and upper arms.

Deep breathing

Lie on your back on the floor in a relaxed position with your knees bent upwards and feet slightly apart, and with your hands resting on your stomach. Breathe in slowly, making the breath as long as you can manage, and expanding the stomach — feel it rise with your fingers. Then breathe out slowly, emptying your lungs, pulling your stomach flat, and pressing the small of your back into the floor. Start by breathing out to a count of five and work up to ten. Repeat the exercise 10–20 times.

Stretch

Sit on the floor with your legs stretched out in front of you, knees together and back straight but relaxed. Breathe in, lowering your chin forward so that

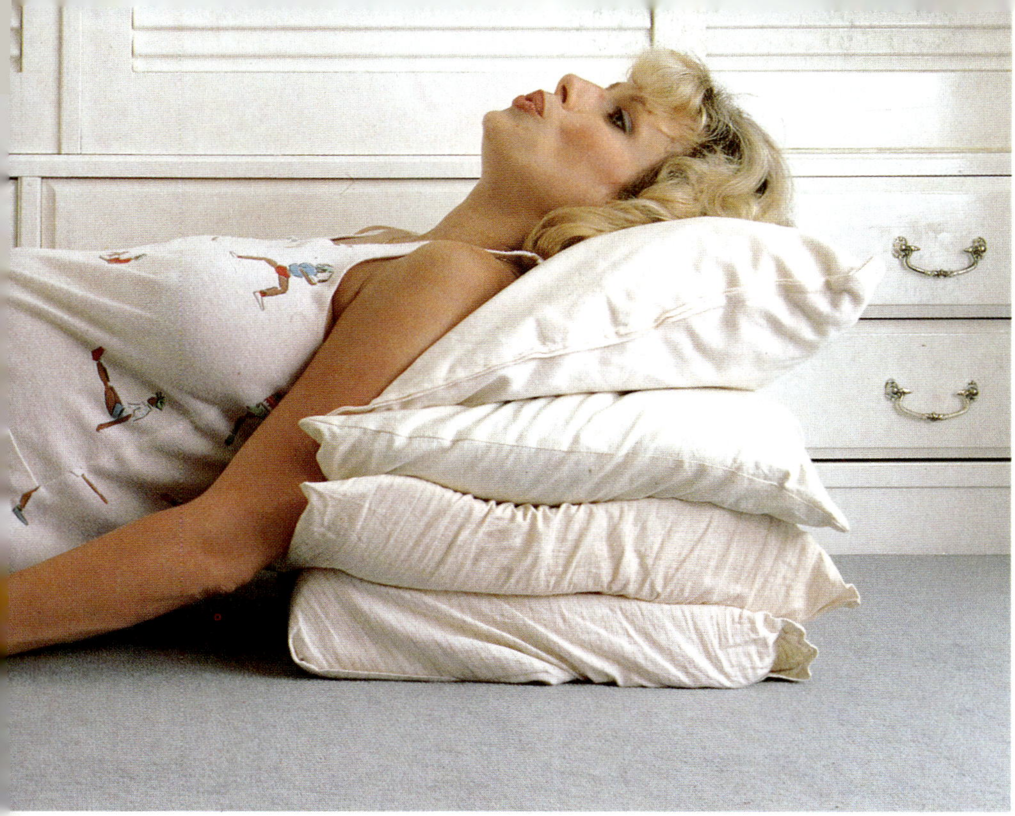

A relaxation programme is simple and involves breathing and basic stretching exercises.

you lengthen your spine, but keep it straight, at the same time reaching upwards with your arms — the palms facing each other and fingers splayed. Keeping your legs straight (knees pressed into the ground) and arms in the same position, stretch out forward from the base of the spine, simultaneously breathing out and pulling in your stomach. Lean as far as you can over your legs and hold it for a few seconds before returning to the upright position. Repeat 10–20 times. This is both a relaxing and stretching exercise; you won't of course be able to reach so far forward during the later stages of pregnancy.

Back stretch

Lie on your back with your knees bent up so that your feet are flat on the floor and slightly apart, and your arms stretched back above your head. Keeping your arms relaxed, breathe in, expanding your stomach and arching your back slightly off the floor. Then breathe out all your air, pulling the back of your waist into the floor so that your tailbone lifts very slightly, and stretching your arms out backwards as far as you can. Repeat 10–20 times. This stretch complements the previous exercise.

TONING UP EXERCISES

The following tone-up exercises are for the pelvis, abdomen, back, legs, arms, bottom and breasts.

Pelvic tilt

To tone up the muscles of the pelvic area and abdomen, lie flat on the floor with your legs bent, knees together, feet slightly apart, and arms by your sides. Arch your back slightly. Then push the small of your back into the floor and tighten your buttock muscles. As you do this you will feel your tummy muscles gently tighten also. Relax back into the first position and repeat 10 times. This exercise is particularly good for relieving backache.

Leg stretch

Using a chair, mantelpiece or doorknob for support, stand sideways to this with your back and legs straight, feet together. Balance your weight on the leg nearest your support and lift the outside leg 10 centimetres from the ground in front of you — or higher if you can — keeping the toes pointed. Bend and straighten the knee six times. Then turn round and repeat with the other leg.

Bottom toner

Lie on the floor with your legs bent, feet apart, and arms by your sides. Raise your bottom slightly off the floor so that the weight of your body is supported by the upper part of your back. Tighten and relax the buttock muscles, 30 times to start with, but try to work up to 100 if you can. This is only a little movement, the hips should not move much, but it is an excellent exercise for toning the pelvic area and stomach.

Breasts

Stand straight and hold your left wrist with the right hand and your right wrist with the left hand, palms facing. Keep your wrists away from your body and raise your arms to chin level — the higher the better. Holding firmly, push the hands towards your elbows in short, sharp movements — 30 times or as many as you can comfortably manage. Move your arms up and down as you do this exercise, from chin to eye level.

Upper arms

Still standing, hold your arms straight out to the sides at right angles to your body. Clench your fists to tense the arms. Then rotate both arms together in small, tight circles backwards 20 times, then 20 times forwards.

Scissors in the air

Lie flat on your back and bend your knees up towards your chin. Hold on to your thighs and curl the top part of your body forward towards your knees so that your head and shoulders come off the floor.

Straighten your legs out completely; let go of your thighs and stretch your arms to the ceiling. You should now be stretching upwards with legs, arms and head.

Keeping your legs very straight (toes either pointed or flexed towards you) make large, slow strides up and down in the air without quite touching the ground. This is a smooth, sweeping scissor action, don't jerk. Start with 10 and see if you can build up to 50 scissors. This exercise is very good for the stomach and legs.

Back arch

Kneel on all fours with your arms straight and directly under your shoulders. Breathe out all your air, humping up your back, pulling your stomach into your backbone, and letting your head drop right forward — try to touch your chest with your chin. Then breathe in deeply, pushing your bottom into the air, arching your back and lifting your head up and back so that you can look at the ceiling. Repeat this whole movement up to six times. This exercise is for the spine, stomach and pelvic area, and is another good one for relieving backache.

YOGA

As with all exercises, you should check with your doctor before taking up yoga when you are pregnant, however simple the poses look. These positions are specially designed for pregnant women and, unless you have a history of miscarriage, will be safe to do throughout pregnancy.

Mountain pose

Stand straight with your feet together. Don't lean over your toes, but keep your weight evenly distributed between the balls of your feet and your heels. Stretch your whole body up towards the ceiling as though the top of your head was attached to it by a string. Keep your chin down slightly and let your shoulders relax, holding them back and down at the same time. Breathe deeply.

Baddha Konasana

Sit on the floor with your back against a wall, and bring the soles and heels of your feet together. Catch hold of your toes with your hands, straighten your back, then press your knees downwards towards the floor so that your thighs open wider. Hold your legs in this position for as long as you can — try to work the time up from say 10 seconds to a few minutes.

Virasana (Hero pose)

Kneel down with your feet on either side of your buttocks, which should be resting on the floor (if necessary support them with a cushion). Make sure your toes are pointing backwards as far as you can so that you feel the stretch along your legs, and keep your back straight. Lift your hands above your head, intertwining your fingers, and hold for a few minutes. This is a lovely open upward stretch that really feels good as well as being excellent for toning the spine and pelvic area and also relaxing for tired legs.

Squatting

Stand with your feet about 45–60 centimetres apart, toes pointing slightly outward. Then crouch down in a squatting position keeping the feet flat (go on to your toes if you can't manage this at first), knees out and the back straight. Hold on to a support (the arms of a low chair, for instance) to begin with if you need to. Stay squatting for about a minute to start with, but try and work up to five minutes, and go into it when you can throughout the day. This 'birth' position helps to stretch the muscles of the pelvic floor in preparation for labour; it is most important to practise it right from the beginning of pregnancy until the very end.

Savasana (Corpse pose)

Lie on your back with your eyes closed (check you are lying in a straight line), legs slightly apart and your arms resting at about an angle of 45° to your body, and with the palms upwards. Your spine should be flat on the floor — if you find this uncomfortable or difficult, try placing a cushion under your thighs.

Now, starting with your feet, go through each part of your body slowly tensing and relaxing it (imagine your tensions and worries disappearing as you do so). Flex your toes up towards you, and relax them so they fall outward. Tighten and relax your calves, knees, thighs, buttocks and stomach — try and make it touch your backbone. Make fists with your hands and relax them, tighten and relax your arms, raise your shoulders and let them sink back, lift your head and let it relax back. Screw up your face and relax it, keeping your mouth slightly open so that the jaw is relaxed.

Having relaxed your body, now concentrate on nice, slow, rhythmical breathing. Breathe in, filling your lungs and expanding your stomach, and breathe out emptying them. Continue to lie in this position for as long as you like or have time for. It is a good way to end an exercise session and is also very useful if sleeping becomes difficult in the later months.

facial foibles

Most pregnant women acquire a definite bloom to their complexion as pregnancy advances beyond the first 12 weeks and any feelings of nausea and sickness subside. In fact, this rosy glow is due mainly to extra blood circulating around the body. By the 34th week of pregnancy the amount of blood in the circulation may have increased by as much as 50 per cent and remains virtually the same until the birth, when hormone levels fall and the body goes back to its non-pregnant state.

On the whole, pregnant women find their skin condition changes during pregnancy — usually for the better. This may be because of the increased blood flow to the skin or possibly because they are eating more sensibly or taking life at a slower pace and therefore are less susceptible to stress. Dry skins tend to become oilier and more supple, oily skins may become drier (although the reverse may also be true). Some women do find that spots appear unexpectedly; this is probably due to the action of progesterone, which increases sebaceous activity. Cleanse the skin thoroughly every night and try to eat more fresh fruit and vegetables rather than chocolate and fatty foods. If, however, you continue to have problems with your skin and nothing seems to work, your doctor may refer you to a dermatologist.

Some rounding of the face is normal during pregnancy — a plumpness of the cheeks and beneath the jaw is due to fluid retention and extra fat deposits. While the face should not become really swollen — a condition associated with excessive fluid retention — that slight extra fullness will help to plump out lines and wrinkles making you look younger and healthier.

A NATURAL MAKE-UP

During pregnancy you want to enhance the new glow in order to focus attention on your face and not on the bulge. But don't overdo it. A natural make-up is best at this time (you may look younger anyway as the cheeks plump out); anything startling or outrageous can look absurd.

Foundation

Choose a foundation that matches your natural skin colour, taking the tone from your neck. This may seem a little pale, but a blusher should give colour, not foundation. Use the back of your hand as a palette (so that you don't put too much on at once) and with your fingertips or a sponge apply the foundation to your face in sections, starting with the cheeks and forehead. Stroke downwards in the direction of the hairs of the face or you will tend to get a matted look. Stipple a little extra foundation over broken veins or blemishes — a natural look is achieved by applying many thin layers rather than one thick one.

Use an eye stick or under-eye cover cream in a lighter shade than your foundation to conceal any dark shadows under the eyes. Again warm and thin it on the back of the hand first. Don't rub the stick under your eye or it will drag the delicate skin.

Natural, soft colours rather than strong, hard colours will enhance your looks.

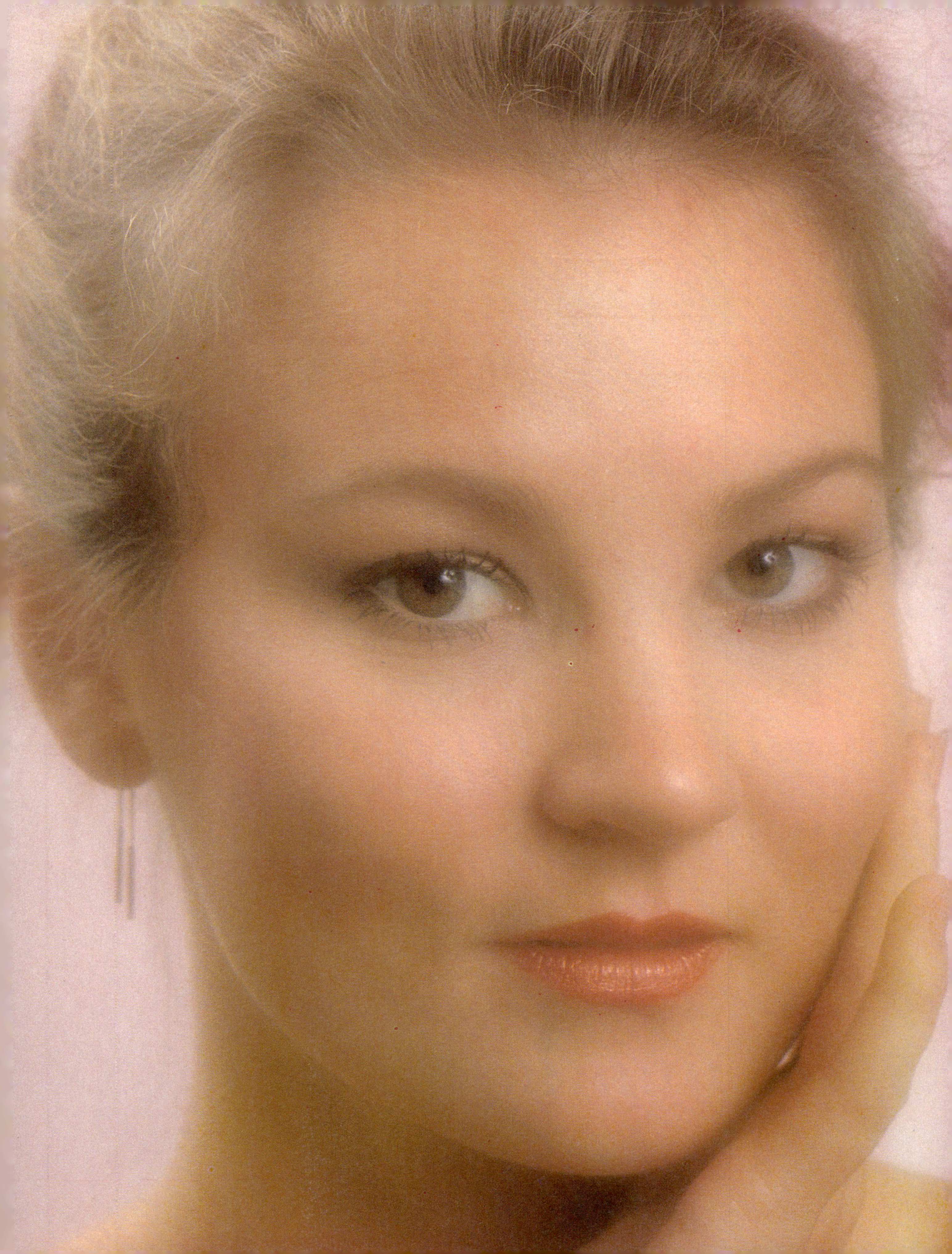

Blusher

If you like to wear a blusher, powder is easier to use than a cream or gel. A pinky tone will look most natural, particularly if you have a high colour or broken veins, since it won't clash with pink cheeks or a sudden flush. Fill the blusher brush with powder, tapping off the excess. Smile, and apply to the cheekbones just below the middle of the eye and outwards towards the hairline.

Powder

Use a translucent loose powder to set your make-up — it needn't look powdery and does help make-up last longer. Don't use a coloured powder on top of a coloured foundation: as your face warms up oils are released that may cause the two colour pigments to react on one another and change — and you could end up with an orange face. Shake some powder onto a wad of cotton wool and press onto the skin. Do not scrub and scrape or your carefully placed make-up will be moved. Turn the cotton wool over and flick any excess powder off the face.

The eyes

Bright hard colours will kill the colour of your eyes and their natural sparkle, so choose soft sludgy browns, greys, and mauves to set them off. Blue and green are hard colours but their effect is softened if used in conjunction with brown, grey or mauve.

Apply eyeshadow all over the eye area from lashes to eyebrow, but fade it out towards the eyebrow and blend well at the edges.

To give extra sparkle to your eyes, take a white frosty shadow and draw an upside down triangle on the centre of the lid, and then outline with a 'V' the innermost corner of each eye. If your lashes are very fair you may find it useful to have them dyed regularly, so that the roots always look dark. Otherwise you can emphasise them by drawing a *very* fine line right at the base of the upper lashes with dark liner, carefully using the edge of the brush.

To achieve a natural silky look to the eyelashes, apply several thin coats of mascara and always wipe the brush on a tissue first to blot off any excess mascara that would clog up the lashes.

Lip colour

Choose soft lip colours to go with your clothes. Glossy colours accentuate small lips; use flatter colours for large lips. Lines drawn round the lips first with a brush will help to define the shape of the mouth, or outline the top lip only with a white frosty shadow (the one used for your eyes).

CAMOUFLAGE MAKE-UP

If at any time during pregnancy the 'bloom' seems to elude you and you find that your face has become puffy, or that hormonal changes or bad sleeping habits are causing skin problems, there are ways to camouflage these bad points and to minimise their effect on your appearance.

Dark circles under the eyes

Dark circles may be emphasised by tiredness during pregnancy. To disguise the dark area, use a good under-eye cover cream that is fine in texture. Rub a small amount between your thumb and finger to warm and thin it before stippling it on with your fingers over a thin layer of foundation. Cover with another thin layer of foundation and blend carefully.

It may not look too appealing, but cucumber slices help reduce puffiness around the eyes.

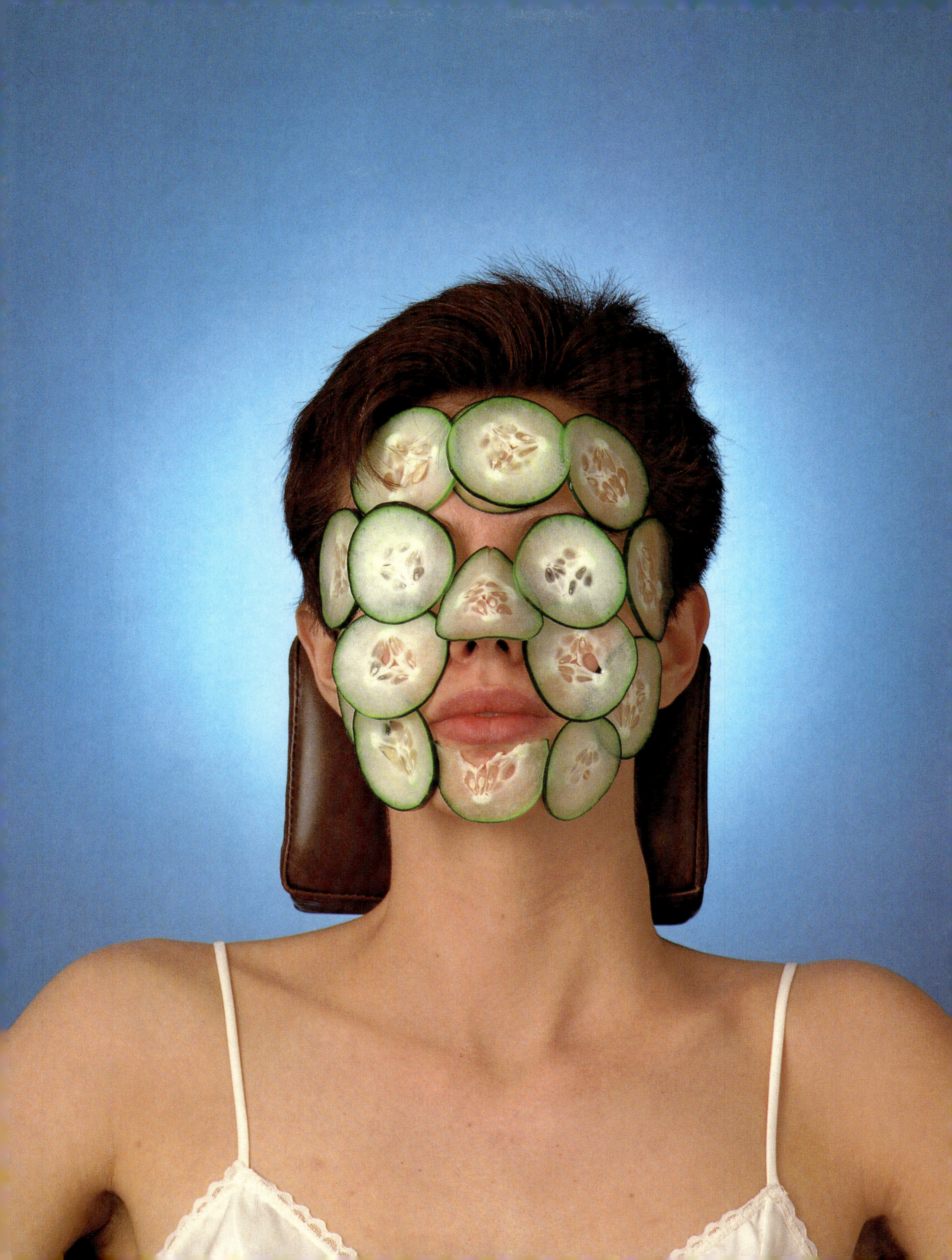

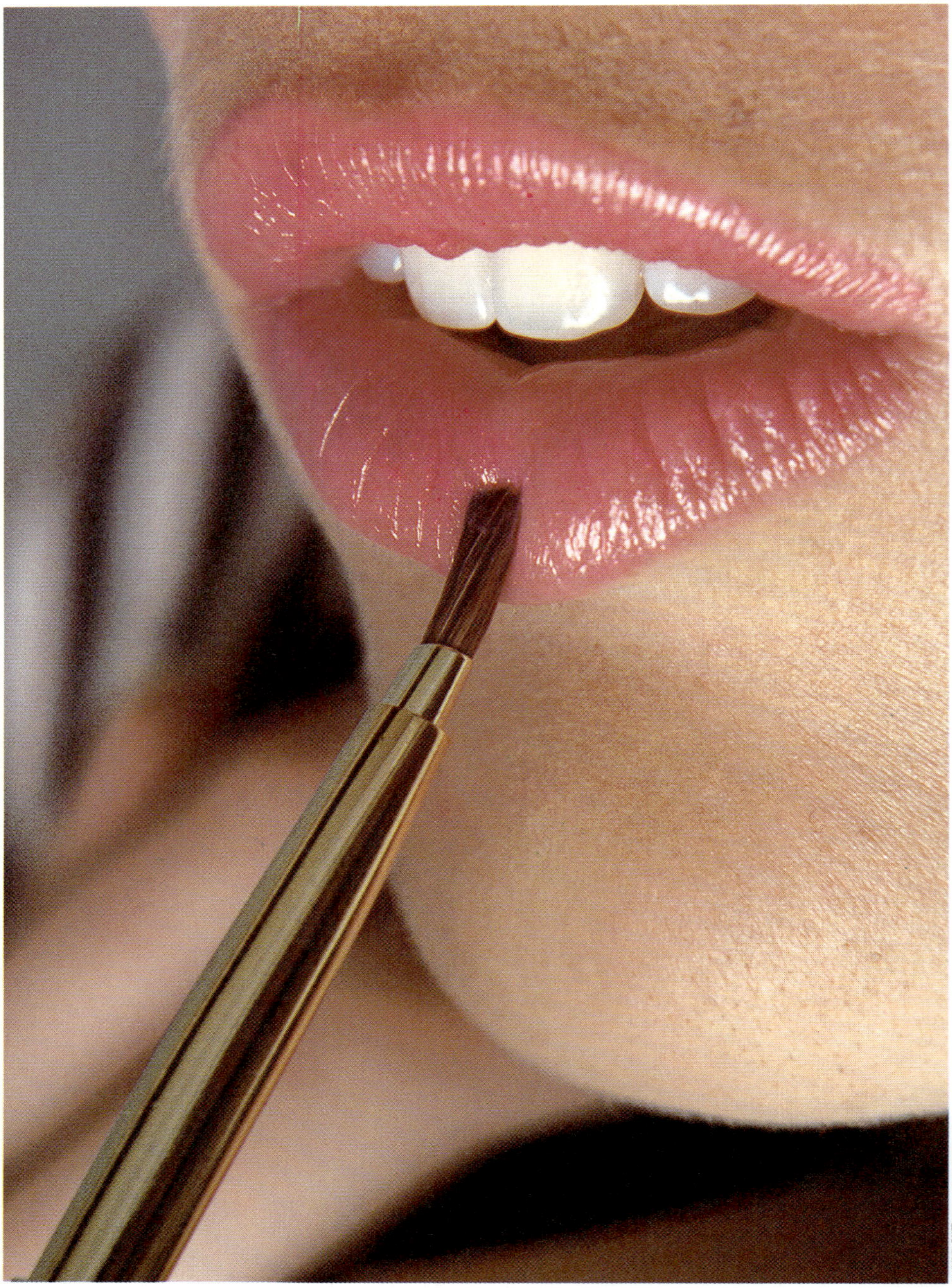

Elle Bache

Look after lips with lanolin or vaseline if they become dry or cracked and use a soft, glossy lip colour.

Puffiness or bags under the eyes

Fluid retention during pregnancy can cause this puffiness, which again is increased by tiredness and strain. Use a good eye mask while resting to reduce the puffiness (cucumber slices are also very good for this). To camouflage, use a very fine eyeliner brush to paint a light-coloured under-eye cover cream along the dark line underneath the 'bag'. The light shade will bring the dark line forward; do not apply it to the puffy area or this will appear to be even more prominent. Blend in carefully and cover with foundation.

Pink eyes

Tiredness or the increased blood in the circulation may make your eyes look bloodshot. Use a gentle eye mask to soothe them while you are resting and safe eye drops to bring back a little sparkle.

Greasy or dry patches

Pregnancy may cause your skin to become greasier or drier than usual. Greasiness is more likely because of the action of progesterone. For greasy patches use only a water-based moisturiser and a fine-textured, non-oily foundation and translucent powder. For dry patches you need an oil-based moisturiser and a sparing amount of foundation and powder. If the skin is flaking use no foundation or powder at all as these will only show up the problem.

Wrinkles and crow's feet

During early pregnancy the skin may become drier than usual, which can make fine lines and wrinkles more apparent. Use a very fine-textured foundation over the problem area and only the finest translucent powder — anything heavy or containing a shine will accentuate the wrinkles. Anti-wrinkle creams can temporarily diguise wrinkles by charging the skin with fluid, but certainly won't cure them.

Spots

A change in the hormone balance can produce spots. As long as you cleanse properly, water-based make-up will not make spots worse (though note that anything with an oil, lanolin or paraffin base probably will) so there is no reason why you shoundn't use it to conceal them. If they are not too bad just stipple a little extra foundation over the spots with a brush or your finger. If this is not sufficient, apply water-based foundation and then stipple with a spot-erase stick or cream in the same shade. Finish with another stipple of foundation, and then translucent powder.

Puffiness under the chin

Puffiness under the chin is probably more likely to occur later on in pregnancy and is again due to fluid retention. Camouflage by subtle shading with a browny shade of blusher or shader. Brush this under the jawline and on either side of the neck. Use the same blusher to emphasise your cheekbones — feel for the bone and then brush up on to it with a flicking movement. Use a pinky blusher on the temples to bring the attention to your eyes and away from the jawline.

High colour in the cheeks

The extra blood circulating is responsible for your 'bloom and an increased metabolic rate may make you feel more heated. To tone down very pink cheeks, use a flat, beige foundation (there should be no hint of pink in it) that is not too thick or greasy — or it will separate on your skin — and apply it in two or three very thin layers, stippling on extra where needed. Green foundation is sometimes advocated for concealing high colour and you could try this under your usual foundation, but it may just make you look green and ghostly. The idea originated from the theatre where the green counteracted the red in the bright lights.

Pigmentation on the face

Brunettes especially may notice increased pigmentation on the face — freckles, birthmarks and moles may get darker especially after exposure to the sun. Sometimes the sun will bring out a butterfly-shaped 'mask' over the cheeks, nose and forehead. This can be camouflaged with an erase stick blended with foundation. Never attempt to bleach.

Dry lips

Breathing through the mouth because of a blocked-up nose during pregnancy may cause one to lick the lips a lot, which can make them very dry. Rub in vaseline and camouflage with a glossy lipstick.

clothes sense

Being pregnant doesn't mean you have to look frumpy, dowdy or unfashionable. Nor does it necessarily mean you have to change your normal style of dress. True, the popular image of a pregnant woman is one who is dressed in an all-enveloping smock and many people do like this kind of comfortable, easy style. But if you have always preferred jeans and sweaters there is no reason to be different now.

ADAPTING YOUR WARDROBE FOR THE FIRST MONTHS

Unfortunately there is just no way of foretelling exactly how large you are eventually going to be, nor when you are actually going to be 'showing' your pregnancy. Some women look pregnant at three to four months, whereas

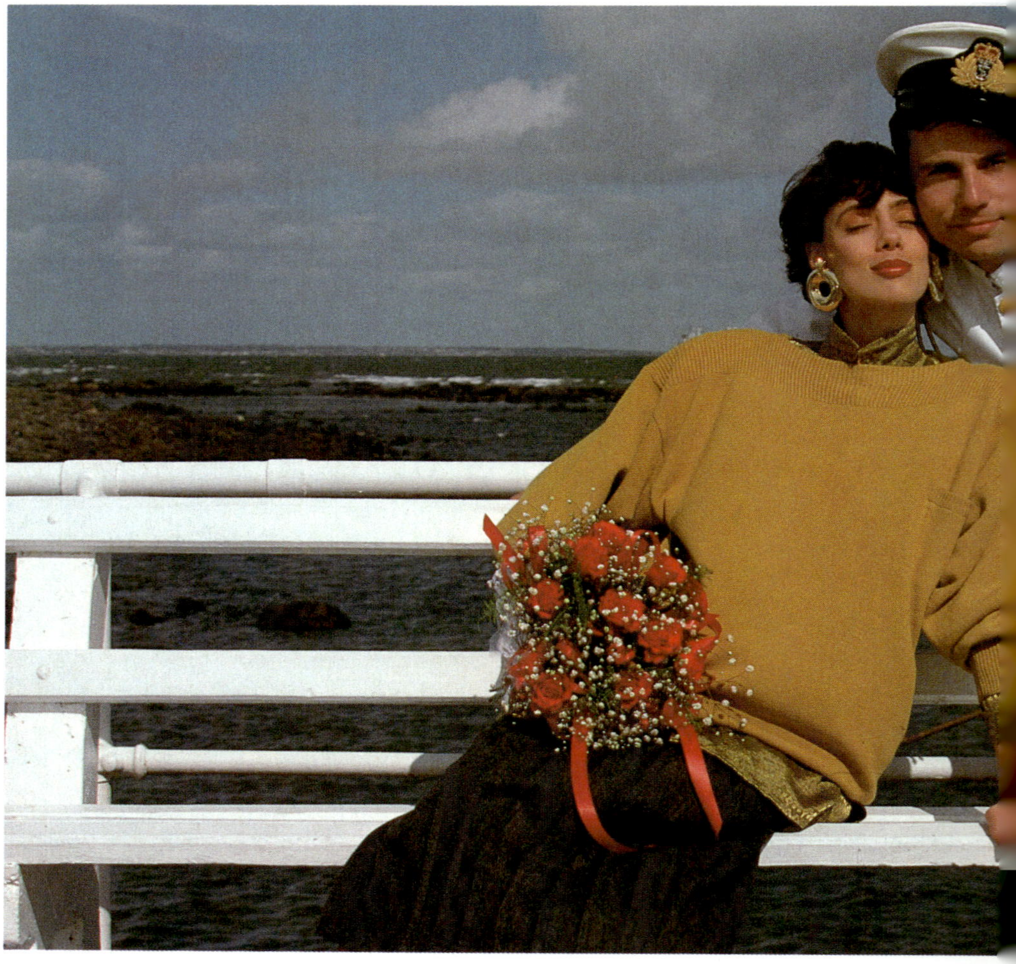

Raphael maternity wear

others go unnoticed well into their sixth month. The most obvious change is of course your tummy, but quite early on you will probably find that your waistline thickens and your breasts become larger. In fact, it is those first few months that are the most awkward. You know that you're pregnant and will feel larger than you look to others. Waistbands will be tight and blouses uncomfortable across the bust. Wearing tight clothes won't harm your baby; the discomfort will merely make you feel bigger than you are. So don't go on struggling into tight jeans, straight skirts and slinky dresses. But before you dash out and panic-buy expensive maternity clothes, take stock of your wardrobe. Have a good look at everything and see what can be altered, adapted or used as it is.

For casual wear at home, jeans can be adapted for a while by clipping a pair of men's braces to the front and back and leaving the zip undone, with a loose, undarted shirt or baggy T-shirt or jumper to hide the gap. If you want to wear trousers throughout pregnancy you can convert them by letting out the darts, taking off the waistband and zip, and inserting bands of wide, soft elastic ribbing in the front, back and side seams.

You can go on wearing boiler suits and dungarees during much of your pregnancy and towelling track suits in primary colours are fun and comfortable. If the elastic at the waist feels too tight, replace it with drawstrings. Wrap-around skirts are useful for the early months and many loose dresses with undarted busts can be worn without belts — or cut down to make baggy tops. When your tummy is only just noticeable, sweater and shirt dresses look elegant with the material 'bloused' up over the belt, which can be worn 1920s-style, low down on your hips.

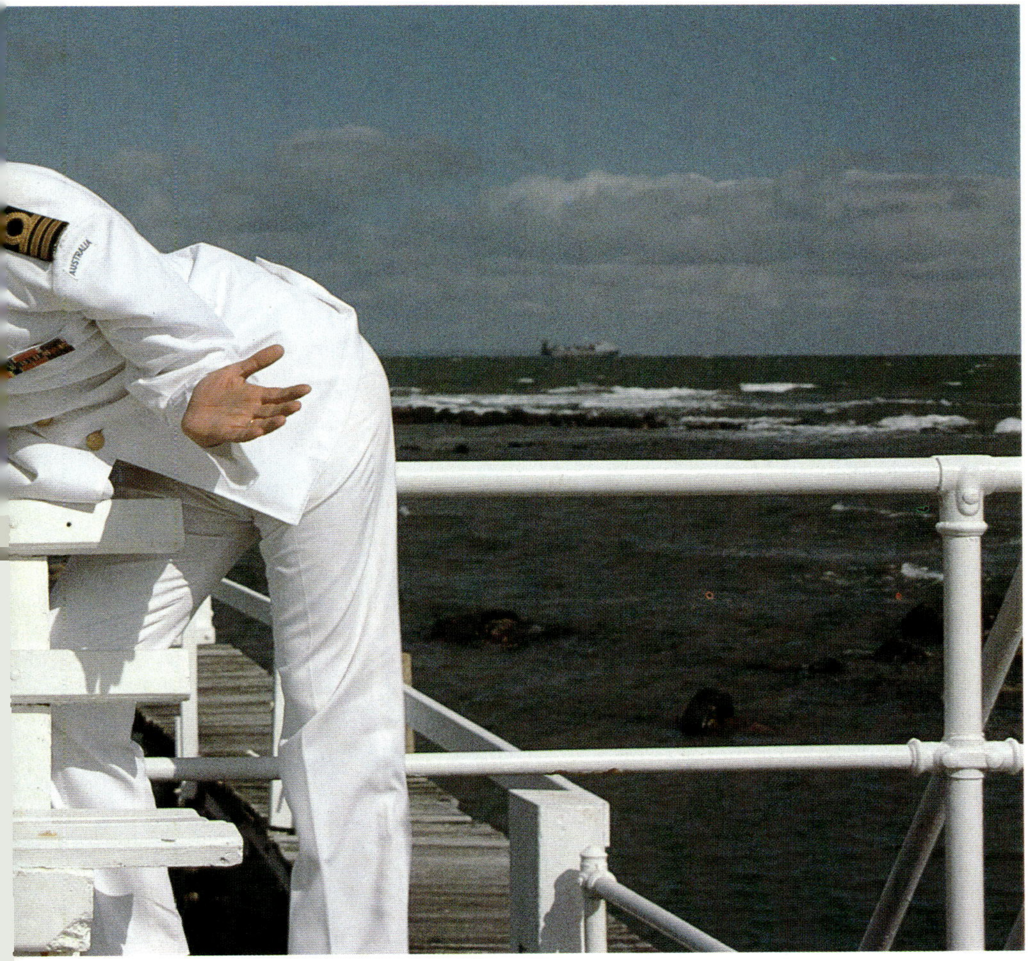

Fashion designers are increasingly extending their range to maternity wear with some very attractive and eye-catching results.

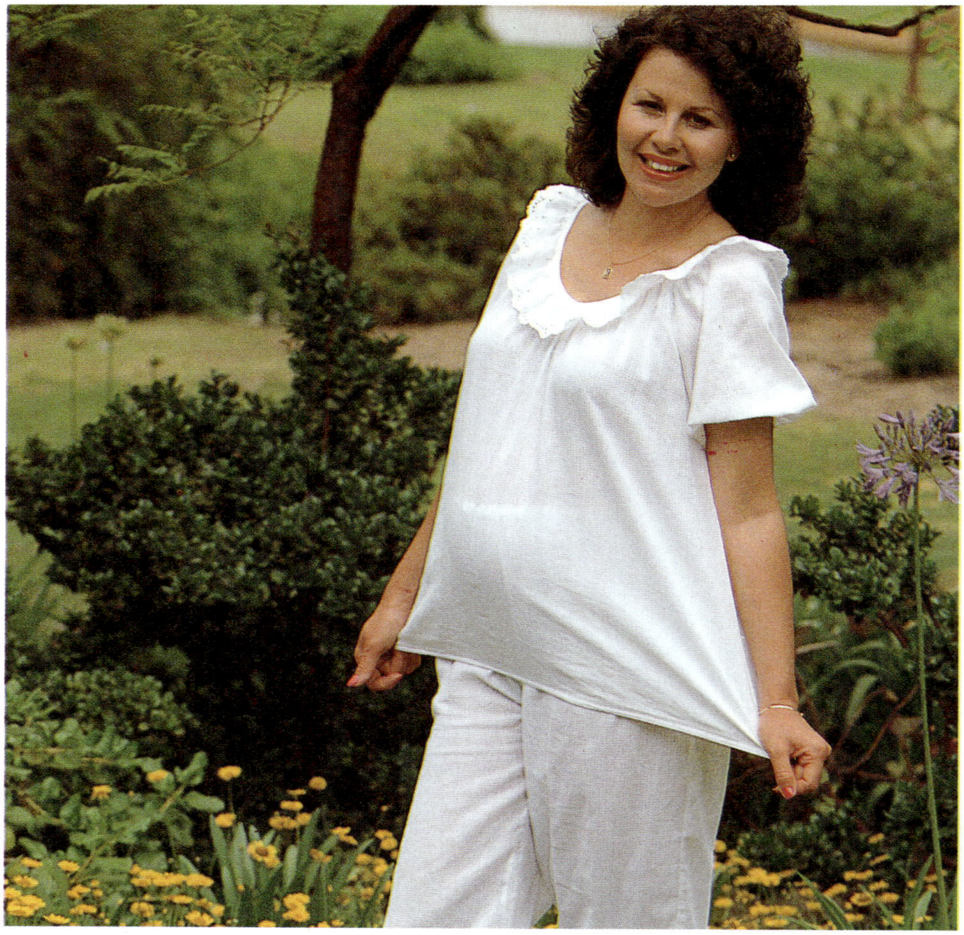

Loose-fitting, natural fibre clothes are comfortable and look good.

MATERNITY AND NON-MATERNITY CLOTHES

When you start to look for new clothes you may find that there isn't a great deal of choice — and what there is could be expensive. However maternity styles are improving and if you hunt around you should be able to come up with some attractive outfits.

If you like to wear jeans, maternity trousers are now becoming more fashionably cut, so look for a good quality pair with a large elastic panel in the front and plenty of give at the back. They may be expensive but you can wear them virtually everyday throughout the second half of your pregnancy with a variety of different tops and T-shirts.

If you can't find what you want among the maternity clothes, look out for dresses that are pin-tucked or pleated from the shoulders, or, in the summer, loose sundresses with a shirred elastic yoke over the bust.

You probably won't want to invest in a new winter coat while you are pregnant, but unwaisted A-line raincoats, capes and hip-length loose or blouson jackets are all useful and concealing — as are unwaisted fur coats if you are lucky enough to have one in your wardrobe!

If you need a new evening dress now may be the time to make the most of an unaccustomed cleavage. Why not boost your morale with a low-cut, glamorous dress in a silky washable fabric. There are quite a few styles that can be gathered in with a belt and so worn afterwards when you have regained your waistline.

Beachlovers can select from either maternity swimwear or ordinary bikinis. The sight of a bare, pregnant stomach on the beach upsets very few people, so you don't have to pass up the opportunity of a tan. If you are self-conscious though, a large T-shirt knotted at the side will cover you up and add style.

Wear bright, cheerful colours if you are happy in them. But remember that large prints and stripes will tend to make you look bigger. If you prefer a more subtle, feminine look, choose soft, muted prints in small patterns. Black and navy blue always look smart but avoid dark browns and greys which can be drab.

Fabrics should be easy to wash and not too thick, since your higher metabolic rate and increased blood circulation will probably make you feel warmer than usual, even in the winter. If natural fibres are too expensive, choose blends such as cotton-polyester or wool-acrylic rather than pure synthetics — and nothing too clingy!

UNDERCLOTHES AND NIGHTWEAR

Pants are most comfortable worn below the tummy, so stretchy bikini briefs are best. Buy cotton briefs rather than synthetic as you are less likely to perspire in this fabric. Pantyhose can be worn throughout pregnancy so long as you find them comfortable; they should have a lot of 'give' so that you can pull the gusset right up under your bust. Stockings tend to become impractical as you grow larger, simply because the suspender belt will feel tight and ungainly. You should never wear garters to keep your stockings up; this will constrict the blood flow in your legs and could cause varicose veins. If you like to wear socks with trousers, make sure the elastic isn't too tight and keep them loosely rolled down if necessary — or better still wear ankle socks in cheerful colours.

Anything loose and airy is suitable for nightwear. If you are not a nightie person, a large T-shirt or ordinary man's shirt with the collar and cuffs removed are comfortable alternatives. But if you are buying with your hospital confinement in mind, two or three nighties or loose-fitting pyjamas with front openings for breastfeeding are essential. Don't be tempted by slinky negligees in synthetic materials as they will make you sweat — hospitals are invariably hothouses.

FOOTWEAR

The combination of your increased weight and the softening of your ligaments during pregnancy means that your feet will need extra support and comfort. Buy new shoes half a size larger than usual to allow for expansion. High heels are bad for your feet and could be dangerous since they affect your balance by throwing your weight forward. So choose from the lower-heeled styles, and preferably shoes with straps, laces or some other fastening. Boots should have chunky heels and be supportive yet wide enough across the instep in case your feet swell. Check that they are not too tight at the ankle or calf. Summer sandals are fine as long as they are comfortable and reasonably supportive. For round the house, wooden exercise sandals, thongs or no shoes are three quite good ways to exercise your feet, but avoid slippers and mules as they are no benefit at all.

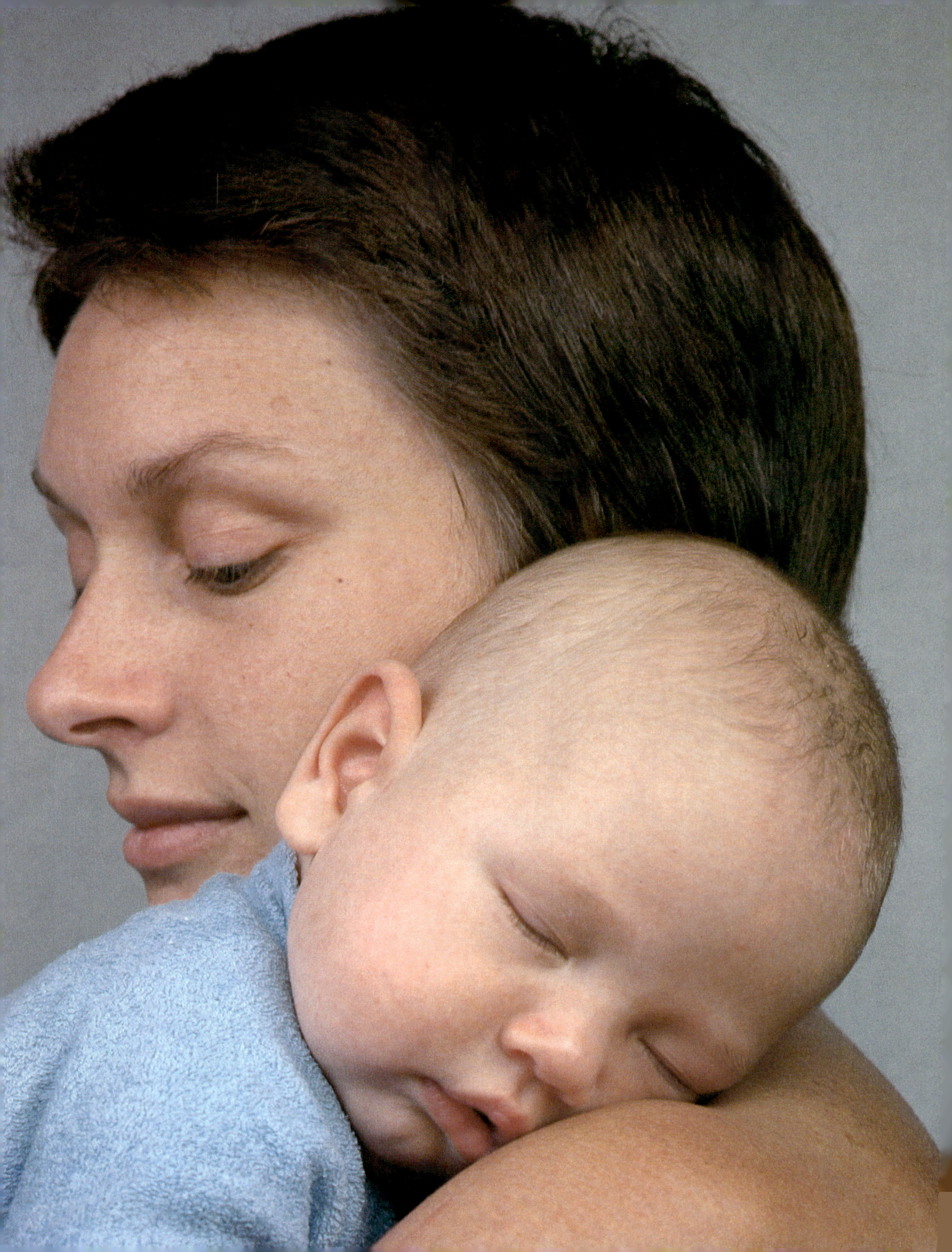

back into shape

After the birth you will find that your former svelte shape will not magically return. In fact, it will take nine months for your body to return to normal. Lithe and supple women might make it in six.

As the postnatal period is extremely demanding for the new mother, it would be wise not to expect miracles in any department. The weight gained during pregnancy will not automatically disappear and, in fact, some women do not return to their normal weight until they have finished breastfeeding. Embark on a gentle exercise programme consisting initially of stretching exercises and graduate on to more energetic techniques as you become stronger.

Changes in breast shape after pregnancy are due to the weight gain and change in shape over the nine months and are not related to the decision to breastfeed. It you opt for this, wear a well-fitting nursing bra to prevent drooping breasts.

It is very important while breastfeeding to maintain awareness of nutrition and health to ensure an optimum level of sustenance for the child and to enable you to cope with your busy schedule. Add vitamin pills to your diet if necessary. Don't smoke and don't drink to excess. Another very important point: if you are on any prescribed drugs, check with your doctor to find out if they are still suitable to take while you are breastfeeding. Remember while breastfeeding you will need plenty of carbohydrate to manufacture the milk.

Your hormone levels have undergone a massive upheaval and they will need time to readapt. One effect is a loss of tone in hair and skin. Hair fallout will increase for about 12 weeks after the birth, and may continue to fall out for another two months. This is a normal reaction to the surge in hair growth caused by hormonal changes during pregnancy. Supplement your diet with B vitamins — found in brewer's yeast or wheatgerm — and your hair condition should improve. Rest is the best panacea — so a supportive friend or family member is a must.

If you take life slowly and quietly after the birth and understand that time is required to enable you and your body to adjust to a new lifestyle, the transition from pregnancy to a fully fledged mother should be accomplished with ease.

Take life slowly and quietly after the birth to give your body a chance to recover and to give you time to enjoy your baby.

index